W0228134

Management of Fecal Incontinence

Massimo Mongardini • Manuel Giofrè
Editors

Management of Fecal Incontinence

Current Treatment Approaches and Future Perspectives

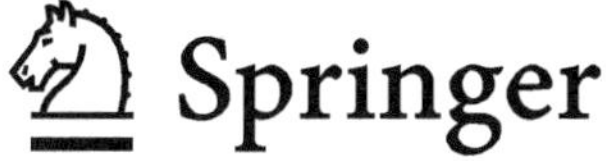

Springer

Editors
Massimo Mongardini
Sapienza - University of Rome
Rome
Italy

Manuel Giofrè
Sapienza - University of Rome
Rome
Italy

ISBN 978-3-319-32224-7 ISBN 978-3-319-32226-1 (eBook)
DOI 10.1007/978-3-319-32226-1

Library of Congress Control Number: 2016950205

Printed on acid-free paper

This Springer imprint is published by Springer Nature
The registered company is Springer International Publishing AG Switzerland

Foreword I

Many resource materials exist for the physician or surgeon evaluating and managing the patient with fecal incontinence. Much of the available information is embedded in the context of an overall textbook or compendium of colorectal surgery. There are a relatively limited amount of focused data for the practitioner who wishes to become familiar or updated with the latest relevant diagnostic and therapeutic information. Professor Mongardini is to be commended for having assembled in a cogent, succinct, and imminently readable textbook all of the abovementioned required details. He has selected 14 chapters each of which was authored by between one and five experts. This book commences with a very surgeon-specific view of pelvic floor anatomy which I found readily comprehensible and clinically relevant. The second chapter which I also very much enjoyed reading is a description of physiology and physiopathology again written from the perspective of the practicing surgeon. Studying this chapter is an excellent prerequisite to digesting the subsequent four chapters each of which delves into a different but important facet of evaluation. Specifically, the chapters on endoanal ultrasound, magnetic resonance, anorectal manometry, and electromyography are all very up to date, highly descriptive, and again immediately useful in daily patient management. Reading these four chapters allows one a comprehensive overview of the optimal available current diagnostic tools. The remaining eight chapters describe virtually every currently available therapeutic modality by which the practitioner can try to assist the patient with fecal incontinence. The chapters include the gamut from pelvic floor rehabilitation and radiofrequency tissue remodeling to stomas and stem cells. In between these extremes are reviews of injectable and implantable agents, sacral neuromodulation, the artificial bowel sphincter and the more "standard" surgical therapies of sphincter repair, post anal repair, and muscle transposition. The easy readability of the material in the textbook is further complimented by the high-quality illustrations and photographs. It is clear that each of the authors commands expertise in his or her respective chapter. It is also quite apparent that Professor Mongardini edited the material to allow for an easy narrative flow between chapters with minimal subject overlap but excellent subject juxtaposition and interplay. I am very grateful to Professor

Mongardini for having invited me to author this Foreword. I highly commend this textbook to all physicians and surgeons who evaluate and/or manage patients with fecal incontinence. This book shall certainly occupy a prominent place in my personal library and will be enjoyed by all of my residents and fellows.

Steven D. Wexner, MD, PhD (Hon), FACS, FRCS, FRCS (Ed)
Chairman, Department of Colorectal Disease
Director, Digestive Disease Center
Cleveland Clinic
Florida, USA

Foreword II

The Management of Fecal Incontinence

Traditional anatomy and most importantly, an anatomy which is advanced and modern, both functional and pathological, of the pelvis and the perineum, has forever incited my non-ephemeral attention and even provoked me, at times, with interpretive difficulties of the mnemonical or terminological nature: much of this due to its intertwined classification and challenging pathophysiological attributes. The awareness of the anthropological and ethical impact, far from pedestrian, and of the consequences deriving from regional pathologies permeates one's understanding and demands the utmost attention. Thus the most dire of fecal incontinence's problematics, often severely debilitating for the patient, have been ever-present throughout my areas of interest in colorectal pathology and surgery, and have led me to seek out and to obtain an understanding of the evolution of knowledge in this field.

Within this area of interest, the need to be kept abreast of the latest research and studies as well learn from the experience of the field's "best" and most "dedicated" experts is paramount; this must be achieved through the objective awareness of personal practice, phenomena causality, and through methodological improvements and opportunities provided by technological achievements. Hence, I have challenged myself with curiosity and commitment, with all there is to acquire within this specific area. Thereby I was able to observe, during my long career as a surgeon, and during not so recent times, how fecal incontinence's identity and frequency were not yet fully explored and valued, further still, they were neglected and resulted in poor and inappropriate therapeutic consequences. Yet a regulated "curative consciousness" has taken form as of late, resulting either from the pressure of social and environmental obligations or due to those of the recognition of patient's rights. We owe surgical research groups, who are taking direct action on this matter, the understanding of contemporary doctrinal and clinical-therapeutic issues.

This monographic work, represented by "schools" and "groups" which are motivated by a strong sense of operational collaboration and remarkable clinical and surgical experience, coupled with a cautious judgment for possible outcomes, undertakes the fundamental duty of describing and assimilating the present state of these discoveries while taking into consideration the elements of its authentic history and enabling future findings.

Fecal incontinence is more common than what is generally believed and is prevalent among females. It mortifies and humiliates its sufferers, most often too embarrassed to communicate their often severely debilitating condition, lest they damage their social individuality.

In the past, many surgical repair techniques have failed, proved inadequate, or have been modified and enhanced in order to achieve success; yet as a whole, only modest progress has been recorded. Today we may rely upon a more precise and critical qualitative assessment of results. Therapeutic options are numerous and address many aspects of the condition: in relation to various causal conditions, clinical presentations, and through the respecting of important and global statistic results.

Naturally, there is no single treatment for fecal incontinence which may be applied unbiasedly to a large series of clinical cases with different pathogenesis, conditions, or severity, as is possible with other more homogeneous diseases. Traditional techniques have been modified and fine-tuned, thus determining through time, a curative value.

For less severe pathological conditions, "conservative" techniques, which may be coupled with a more invasive approach, have been implemented. The evolution of biotechnology has led to the creation of new generations of artificial sphincters. New methods such as sacral neuromodulation have been introduced and have been legitimized due to their "flattering" results. Progress has been made in the research and development of new biocompatible materials which produce different types of "bulking agents," and stem cells have been studied as of late for reconstructive purposes. Now more than ever, a scrupulous diagnostic conduct is required in order to allow for the planning of adequate "individual" therapy.

The aforementioned information is presented and compiled in an orderly, systematic, and illustrative manner in this text, and may be used both as a guide and a handbook. I wish to see this book browsed, annotated, read, and reread, its passages and concepts reflected upon and brought to everyday practice in the hands of the young and affirmed surgeon, the "generalist" and "specialist" surgeon, scholars, researchers, clinicians, physiopathologists, radiologists, psychologists, and non-medical specialized hospital personnel. This volume greatly deserves to be dealt with thusly, thanks to its acculturation characteristics and its practical guidance: I profoundly hope and strongly believe that this will transpire.

Giorgio Di Matteo
Professor Emeritus of Surgery
Sapienza - University of Rome
President Emeritus and Honorary
Member of the Italian Society of Surgery
Rome, Italy

Foreword III

Fecal Incontinence Management

Fecal incontinence, though it be an unfamiliar area of expertise to most physicians, is of paramount importance physically, socially, and psychologically to those who suffer from it.

The following is a book which reads like a treatise, while retaining the nimble nature of a reference manual. The editor wished that its chapters be entrusted to individual experts or teams of devoted specialists who represent the best that the field has to offer today. Upon first glance, the text is not falling in value of a monograph written by a single scholar, due to the homogeneous manner in which the work develops, and due to its broad range of clinical and therapeutic concepts shared by specialists in the field. This work presents strategies currently in use as well as future goals, offering those who wish to devote themselves to this discipline a scientific approach which is the fruit of debates and experience spanning several decades. These concepts are presented in an area of research that, despite having originated in the nineteenth century, has just recently emerged from its experimental phase. The future goal, unattainable without the participation of some of the most prominent institutions, is to implement ratiocinative protocols within the field, as well as in the area of anatomical and functional surgery of the anus and the rectum, which have until very recently raised substantial doctrinal conflicts in congresses.

As this book is hereby presented by two of the utmost experts of surgery, I leave to them the task of delving into the most meaningful aspects of diagnosis and therapy. It is my good pleasure, however, to recall our long experience in treating these pathologies: having been quite fortunate at the time to have had the editor himself by my side in his young years. At that time, the initial obstacle to overcome before delving into a case was the difficulty in understanding the subtleties of anatomy, above all of the pelvic floor: a query which was subsequently clarified and defined by several colleagues. The pathophysiological and diagnostic definition of the determining causes of fecal incontinence was in and of itself quite controversial and arduous, as it encompasses numerous pathological conditions. Thus, it was difficult to carry out diagnostic procedures which would have consistently adhered to the rigorous methodology set forth. I think back to the discussions we had long ago, and how the need to clearly identify effective diagnostic protocols was often at the heart of our debates.

Therefore, it is opportune that this book opens with the topic of anatomy, which in this case is not a mere "rappel" but a crucial part of the technical mastery of the surgeon.

The improvement of diagnostics is inherently related to the detailed study of complex pathophysiology, and to the collaboration and joint effort of various specialists in their struggle to avoid superficial and inaccurate diagnosis which in turn leads to inadequate therapeutic plans.

This text concludes with surgery. Therapeutic options have remarkably increased in recent years. This demonstrates that the various available approaches are not univocal. Time, experimentation, and the exchange of ideas will lead us to establish guidelines and techniques, while consistently referring back to our shared experiences.

I remind the reader that this text reviews the most common medical and surgically conservative techniques, which have produced favorable results in well-selected cases.

We await further technological developments, above all a possible use of stem cells.

I wish the authors that proctologists may study from this book and as a result bring about a further evolution of this highly practiced surgical discipline.

Filippo Custureri
Full Professor of Surgery
Sapienza - University of Rome
Rome, Italy

Preface

Fecal incontinence is an extremely common condition, whose true prevalence is difficult to assess. Until a few years ago in non-specialized centers, care was confined on the use of restraint principals such as absorbent pads.

The loss of the ability to hold gas and feces is an outcome of a dysfunctional sphincter whose orderly ability to voluntary release stool and evacuating bowel contents in socially appropriate moments is damaged. This ability is related to the normal functioning of the involved structures (rectum, pelvic floor, and anal sphincters) and is associated with the integrity of their neurosensory components. Incontinence is the result of irregularity of any of these systems together with other systemic diseases, which may have altered intestinal motility and stool consistency as well as diseases that affect superior cerebral capability.

Incontinence can have features of enhanced disability that reduces significantly the patient's quality of life and, in severe cases, leads patients to renounce all forms of social life.

The prevalence increases significantly with age coupled with the ordinary aging process of the connective tissue, of the smooth and the striated muscle component and of the pelvic district fascia, which anatomically and physiologically guarantee its functionality. Therefore, the elderly are affected the most by this pathology, that even if found to be benign it still becomes debilitating, not only for the patient but for his caregiver as well, with a considerable social and health impact.

In most cases, the diagnosis of the disease is made belatedly, not only due to its increased prevalence in elderly subjects, but also due to the habitual patient's reticence in dealing with the problem since it troubles one's most intimate and personal sphere.

The psycho-emotional effects, namely, stress, anguish, tears, anxiety, fatigue, fear of public humiliation and the sensation of been unclean, are devastating. Limited sexual activity is inevitable as also fear of the anticipated incontinence (which itself often increases the probability of an episode), anger, humiliation, depression, isolation, secrecy, frustration, and embarrassment. In addition, physical activity is severely undermined; for many patients, simply walking can become a trigger for incontinence to the extent that part of people avoid any movement and as a result have inevitable difficulties in carrying out basic daily and working activities.

Fecal incontinence is not a diagnosis, but a symptom. Its causes are numerous and often multifactorial. Consequently, therapeutic strategies are manifold.

Respecting the above considerations, we intend to clarify at what point this pathology is fund today by analyzing, with the help of leading experts in the field, all its pathological details and implications. The aim of this volume is to evaluate every aspect of this disease in detail: the anatomical description of the pelvic floor, the pathophysiology of different noxae, and the structured diagnostic iter of the possible conservative and surgical therapeutic strategies. We wish to propose eventually the one method that represents the therapeutic approach, currently as well as in the near future, by exploiting all the new curative measures and biotechnological innovations.

In conclusion, we would like to express our gratitude to all those who, with their invaluable contribution, made the accomplishment of this work possible.

Rome, Italy

Massimo Mongardini
Manuel Giofrè

Contents

1 **Pelvic Floor Anatomy** 1
Menelaos Karpathiotakis

2 **Physiology and Physiopathology** 11
Paolo Urciuoli, Dimitri Krizzuk, and Giada Livadoti

3 **Endoanal Ultrasound** 23
Domenico Mascagni, Gianmarco Grimaldi, and Gabriele Naldini

4 **Diagnosis and Imaging: MR** 33
Gianfranco Gualdi and Maria Chiara Colaiacomo

5 **Anorectal Manometry** 43
Danilo Badiali

6 **Electromyography** 51
Maurizio Inghilleri, Maria Cristina Gori, and Emanuela Onesti

7 **Pelvic Floor Rehabilitation** 59
Lucia d'Alba and Margherita Rivera

8 **Radiofrequency (SECCA® Procedure)** 69
Marco Frascio and Francesca Mandolfino

9 **Sacral Nerve Stimulation in Fecal Incontinence** 75
Marileda Indinnimeo, Cosima Maria Moschella,
Gloria Bernardi, and Paolo Gozzo

10 **Injectable and Implantable Agents: Current Evidence and Perspective** 91
Carlo Ratto, Angelo Parello, Lorenza Donisi, and Francesco Litta

11 **Artificial Bowel Sphincter** 107
Filippo La Torre, Giuseppe Giuliani, Diego Coletta,
Francesco Guerra, and Marco La Torre

12 **Surgical Treatments** 113
Massimo Mongardini and Manuel Giofrè

13 **Ostomy in Fecal Incontinence** 127
Livia de Anna, Raffaele Merola, and Claudia Donello

14 **Stem Cells** 133
Mario Ledda, Antonella Lisi, and Alberto Giori

1 Pelvic Floor Anatomy

Menelaos Karpathiotakis

1.1 Introduction

The pelvis is a complex structure made up of bones, muscles, ligaments, and fascia and contains organs such as the bladder, urethra, uterus, prostate, and rectum. The pelvic floor is separated into three compartments (anterior, middle, and posterior) and consists of muscles and connective tissue that work as a coordinated system to support the organs and to prevent dysfunctions [1, 2].

This chapter attempts to provide an essential description of those structures and organs of pelvic floor that contribute to the complex mechanism of anal continence. The pelvic cavity, the anterior and middle compartment of the pelvic floor, and the ischioanal fossae are anatomic structures beyond the scope of this section.

Fecal incontinence is described mostly as a disorder of the posterior compartment of pelvic floor [2], managed traditionally by colorectal surgeons. Therefore, in order to make easier to understand the physiology of continence mechanism, we concentrated our attention to the anatomical aspects regarding the muscles of pelvic floor and the structure of the anorectum.

With the contribution of Giovanni Tortorelli.

M. Karpathiotakis
Department of Surgery R. Paolucci, Sapienza – University of Rome, Rome, Italy
e-mail: enimdisify@hotmail.it

1.2 Pelvic Floor Muscles: Overview

Pelvic floor is a funnel made up of a striated muscular sheet (pelvic diaphragm) that delimits inferiorly the abdominopelvic cavity providing enclosure and support at the pelvic organs throughout its midline hiatuses [1, 3, 4]. The pelvic diaphragm extends from pubic symphysis anteriorly to coccyx posteriorly and between the two ischiatic spines laterally [1, 5].

The pelvic floor muscles (Figs. 1.1 and 1.5) may be organized in superficial and deep muscles [6–8]. The superficial muscles include the anal sphincter complex, perineal body, and transverse perinei muscles, whereas the deep pelvic floor muscles include the levator ani muscle, the ischiococcygeus (coccygeus), and the obturator internus muscle. Between these two layers of muscles is described the conjoint longitudinal muscle of the anus [9].

1.3 The Anorectum

1.3.1 Embryological Development

The origin of the rectum and the anal canal occurs through the division of the cloaca that represents the caudal end of the hindgut [10, 11]. The cloaca is connected to the allantois ventrally. The mesoderm at the angle between the allantois and the hindgut proliferates and invaginates the endoderm of the cloaca forming

M. Mongardini, M. Giofrè (eds.), *Management of Fecal Incontinence*,
DOI 10.1007/978-3-319-32226-1_1

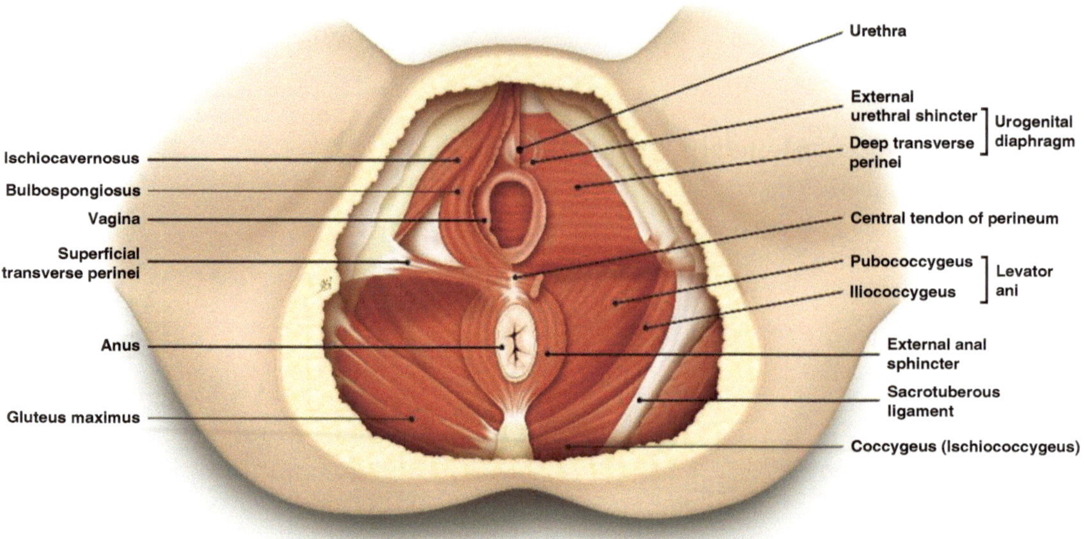

Fig. 1.1 Pelvic floor muscles (Inferior view, female)

a septum, called urorectal septum. The septum extends caudally composing, anteriorly, the primitive urogenital sinus and the anorectal canal, posteriorly [10, 12]. Further extension of the urorectal septum caudally divides the cloacal membrane into two parts: anterior part called urogenital membrane and posterior part called anal membrane which are separated by the perineal body (ectoderm).

At the 9th week of development, proliferation of the mesenchyme around the anal membrane creates an ectodermal depression around it, called proctodeum that forms the lower part of the anal canal [10, 12, 13]. The upper part of anal canal and the mucosa of rectum is formed from the anorectal canal (endodermal in origin). The proctodeum raises the anal membrane and finally it ruptures so that the two parts of anal canal become continuous. At the same time, mesenchyme surrounding the anorectal canal proliferates, forming the musculature of rectum and anal canal [11].

At the 16th week of development, the levator ani muscle is completely formed and delimits the ischiorectal fossa and the pelvic floor [13].

1.3.2 The Rectum

At the level of the 2nd–3rd sacral vertebra begins anatomically the rectum which is the last part of the large intestine and connects the sigmoid colon to the anal canal. The rectum is about 12–16 cm long, ends at the perineum, and may be subdivided into two segments: pelvic segment and perineal segment [7, 8, 13].

The pelvic segment of the rectum presents a much larger lumen than its intraperitoneal segment, and it is known as the rectal ampulla; it is quite stretchable and serves as a reservoir during defecation [14]. The perineal segment of the rectum (lied under the pelvic diaphragm) is known as anal canal. The point of transition (anorectal junction) results from the encirclement of the rectum by the levator ani muscle (puborectalis muscle sling) (Fig. 1.2) [1, 2, 8].

Below the rectosigmoid junction, the muscular tenias are replaced by the continuous longitudinal muscle layer which is enveloped around the entire rectum. Caudal extension of the circular layer of smooth muscle of rectum into anal canal forms the internal anal sphincter, while the

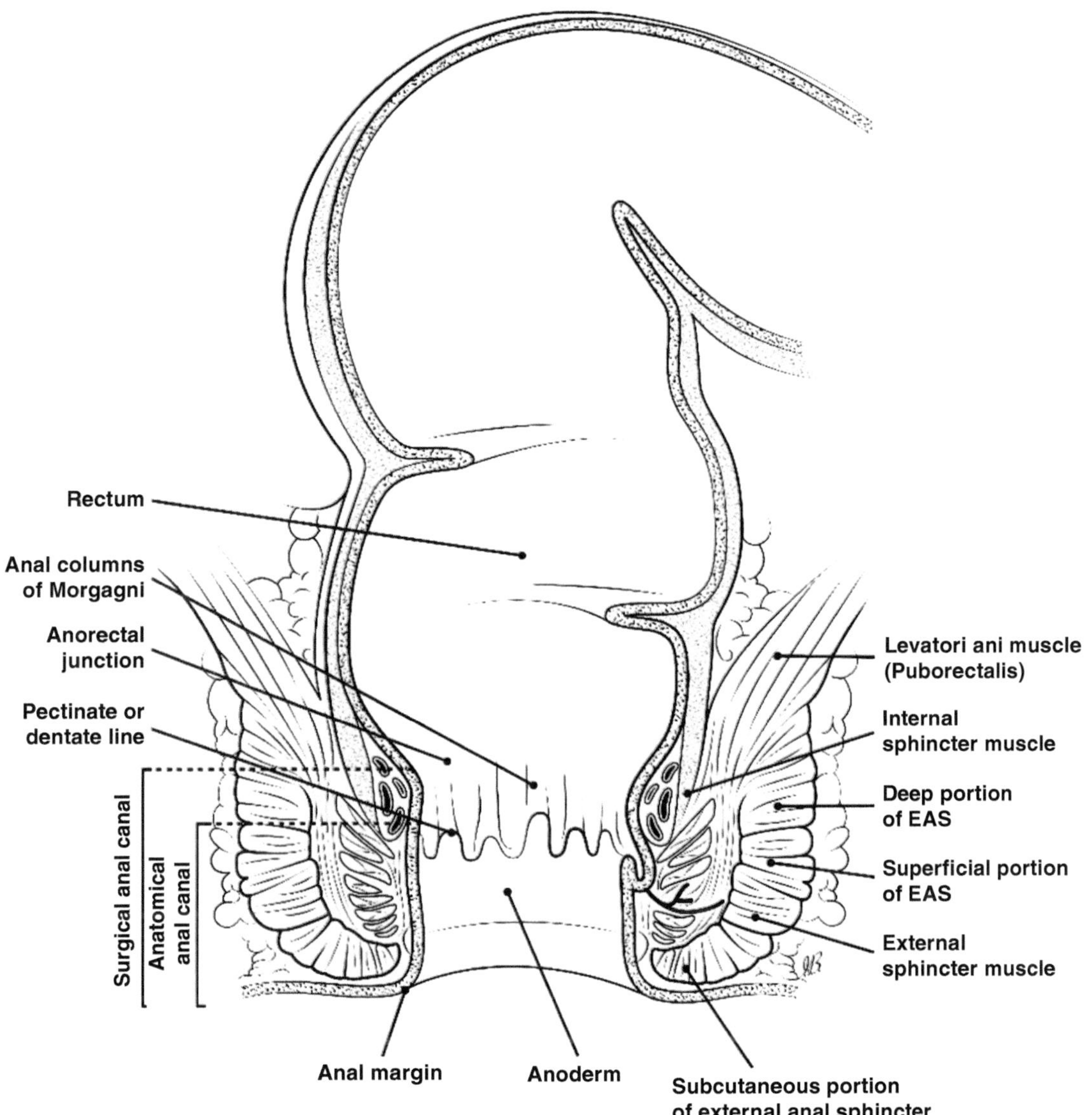

Fig. 1.2 Coronal section of the anorectum

extension of longitudinal layer of smooth muscle of rectum forms the external anal sphincter of the anal canal [5, 15].

1.3.3 The Anal Canal (Fig. 1.2)

The anal canal, approximately 3–4 cm long, is the terminal part of the colon and is a close tube surrounded throughout its length by the sphincter muscles which contribute significantly to the regulation of defecation and continence [3, 7, 14].

Anatomically (Fig. 1.2), the anal canal extends for a distance of 1.5–2 cm from the pectinate line to the anal margin (anatomic anal canal). From a surgical point of view, the anal canal begins at the anorectal ring and ends at the anal margin (surgical anal canal) extending for 3–4 cm [7, 9, 15, 16].

The pectinate line (also known as the dentate or mucocutaneous line) lies at the inferior level of the anal columns and indicates the junction of the superior part of the anal canal (derived from the embryonic hindgut) and the inferior part (derived from the embryonic proctodeum) [7, 15]. The mucosa of the upper anal canal is lined by columnar epithelium, whereas the mucosa distal to the dentate line is lined by squamous epithelium. However, a transitional zone lies immediately above the pectinate line and consists of mucosa covered by cuboidal epithelium.

The anorectal ring which makes up the upper limit of the surgical canal is constituted by the puborectalis muscle which is the deepest fascicle of the levator ani muscle and forms a true sling surrounding the rectum posteriorly. The anterior pull of the puborectalis sling around the anorectal ring maintains the normal anorectal angle between 80° and 120° at rest (Fig. 1.3) [10, 13, 17].

The anal canal plays an important role in fecal continence and is normally kept closed by the tonic contraction of the anal sphincters. The anal canal can be conceptualized as three tubular structures overlying each other (Fig. 1.3). The inner component is mucosa surrounded by the other two outer components which form the sphincter complex [13, 15, 18].

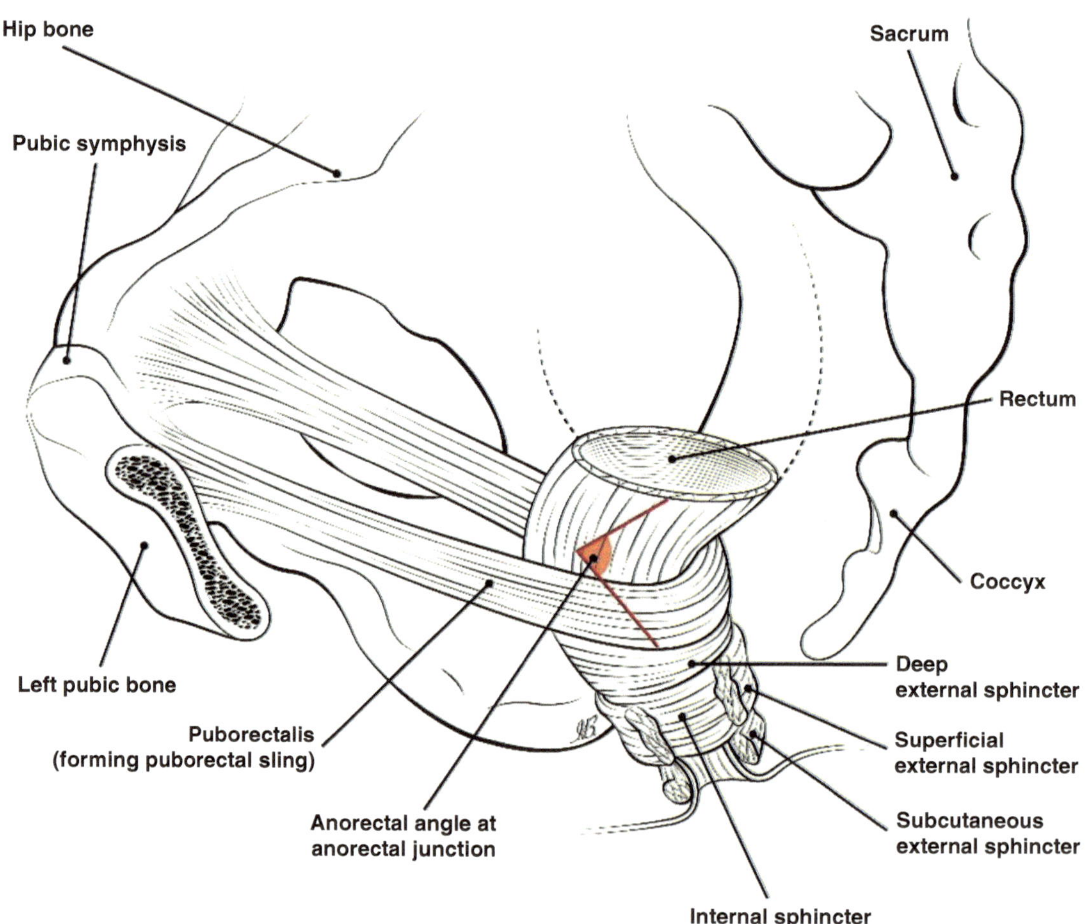

Fig. 1.3 Muscles of the anal canal. The normal anal canal is a closed tube surrounded throughout its length by the sphincter complex muscles. The fibers of puborectalis muscle are in close relation with the deep portion of the EAS, which is partially overlapped. Puborectalis muscle surrounding the anorectal junction, maintain with its pull the anorectal angle between 80° and 120° at rest (mean 90°)

1.3.4 Muscles of the Anal Canal (Fig. 1.3)

The sphincter muscle complex of the anal canal is composed from the inside toward the outside of the internal anal sphincter and the external anal sphincter related posteriorly to the puborectalis portion of the levator ani muscle. Immediately under the skin of the anal margin is found a thin layer of smooth involuntary muscle, the corrugator cutis ani, unimportant for the continence [5, 7, 8, 18, 19].

The internal anal sphincter (IAS) is a circular layer of involuntary smooth muscle that surrounds the mucosa layer of the anal canal. With a thickness of 2 mm and about 25–35 mm long, it ends approximately 1.5 cm below the pectinate line, delimiting a plane with the external sphincter easily perceptible in clinical practice, the intersphincteric groove [6, 9, 20].

The internal anal sphincter is the continuation of the smooth circular muscle layer of the rectum and although is separate from the external sphincter, some elastic fibers reinforced by connective tissue may intersect across the space between the two muscles [3, 7, 21].

The external anal sphincter (EAS) is a voluntary striated muscle approximately 3–5 cm long that forms the outer circular component of the anal canal and may be divided in three portions commonly known as the subcutaneous, superficial, and deep part of the external sphincter, which can be regarded as one functional unit [5, 8, 16, 19, 20].

The subcutaneous portion is defined by the lower fibers of EAS and lies below the internal anal sphincter and the skin of the anal margin.

The superficial portion with its middle fibers constitutes the main part of the muscle which encircle the lower part of the internal anal sphincter. This component of EAS joins posteriorly the anococcygeal raphe and the coccyx and anteriorly, through decussation of some of its fibers, inserts to the perineal body, joining with the superficial transverse perinei, the levator ani muscle and the bulbocavernosus muscle [4, 5, 17, 20].

The deeper portion of the EAS with the upper fibers intermingle anteriorly with the fibers of the puborectalis fascicle of the levator ani muscle.

1.3.5 The Levator Ani Muscle (LAM)

The levator ani muscle in association with its fascial layer forms the main part of the pelvic diaphragm with a form of a funnel trough which passes the urethra, the vagina, and the rectum (levator hiatus). The levator ani is a paired thin muscle made up of the following three muscle components (Fig. 1.4) [22–24]:

- The puborectalis muscle consists the deepest portion of the levator ani muscle. It originates lateral from both sides of the symphysis pubis and surrounds the posterolateral plane of the anal canal (anorectal junction) forming a sling behind the rectum. Some of its fibers are partly intertwined with the deepest portion of the external anal sphincter.
- The pubococcygeus muscle arises in the posterior portion of the pubis, lateral of the origin of puborectalis muscle, and runs horizontally backward to the tendinous center of the perineum to insert into the coccyx.
- The iliococcygeus muscle is a thin muscle that arises more laterally, from the ischial spine and from the posterior part of the tendineus arch of the obturator fascia, and it inserts to the coccyx and the anococcygeal raphe [6, 13, 15, 16, 23, 24].

As a whole, the levator ani muscle forms a U-shaped structure, a muscular diaphragm, in which there is a triangular opening (hiatus) through which passes the anorectal junction (Fig. 1.5). The levator hiatus is bounded by the pubococcygeus and puborectalis muscle and is divided by connective tissue, fibers, and ligaments into the urogenital hiatus (ventral) and anal hiatus (dorsal) which are the pathway for the urethra, the vagina (in women), and the rectum, respectively. The mean diameter of the levator hiatus is approximately 4 cm at rest [4, 5, 13, 25].

The baseline tonic activity of the levator ani muscle keeps the levator hiatus closed by compressing the urethra, vagina, and rectum against the pubis as they exit through this opening [16, 20].

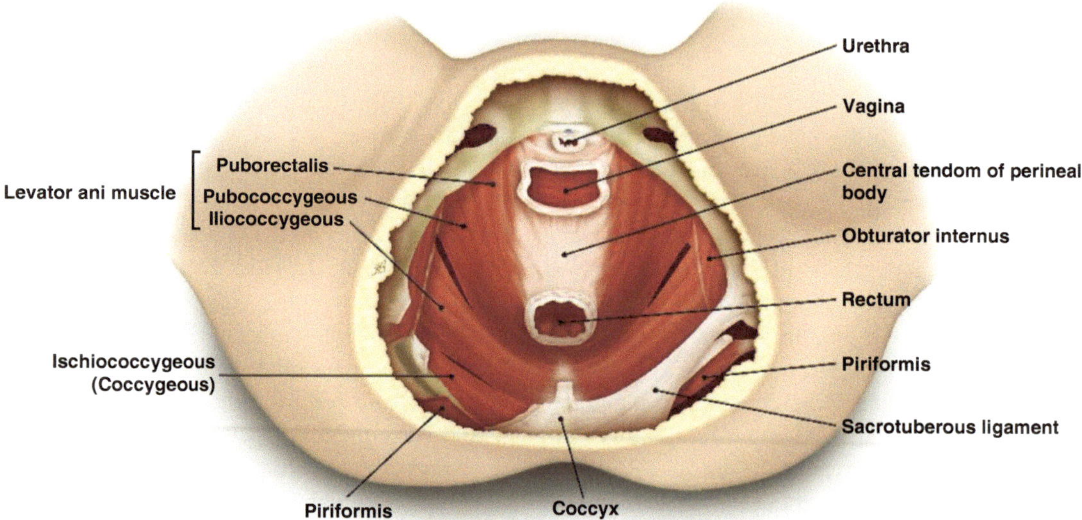

Fig. 1.4 Inferior view of female pelvis. The levator ani muscle

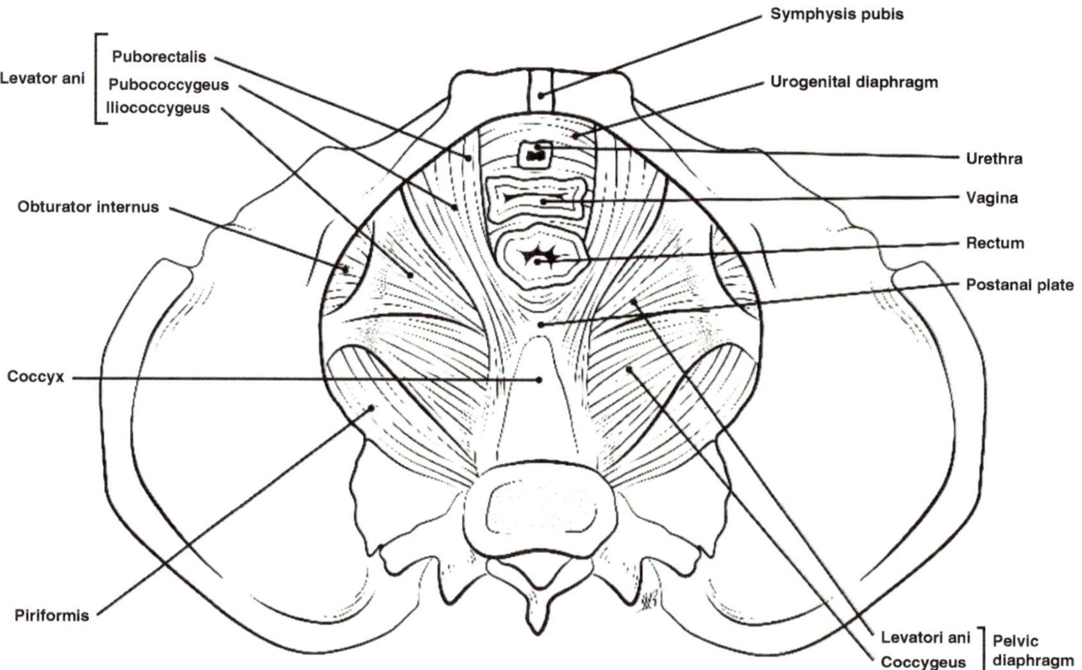

Fig. 1.5 Superior view of female pelvis showing the relation between the muscles of the pelvic diaphragm and the pelvic organs

1.3.6 The Muscular Supports of the Anorectum (Figs. 1.1, 1.4, and 1.5)

The anorectum is supported posteroinferiorly by the levator plate and anteriorly by connective tissue attachments to the vagina (in women, rectovaginal fascia). The levator ani fibers converge behind the rectum and insert directly into his posterior wall to form the levator plate (LP) which contraction forms a horizontal shelf over which the pelvic organs rest [6, 8, 15, 25].

The smooth longitudinal muscle of the rectum inserts into striated muscle arising from the levator plate, the lateral part of pubococcygeus muscle and puborectalis muscle to become the conjoint longitudinal muscle of the anus (LMA) [4, 9].

The puborectalis muscle (PRM) anchors the posterior wall of the anorectum and with its contraction accentuates the anorectal angle [13].

The perineal body is a central insertion point of the perineum for the external anal sphincter, the bulbospongiosus muscle, and the deep and superficial transverse perinei muscles. This important fibromuscular node interposes between the anal canal and the urogenital diaphragm anteriorly. The external anal sphincter acts as a tensor of the perineal body [4, 25, 26].

Between the external anal sphincter and the coccyx lies the postanal plate, a tendinous structure which also contains striated muscles inserting into the external anal sphincter. Contraction of the anterior part of the pubococcygeus muscle, perineal body, external anal sphincter, and postanal plate anchors the anus distally [2, 26].

Because the pelvic muscles (PCM, LP, LMA) insert into the pelvic ligaments (pubourethral, uterosacral, pubovesical ligaments), laxity in these ligaments may cause fecal incontinence and evacuation disorders [2, 17].

1.3.7 Vascularization

The rectum and the anus are supplied by the superior rectal artery (branch of the inferior mesenteric artery) as well as the middle and inferior rectal arteries [8, 14, 27].

The superior rectal artery supplies the portion of the anal canal that is superior to the pectinate line.

The middle rectal artery arises mostly from the internal iliac artery and reaches the rectum at the level of the levator ani muscles through the lateral rectal ligaments (the middle rectal artery anastomoses with the superior rectal artery).

The inferior rectal artery originates from the internal pudendal artery and supplies the most part of the anal canal below the pectinate line and the muscles of the anal sphincter complex. The three arteries anastomose with each other between rich arterial systems.

The veins of anorectum follow the same course as the arteries and form two plexus of veins. The internal hemorrhoidal plexus drains into the superior and middle rectal vein, emptying into the inferior mesenteric vein and the internal iliac vein, respectively. The external hemorrhoidal plexus drains into the inferior rectal vein and the internal pudendal vein.

1.3.8 Innervation

The innervation of the anorectum is made up by the autonomous nervous system with its sympathetic and parasympathetic component. The nerves follow the course of the blood vessels [8, 28].

The fibers of the sympathetic innervation come from neurons of the 1st, 2nd, and 3rd lumbar sympathetic ganglia and are distributed mainly via the hypogastric plexus. The parasympathetic innervation arises from neurons of the 2nd, 3rd, and 4th sacral nerves and is distributed through the nervi erigentes [8, 28].

The levator ani muscle is supplied by fibers of both the 4th sacral nerve and the perineal nerves (coccygeal plexus). The LAM receives branches of the levator ani nerve and of the inferior rectal nerve, both collaterals of the internal pudendal nerve (S3, S4) [8, 29].

The external anal sphincter is a voluntary muscle and has a nerve supply from the inferior rectal nerve (subcutaneous portion), the 4th sacral nerve (superficial portion), and the branches of the pudendal nerve (deep portion). The pudendal nerves provide both the sensory afferents of the anal canal and the motor efferents (somatic innervation) to the voluntary muscles of the anal canal [8, 29–31].

The internal anal sphincter is an involuntary muscle with the same autonomic innervation as the rectum. The parasympathetic nerve fibers have inhibitory action causing relaxation whereas the sympathetic nerve fibers from the superior rectal and hypogastric plexus, have stimulating action causing contraction [8, 28, 29].

Above the pectinate line, the nerve supply is visceral, coming from the inferior hypogastric plexus, so this part of the anal canal is only sensitive to stretch. Below the pectinate line, the nerve supply is somatic, receiving fibers from the inferior rectal nerves (branches of the pudendal nerve). As it is somatically innervated, it is sensitive to pain, temperature and touch [13, 28, 29].

Conclusions

In conclusion, any kind of damage or structural modification of the muscles, fascia, and ligaments that implicated in the mechanism of fecal continence are associated with anorectal dysfunction. Therefore, it is highly important for the surgeons to have a thorough knowledge of the anatomy and physiology of the anorectum and the associated pelvic floor muscles, in order to obtain an appropriate management of fecal incontinence and defecatory disorders, resulting from the loss of anatomical integrity of these structures.

The images were created by Ilaria Bondi.

Acknowledgment The authors thank Prof. Francesco Ruotolo for his valuable contribution.

References

1. Lawson JO. Pelvic anatomy. Ann R Coll Surg. 1974;54:244–52.e288–300.
2. DeLancey JOL. Structural anatomy of the posterior pelvic compartment as it relates to rectocele. Am J Obstet Gynecol. 1999;180:815–23.
3. Bharucha AE. Pelvic floor: anatomy and function. Neurogastroenterol Motil. 2006;18(7):507–19.
4. DeLancey JO, Delmas V. Gross anatomy and functional anatomy of the pelvic floor. Philadelphia: Elsevier Saunders; 2004.
5. Courtney H. Anatomy of pelvic diaphragm and anorectal musculature as related to sphincter preservation in anorectal surgery. Am J Surg. 1950;79:155–73.
6. Lawson JO. Pelvic anatomy. I. Pelvic floor muscles. Ann R Coll Surg Engl. 1974;54:244–52.
7. Pl W, Warwick R, Dyson M, Bannister LH. Gray's anatomy. 37th ed. London: Churchill Livingstone; 1989.
8. Sabiston Jr DC. Textbook of surgery: the biological basis of modern surgical practice. 15th ed. Philadelphia: Saunders; 1997.
9. Morgan CN, Thompson HR. Surgical anatomy of the anal canal, with special reference to the surgical importance of the internal sphincter and conjoint longitudinal muscle. Ann R Coll Surg Engl. 1956;19:88.
10. Tench EN. Development of the anus in the human embryo. Am J Anat. 1936;59:333.
11. De Vries PA, Friedland GW. The staged sequential development of the anus and rectum in human embryos and fetuses. J Pediatr Surg. 1974;9:755–69.
12. Nobles VP. The development of the human anal canal. J Anat. 1984;138:575.
13. Shafik A. A new concept of the anatomy of the anal sphincter mechanism and the physiology of defecation II. Anatomy of the levator ani muscle with special reference to pubo-rectalis. Invest Urol. 1975;13:175.
14. Tagart REB. The anal canal and rectum: their varying relationship and its effect on anal continence. Dis Colon Rectum. 1966;9:449.
15. Hugues ES. Surgical anatomy of the anal canal. Aust NZ J Surg. 1957;26:48–55.
16. Milligan ETC, Morgan N. Surgical anatomy of the anal canal: with special reference to anorectal fistulae. Lancet. 1934;2:1150.
17. Shobeiri SA, Leclaire E, Nihira MA, Quiroz LH, O'Donoghue D. Appearance of the levator ani muscle subdivisions in endovaginal three-dimensional ultrasonography. Obset Gynecol. 2009;114:66–72.
18. Fritsch H, Brenner E, Lienemann A, et al. Anal sphincter complex: reinterpreted morphology and its clinical relevance. Dis Colon Rectum. 2002;45(2):188–94.
19. Shafik A. A new concept of the anatomy of the anal sphincter mechanism and the physiology of defecation I. The external anal sphincter: a triple-loop system. Invest Urol. 1975;12:412–9.
20. Fernandez-Fraga X, Azpiroz F, Malagelada JR. Significance of pelvic floor muscles in anal incontinence. Gastroenterology. 2002;123:1441–50.
21. Liu J, Guaderrama N, Nager CW, et al. Functional correlates of anal canal anatomy: puborectalis muscle and anal canal pressure. Am J Gastroenterol. 2006;101:1092–7.
22. Kearney R, Sawhney R, DeLancey JO. Levator ani muscle anatomy evaluated by origin-insertion pairs. Obstet Gynecol. 2004;104:168–73.
23. Li D, Guo M. Morphology of the levator ani muscle. Dis Colon Rectum. 2007;50:1831–9.
24. Guo M, Li D. Pelvic floor images: anatomy of the levator ani muscle. Dis Colon Rectum. 2007;50:1647–55.
25. Shobeiri SA, Rostaminia G, White DE, Quiroz LH. The determinants of minimal levator hiatus and

their relationship to the puborectalis muscle and the levator plate. BJOG. 2013;120(2):205–11.
26. Petros PE. The female pelvic floor. Function, dysfunction and management according to the integral theory. Berlin/Heidelberg: Springer; 2010.
27. Patricio J, et al. Surgical anatomy of the arterial blood supply of the human rectum. Surg Radiol Anat. 1988;10:71–5.
28. Dyck PJ, Thomas PK. Autonomic and somatic systems to the anorectum and pelvic floor. 4th ed. Philadelphia: Elsevier Saunders; 2005.
29. Guaderrama NM, Liu J, Nager CW, et al. Evidence for the innervation of pelvic floor muscles by the pudendal nerve. Obstet Gynecol. 2005;106:774–81.
30. Laeson J. Motor nerve supply of the pelvic floor. Lancet. 1981;i:999.
31. Gagnard C, Godlewski G, Prat D, et al. The nerve branches to the external anal sphincter. Surg Radiol Anat. 1986;8:115–9.

2 Physiology and Physiopathology

Paolo Urciuoli, Dimitri Krizzuk, and Giada Livadoti

2.1 The Physiology of Human Defecation

Defecation involves an integration of coordinated and complex sensory and motor functions, controlled by the central, spinal, peripheral, and enteric neural system activity and acting on a morphologically intact gastrointestinal tract [1].

The concepts of continence and defecation are inextricably linked, since their balance is based on common anatomical, physiological, and neurological aspects [2].

The motoric mechanism at the root of defecation uses voluntary and involuntary muscles. Therefore, a delicate collaboration between the sphincter complex, rectum, and pelvic floor is held. Pelvic nerves, which carry out both somatic and visceral functions, mediate the sensory component. Moreover, muscles and nerves of the pelvis mediate the connection between sensory and motor functions [3].

It is widely agreed that the normal defecation frequency in adults varies between maximum of three times a day and a minimum of three times a week. However, we can define evacuating three times a week as a normal condition only if there is no discomfort for the patient [4, 5].

It is acknowledged by now that a variety of psychological and behavioral factors can influence gastrointestinal functions. The influence of the psychological sphere has been approved by studies revealing an increased incidence of constipation in patients with psychological impairments due to a trauma or sexual abuse as well as anxiety or stress [6, 7].

Even posture plays an important role in the dynamics of defecation. Defecography has shown that the anorectal angle becomes more obtuse (open) due to an increased flexion of the hips, thus facilitating evacuation. A study that examined how duration of evacuation and sense of satisfaction is related to the position taken during defecation found that assuming a squatting posture makes evacuation faster and provides greater feeling of complete emptying in comparison with a sitting position (according to Western usage) [8, 9].

Stool's volume and consistency are other factors that affect intestinal transit duration and consequently the defecation [9]. The transit time and the velocity with which the content reaches the rectum are depending on the coordinate motor activity of the colon. Similarly, the physical and chemical nature of the stool comes into consideration [10, 11]. Indeed, the intestinal prolonged transit allows the colon to perform his functions: to absorb water, electrolytes, and nutritive elements as well as to store and control the evacuation of feces. Intuitively, the reduced motor

P. Urciuoli (✉) • D. Krizzuk • G. Livadoti
Department of Surgery R. Paolucci, Sapienza – University of Rome, Rome, Italy
e-mail: paolo.urciuoli@uniroma1.it

M. Mongardini, M. Giofrè (eds.), *Management of Fecal Incontinence*,
DOI 10.1007/978-3-319-32226-1_2

activity of the colon and therefore a delayed transit allow for a greater absorption of water from the intraluminal content and reduce the volume of stool, making defecation more challenging [12, 13]. The motor activity of the colon has a circadian rhythm. It increases after awakening and is more active during daytime than at night. Ingestion of a meal is considered the most powerful physiological stimulus that can affect gastrointestinal transit and motor activity. In fact, during alimentation, an increased motor activity is observed in the transverse and descending colon [14, 15].

The muscular apparatus of the colon and the rectum is formed of a smooth muscle tissue, and its contractile function is guaranteed due to interstitial cells (cells of Cajal) with a pacemaker function. Four types of terminations ensure the innervation: the enteric nervous system, the sympathetic nervous system, the parasympathetic nervous system, and the extrinsic sensory innervation [2, 16].

The motor activity of the colon is supported by phasic and tonic contractions [17]. Phasic contractions are divided further into propagating and non-propagating contractions, depending on the generated colonic transit. The non-propagating type is more frequent, since they contract with 2–4 cycles per minute, exert compressed pressure between 5 and 50 mmHg, and can have either a short (15 s) or long (15–60 s) duration. It is believed that the function of these contractions is to facilitate the mixing of the intraluminal contents through the propulsion and retropulsion of the fecal bolus [18, 19].

The peristaltic activity of the colon can propagate the intestinal contents in a retrograde (oral propagation) or anterograde (aboral propagation) sense. The first type is less common. It appears confined to the proximal colon, and its frequency may be higher in patients with constipation [19].

Among the peristaltic waves which ensure the propagation of the colonic contents, there are patterns of waves with high amplitude. These are better known as high-amplitude propagated sequences (HAPSs) or high-amplitude propagated contractions (HAPCs) and exert a pressure of 100 mmHg. They commonly arise in the proximal colon then migrate distally for a variable distance [20, 21].

A recent study found that only a third of HAPSs reach the anus, while the rest ends at the rectosigmoid junction. The importance of this type of colic contractions lies in the fact that these are often temporally associated with defecation or intestinal gas leakage. Generally, 15–60 min before defecating, there is a distal progressive migration of the HAPSs that go from the transverse colon or splenic flexure to the descending colon. The HAPSs guarantee the propulsion of fecal material and give rise to what radiologists define as mass movements (that is to say a rapid displacement of a considerable volume of intraluminal contents) [22–24].

Most of the colon activity is characterized by waves of low amplitude, the so-called low-amplitude propagated contractions (LAPCs). These typically exert a pressure of 50 mmHg, with a frequency of 40–120 cycles per 24 h and propagate for a distance of 22.5 cm [21, 25].

When stool reaches the sigma, it is pushed into the rectum by contractions of 15–60 mmHg called motor complexes (MC) [26]. Among this, only 18 % propagate the stool in an aboral sense. When the sigma receives fecal material, its walls are stretched; this triggers a reflex, which leads to contraction of the walls with concomitant relaxation of the rectosigmoid junction. This mechanism probably facilitates the progression of stool into the rectum [27]. The existence of a sphincter between the sigmoid colon and the rectum (the sphincter of O'Beirne) has long been debated. This, in effect, does not result in an anatomical structure but in a high-pressure zone located distally to the sigma that maintains exclusive contractile properties [28].

Inside the rectum, the contractile activity is similar to that of the sigma; contrary to the normal direction of transit, the motor complexes (MCs) guarantee a retrograde propagation. These movements are probably acting to keep the rectum empty, functioning as a braking mechanism, thus avoiding the premature flow of fecal material coming from the colon [29].

At rest, the levator ani, the puborectalis, and the external anal sphincter remain in continuous contraction, guaranteeing the so-called postural reflex that allows maintaining the weight of the hollow viscera. The puborectalis muscle is the most implicated in the control of defecation and receives innervation directly from the anterior roots of S3 and S4 [30, 31]. The traction that exerted during rest by the puborectalis maintains the anorectal angle (angle between the axis of the rectum and the longitudinal axis of the anal canal) at about 90° [13, 32].

In order to preserve continence, the sphincter complex normally remains closed, thanks to the tonic contraction of the external and internal anal sphincter muscle, as well as to the hemorrhoidal cushions [33]. The internal anal sphincter (IAS) is a smooth muscle with high resistance; it is mainly responsible for continence at rest, and its contraction is maintained by slow waves at a frequency of 20–40 cycles per minute. The IAS exerts a pressure ranging from 50 to 120 mmHg [13].

The external anal sphincter (EAS) maintains a constant tonic activity as well; however, it affects only 30 % of the global anal tone at rest. The external anal sphincter is a voluntary muscle, which receives its innervation from the pudendal nerve. It can exert a pressure that ranges from 50 to 200 mmHg [13]. The anal cushions, formed by the hemorrhoidal plexus, are too contributing 15 % of anal tone at rest, providing the "hermetic seal" to the anal canal, which cannot be guaranteed solely by the sphincter muscle tone [3, 34].

The activity of the anal canal is intermittent. It is characterized by a temporary relaxation of the internal anal sphincter muscle that allows the contents of the rectum to descent into the anal canal, thus enabling a conscious perception of their physical nature. This phenomenon is called sampling reflex; it occurs about seven times an hour in healthy subjects and is less frequent in patients suffering from incontinence [35].

Distention of the rectum causes a reflex relaxation of the internal anal sphincter muscle and a concomitant contraction of the external anal sphincter muscle. This occurrence is called recto-anal inhibitory reflex (RAIR). Consequently, the pressure in the upper segment of the anal canal decreases so the rectal pressure becomes greater than or equal to the medium anal pressure. However, in order to preserve continence, the pressure of the lower portion of the anal canal remains virtually unchanged and thus greater than the intrarectal pressure [36, 37].

The net effect of the change in pressure that occurs during the sampling reflex briefly exposes the sensory anal zone to rectal content in order to allow its recognition. The integrity of the epithelium of the anal canal guarantees discrimination and is, in fact, covered with high-sensitivity receptors, including corpuscles of Krause, Golgi-Mazzoni bodies, genital corpuscles, Meissner and Pacinian corpuscles, and sensory, motor, and autonomous nerve endings, as well as the enteric nervous system. The reflex is controlled by the enteric nervous system and affected by the spinal cord and is therefore absent in patients with Hirschsprung's disease. Simply said, the RAIR allows discriminating the fecal content distinguishing the solid, liquid, and gaseous nature of fecal material [38].

The need to defecate originates in the rectum. When HAPSs push fecal material in the sigmoid colon and subsequently to the rectum, its gradual distention produces a sensory response, which is translated into rectal filling sensation [39, 40]. Subsequent to the distension, a constant urge to defecate is felt. Delayed defecation causes a sense of discomfort and an intense need to evacuate which related directly to the volume and the maximum tolerable pressure [41].

A similar feeling to the desire to defecate may be evoked by manometry using a balloon at a distance of 15 cm from the anal margin. Stretching the rectum at a greater distance leads to a suprapubic pain. There are extra-rectal causes for the need to defecate. If in fact the nerve endings, the receptors of the pelvic muscles, and the adjacent structures of the rectum are stimulated, it can induce a sense of defecation urgency [42].

It is now known that stool, transported into the rectum through the HAPSs, stretches and deforms the rectum and stimulating mechanoreceptors, which in turn induce reflex rectal contraction [21].

The rectum has an important compliance that allows tolerating increases in volume with little change in pressure. This function triggers an adaptive relaxation of the rectum, which gives it reservoir characteristics. This ability is guaranteed by its rich in collagen elastic walls and the relaxation of its smooth musculature [13].

The extent of the rectal walls' contraction increases with augmentation of fecal volume. Studies report that the sensation of defecation cannot be verified without the musculature contraction and that the duration of the rectal contraction appears to be directly correlated with the duration of the perception [41].

Several studies have led to the conclusion that the rectal sensation does not depend on the weight or the volume of the contents, while it is strictly related to the change in pressure that is exerted on the stretch receptors. On the other hand, latest studies found that the defecation stimulus depends on the circumferential wall deformation arising from the increase in pressure [43–45].

Our knowledge of defecation's neurophysiology is based on studies conducted on animals. Along the myenteric plexus, the nerve endings have a lamellar aspect with branching ends named rectal intraganglionic laminar endings (rIGLEs) that have been identified as low-threshold sensitive-to-traction mechanoreceptors [46, 47]. There are also other mechanoreceptors, which are sensitive to medium-/high-intensity compression, located at the vicinity of the intra- and extramural vessels along most of the viscera including the colon [48].

The sacral plexus plays a key role in the sensory perception of the rectum, while the thoracolumbar is secondary. The rectal sensory perception is in fact preserved after bilateral pudendal nerve block. However, low spinal anesthesia (L5–S1) abolishes rectal sensation, so that the rectal distension results only in a vague abdominal discomfort. High spinal anesthesia (T6–T12) is able to abolish not only rectal perception but also that of the abdomen [49]. It was also demonstrated that the feeling of rectal distension is impaired in patients with bilateral lesions of the sacral nerve roots (preserving bilaterally S1–S2) [50]. However, some of the rectal sensory perception information follows the lumbar afferents from the inferior mesenteric ganglion and continue to the hypogastric nerve through the pelvic ganglia and reaching the rectum through the rectal nerves. This innervation is probably responsible for the abdominal discomfort that is associated with the distension of the rectum [49].

Currently, neurophysiologists' common belief is that the nerve pathways related to the rectum is working in parallel to the sacral sympathetic and parasympathetic system, following neural structures in the lateral ligaments, through the pelvic plexus and pelvic splanchnic nerves (nervi erigentes), and then reaching the sacral segments of the spinal cord through nerve roots S3 and S4 [50, 51].

Recent studies on the central nervous system showed that the spinal afferents from the abdominal viscera follows a spinal-thalamic-cortical tract [52]. On the insular cortex, in fact, sensitive pathways that encode painful stimuli seem to end, while on the cingulate cortex the autonomic, emotional, and motivational responses to the visceral stimulus are elaborated [53]. Therefore, when the sensation of rectal filling becomes conscious and the act of defecation is socially appropriate, evacuation begins.

The intrarectal pressure must exceed that of the anal canal and is sustained by colorectal contraction and pelvic relaxation.

During rest, the pelvic floor remains in a continuous contraction, thus preserving continence. The increase in the abdominal pressure, perceived by the pelvic floor due to neuromuscular spindles, induces an initial contraction of the muscles. In case this pressure exceeds a certain critical value, an inhibitory reflex enables relaxation of the pelvic musculature [54].

At the same time, the puborectalis muscle branches relax and open a 90° angle between the rectum and the anal canal. In addition, the pubococcygeus muscles "squeeze" the perineum, thus recalling tension on the anterior wall of the anal canal and moving backward the posterior wall. An adequate relaxation of the pelvic floor is essential for effective evacuation; otherwise, dyssynergic defecation occurs [55].

The involuntary relaxation of the internal anal sphincter muscle follows the distension of the rectum so that it is directly proportional to the intrarectal pressure.

After assuming an optimal position, the defecatory "push," which is associated with synergistic contraction of the abdominal muscles, diaphragm, and a closed glottis (Valsalva maneuver), allows, by voluntarily relaxing the anal sphincter muscle, to produce a posteriorly and inferiorly directed vector [55].

The hemorrhoid cushions are flattened by the contraction of the sphincter muscles and the passage of stool. All of this induces changes in pressure that define a gradient between the rectum and the outside that allows the expulsion of feces. It has been suggested that once defecation started, the input generated in the anal canal continues until the rectum is completely empty [56].

In case defecation is postponed, the external anal sphincter is contracted while resisting the increased pressure of the rectum for a sufficient period that allows the adaptation of the rectum to the new volume. There is a further contraction of the pelvic floor, including the puborectalis muscle. During this phase, the anorectal angle acuity is increased, the pelvic floor is elevated, and the high-pressure area of the anal canal extends [3].

The end of defecation is a semi-voluntary phenomenon mediated by the involuntary contraction of the external anal sphincter and the pelvic floor that closes the anal canal and reverses the pressure gradient. In fact, when we apply a traction to the anus which we then subsequently release (similar to passage of stool), a momentary increase of activity in the external sphincter muscle occurs, leading to a closure of the anal canal. This occurrence, called the closing reflex, allows the internal anal sphincter muscle to restore its basic tone. This reflex is mediated by cerebral cortex; therefore, it results in compromised patients with spinal injuries [13, 30, 57].

When defecation ends, the puborectalis muscle regains its tone increasing the traction on the anorectal junction and the anorectal angle. Simultaneously, the longitudinal muscles of the anal canal relax and thus lengthen, allowing the distention of the hemorrhoid cushions [57].

2.2 The Physiopathology of Fecal Incontinence

The principal factors for fecal continence depend on the enteric content, which is essentially stable and voluminous, and on the presence of a passively stretchable, capacious, and evacuable "Rectal Reservoir" and an effective anti-reflux pelvic barrier. Therefore, variations in the quantity and quality of stools reaching the sphincter, the inability of the rectum to receive and retain fecal material, and the mechanical and/or sensory damages of the internal and external anal sphincter can cause fecal incontinence [58]. Most common causes include diarrhea, fecaloma with "overflow" mechanism, defective rectal stool storage, rectal distension sensitivity loss, isolated or combined sphincter, and puborectalis muscle weakness or impairment [58]. The suggested classification is based on a study of fecal incontinence performed by the "Guideline Development Group" (GDG), a multidisciplinary group at the "The Royal College of Surgeons of England," which was published by the "National Institute for Health and Clinical Excellence" in 2007 [59].

The study was based on information obtained regarding fecal incontinence (defined as the "involuntary loss of liquid or solid feces") in patients over 18 years of age. According to the GDG, the majority of patients with fecal incontinence can be classified into one or more of the following groups:

- Patients with abnormal anorectal complex (sphincter trauma, sphincter degeneration, rectal prolapse, perianal fistula)
- Patients with neurological disorders (e.g., multiple sclerosis, spinal cord injury, spina bifida, stroke, etc.)
- Patients with constipation or fecal overload (e.g., diet, drugs, megarectum)
- Patients affected by cognitive and/or behavioral issues (such as dementia, learning disabilities)
- Patients with loose stools or diarrhea from any cause (e.g., gastrointestinal problems such as

inflammatory bowel disease (IBD) or irritable bowel syndrome (IBS))
- Patients with disabilities (frail patients with acute illness or chronic/acute disabilities)
- Idiopathic conditions (e.g., adult patients with fecal incontinence with none of the previous cases)

According to the study performed by GDG, we can assign each case to a group by dividing patients into classes in order to ease the study and the subsequent therapeutic evaluation of the pathology.

2.2.1 Local Primary Lesions

This group includes the most frequent causes of fecal incontinence. First subdivision distinguishes structural anorectal alterations from diseases that lead to fecal incontinence (such as IBDs, intestinal infections, and other diseases that can cause diarrhea like colitis and proctitis) [60].

Among the structural anorectal lesions, traumatic lesions of the anal sphincter are most significant and most frequently observed. This group includes obstetric lesions, postoperative iatrogenic lesions, and accidental traumatic lesions. Obstetric trauma has the highest incidence, both following a surgical procedure (episiotomy) and a sequel of traumatic delivery (prolonged labor, a disproportion between the size of the baby and the pelvis, breech delivery, forceps use).

The correlation between obstetric lesions and incontinence is now well documented in global literature. Incontinence is a complication that can occur either immediately after birth and resolve within a few months representing a temporary consequence of vaginal traumatic childbirth or may be the sequel of a major pelvic floor laceration resulting in a long-term condition. The latter may also predispose to the onset of conditions such as rectal prolapse [61].

The following classification described by Sultan [83] has been adopted by the International Consultation on Incontinence [84] and the RCOG:

- First-degree tear: Injury to perineal skin and/or vaginal mucosa
- Second-degree tear: Injury to perineum involving perineal muscles but not involving the anal sphincter
- Third-degree tear: Injury to the perineum involving the anal sphincter complex:
  - Grade 3a tear: Less than 50 % of external anal sphincter (EAS) thickness torn
  - Grade 3b tear: More than 50 % of EAS thickness torn
  - Grade 3c tear: Both EAS and internal anal sphincter (IAS) torn
- Fourth-degree tear: Injury to perineum involving the anal sphincter complex (EAS and IAS) and anorectal mucosa

Clinical incidence of third- and fourth-degree lacerations varies greatly. The prevalence is of 0.5–3 % in Europe and 6–9 % in the USA [61]. Large prospective studies have clearly shown that about 25 % of primiparous women undergo changes in fecal continence in the postpartum period. Approximately a third of these women have evidence of traumatic lesions of the anal sphincter after their first vaginal delivery. In most cases, these symptoms and lesions are relatively moderate and transient; however, persistent gas incontinence and defecation urgency is an emotionally and socially debilitating factor [61, 62].

Most frequent and significant predisposing factors for third- or fourth-degree perianal lesions are premature birth, Asian ethnicity, increased duration of labor, abstention of vacuum during delivery, and increased weight of the newborn [63]. A large newborn head circumference is another important risk factor for lesions of the levator ani [64].

Eder et al. (2012) in a large female population-based study compared symptoms and their impact on the quality of life. Women with anal sphincter lacerations due to childbirth, women who had a vaginal birth without sphincter lacerations, and women who have undergone a caesarean were included in this study. Women suffering from anal sphincter laceration reported anal incontinence, and their test results showed a higher negative impact on their quality of life [65].

Anal incontinence and quality of life among the two latest categories of women were reported similar. In conclusion, the laceration of the anal sphincter is associated with anal incontinence within 5–10 years after delivery. Women who had lesions of the levator ani muscle will be subject to pelvic organ prolapse (POP 35.3 % vs 15.5 %) [63].

When it comes to episiotomy, the arguments are contradicting. Several studies support the theory stating that episiotomy reduces the risk of pelvic floor dysfunction compared to vaginal birth that is frequently complicated by significant lacerations [66]. Most gynecologists support this theory and therefore recommend it in predefined cases or even as a routine procedure.

Recent studies have established an effective combination between the geometric properties of episiotomy and obstetric anal sphincter lesions. Incision made starting from the posterior margin of the vulvar commissure, tilting it by 40–60°, decreases sphincter's obstetric lesions in comparison to episiotomy with acute angles [67].

On the other hand, the world literature supports a diametrically opposite position; through proctologists and surgeon's experience, it is witnessed that the relationship between fecal incontinence and an episiotomy is more than frequent [68]. Women with lesions in the internal anal sphincter or in the rectal mucosa due to episiotomy are more predisposed to future continence problems [60]. In fact, episiotomy, which in the past was frequently used not only in cases of complicated labor but as a routine technique, had a higher risk of anal incontinence, almost twice then a more restrictive episiotomy policy [69].

Farther, hysterectomies performed especially in cases of uterine cancer increase the risk of fecal incontinence since the anatomical relationship with the rectum is altered by the surgical resection [70].

Abandoning the obstetric argument, it is important to analyze another important pathological field of incontinence: a significant risk factor represented by anorectal diseases. Among the related diseases are hemorrhoids, anal fistula, and rectal prolapse in which the exuberant mucosa at first occlude the anal canal, then dilate it, and subsequently stretch the sphincters, leading to their dysfunction [71].

Chronic inflammatory bowel disease, anorectal cancers, infectious diseases, proctitis, and colitis can represent other colorectal conditions. Moreover, surgical procedures for these pathologies represent a common risk factor for fecal incontinence. A high incidence of soiling following an internal sphincterotomy and fistulotomy (35–45 %), in which the muscle continuity is interrupted, has been historically noticed [72].

The incidence of this surgery's side effect depends on many factors, although a correct procedure performed on a suitably selected patient may lead to better results and reduce consequences.

Incontinence can also result from incorrect surgical procedure during hemorrhoidectomies. Other procedures that place patients at high risk of fecal incontinence include low anterior resection of the rectum (LAR) often performed following rectal cancer diagnosis. Incontinence after LAR results from the post-resection loss of rectal physiological reservoir, an anatomical ampoule adapted to receive feces. This procedure results in the inability of the neorectum to contain feces, thus causing a "passive" loss. The deviation of fecal transit isolating the lower intestinal tract by having a temporary cutaneous stoma led to better functional outcomes [72].

To conclude, it is important to note the existence of anorectal structural alterations due to congenital anomalies such as the imperforate anus and Hirschsprung's disease, which become symptomatic in childhood [71].

2.2.2 Neurological Causes

Neurological causes may be related to central or peripheral nervous system. Among the causes related to the CNS, the vascular pathology, consistent of stroke, is worth mentioning as a cause leading to fecal incontinence even during rehabilitation [73].

It is important as well to mention brain tumors, dementia, and Alzheimer's and Parkinson's disease, which all alter normal neural transmission coming from the proximal motor neuron [74, 75]. Spina bifida has an incidence of 1:1000. It can cause fecal incontinence with a prevalence of 34.1 % and may appear isolated or associated with urinary incontinence present in 26.3 % of cases [76].

The most frequent causes remain those affecting the distal motor neurons originating from the sacral segments of the spinal cord, as in meningocele, the surgical treatment of teratoma and chordoma, compression of the cauda equina, arachnoiditis, and tumors of the sacrum and sacral roots. Anorectal sensitivity and voluntary control of the external anal sphincter are reduced or completely lost in cases of both traumatic and nontraumatic spinal cord lesions, especially when affecting the sacral segments of the spinal cord and cauda equine [77]. The severity of the colon-rectal dysfunction and sphincter control depends on the extent and the severity of the lesions. In these cases, there is a loss of anal tone due to paralysis of the internal and external anal sphincters and lack of fecal loss perception, determined by the lack of sensitivity of the entire perineum.

Peripheral neuropathies are numerous and correspond to primary pathologies (such as pudendal nerve neuropathy) or secondary.

Above all, there is diabetic neuropathy. The elevation of the sensory threshold of the anal canal is an early anomaly in development of fecal incontinence in patients with diabetes [78]. It was found in these patients, by using electrostimulators, that the autonomic neuropathy causes a significant increase in the sensory threshold in the upper and medium part of the anal canal, compared with nondiabetic patients. Fecal incontinence as a result of multiple sclerosis is also worth mentioning. In these young patients, the manometric study shows a decrease of the "squeeze maximal sphincter pressures," decrease of the anal inhibitory reflex, and the presence of paradox contractions of the puborectalis muscle and inferior anal sphincter [79].

2.2.3 Secondary Pathologies

This group includes several morbid conditions that can cause incontinence. Constipation and fecal overload due to megacolon are relatively frequent causes. Fecaloma is one of the constipating pathologies that after a primary obstructive syndrome can cause incontinence due to an "overflow" mechanism [58].

The elderly, without adequate care or suffering from debilitating diseases, can manifest their "fragility" through fecal incontinence, which is senescence dependent or due to a specific disease.

Any form of disability that limits the autonomy of the patient can cause incontinence because of the difficulty in reaching the toilet [80]. This symptom is also common in cognitive/behavioral disorders.

Patients treated with pelvic radiotherapy reported events of fecal incontinence as a real side effect of the treatment. The same can be said about changed consistency of the stool due to laxative drug abuse [71].

2.2.4 Idiopathic Causes

All patients with documented fecal incontinence and without any attributable cause are included in this group. Within these patients, a recent imaging study showed increased volume of the anorectal tract due to a three-directional vector acting on the walls of the rectum, doubling its diameter during defecation [81].

The anterior rectal wall is subject to an anterior traction, while the posterior wall is subject to a posteroinferior traction that increases the anorectal angle. These findings are consistent with relaxation of some of the pelvic floor muscles during defecation and the contraction of others. In fact, the relaxation of the puborectalis muscle defines the so-called syndrome of descending perineum. The relaxation of the puborectalis muscle releases the posterior wall of the rectum so that it can be outstretched and dilated by the contraction of the anterior extremity of the levator ani muscles, aligning longitudinally the rectal channel with the anus.

Subsequently, the contraction of the pubococcygeus muscle draws forward the anterior wall of the rectum, increasing further its diameter [81]. When fecal material enters the rectum, the external anal sphincter relaxes, and a rectal contraction expels the stool. These results are coherent with the assumption that in patients with idiopathic fecal incontinence, the pelvic muscles, by actively tractioning the rectal lumen, dilate it and thus reduce the anorectal resistance to the expulsion of stool.

Idiopathic fecal incontinence can be also associated with the anatomical features of the anal canal [81]. Thekkinkattil et al. (2009) compared, studied, and correlated the diameter of the anal canal and the thickness of the mucosal cushions in women with idiopathic fecal incontinence and in an asymptomatic control group [82]. The rectal mucous cushion volume and the anal canal diameter (C/C) ratio resulted lower in women with idiopathic fecal incontinence compared to the control group. However, according to other studies, a greater latency is observed in both pudendal nerves in women with idiopathic fecal incontinence, supporting the hypothesis claiming that a pudendal nerve neuropathy is at the basis of the pathology [80].

Bibliography

1. Cook IJ, Talley NJ, Benninga MA, Rao SS, Scott SM. Chronic constipation: overview and challenges. Neurogastroenterol Motil. 2009;21:1–8.
2. Brookes SJ, Dinning PG, Gladman MA. Neuroanatomy and physiology of colorectal function and defaecation: from basic science to human clinical studies. Neurogastroenterol Motil. 2009;21:9–19.
3. Palit S, Lunniss PJ, Scott SM. The physiology of human defecation. Dig Dis Sci. 2012;57:1445–64.
4. Heaton KW, Radvan J, Cripps H, Mountford RA, Braddon FE, Hughes AO. Defecation frequency and timing, and stool form in the general population: a prospective study. Gut. 1992;33:818–24.
5. Schaefer DC, Cheskin LJ. Constipation in the elderly. Am Fam Physician. 1998;58:907–14.
6. Dykes S, Smilgin-Humphreys S, Bass C. Chronic idiopathic constipation: a psychological enquiry. Eur J Gastroenterol Hepatol. 2001;13:39–44.
7. Leroi AM, Bernier C, Watier A, et al. Prevalence of sexual abuse among patients with functional disorders of the lower gastrointestinal tract. Int J Colorectal Dis. 1995;10:200–6.
8. Tagart RE. The anal canal and rectum: their varying relationship and its effect on anal continence. Dis Colon Rectum. 1966;9:449–52.
9. Sikirov D. Comparison of straining during defecation in three positions: results and implications for human health. Dig Dis Sci. 2003;48:1201–5.
10. Degen LP, Phillips SF. How well does stool form reflect colonic transit? Gut. 1996;39:109–13.
11. Davies GJ, Crowder M, Reid B, Dickerson JW. Bowel function measurements of individuals with different eating patterns. Gut. 1986;27:164–9.
12. O'Donnell LJ, Virjee J, Heaton KW. Detection of pseudodiarrhoea by simple clinical assessment of intestinal transit rate. BMJ. 1990;300:439–40.
13. Bajwa A, Emmanuel A. The physiology of continence and evacuation. Best Pract Res Clin Gastroenterol. 2009;23:477–85.
14. Rao SS, Kavelock R, Beaty J, Ackerson K, Stumbo P. Effects of fat and carbohydrate meals on colonic motor response. Gut. 2000;46:205–11.
15. Ford MJ, Camilleri M, Wiste JA, Hanson RB. Differences in colonic tone and phasic response to a meal in the transverse and sigmoid human colon. Gut. 1995;37:264–9.
16. Sanders KM, Koh KC, Ward SM. Organization and electrophysiology of interstitial cells of Cajal and smooth muscle cells in the gastrointestinal tract. In: Johnson LR, editor. Physiology of the gastrointestinal tract. San Diego: Elsevier Press; 2006. p. 533–76.
17. Camilleri M, Bharucha AE, di Lorenzo C, et al. American Neurogastroenterology and Motility Society consensus statement on intraluminal measurement of gastrointestinal and colonic motility in clinical practice. Neurogastroenterol Motil. 2008;20:1269–82.
18. Scott SM. Manometric techniques for the evaluation of colonic motor activity: current status. Neurogastroenterol Motil. 2003;15:483–513.
19. Rao SS, Sadeghi P, Beaty J, Kavlock R, Ackerson K. Ambulatory 24-h colonic manometry in healthy humans. Am J Physiol Gastrointest Liver Physiol. 2001;280:G629–39.
20. Cook IJ, Furukawa Y, Panagopoulos V, Collins PJ, Dent J. Relationships between spatial patterns of colonic pressure and individual movements of content. Am J Physiol Gastrointest Liver Physiol. 2000;278:G329–41.
21. Bampton PA, Dinning PG, Kennedy ML, Lubowski DZ, de Carle D, Cook IJ. Spatial and temporal organization of pressure patterns throughout the unprepared colon during spontaneous defecation. Am J Gastroenterol. 2000;95:1027–35.
22. Bassotti G, Chistolini F, Nzepa F, Morelli A. Colonic propulsive impairment in intractable slow-transit constipation. Arch Surg. 2003;138:1302–4.
23. Torsoli A, Ramorino ML, Ammaturo MV, Capurso L, Paoluzi P, Anzini F. Mass movements and intracolonic pressures. Am J Dig Dis. 1971;16:693–6.

24. Ritchie JA, Truelove SC, Ardan GM, Tuckey MS. Propulsion and retropulsion of normal colonic contents. Am J Dig Dis. 1971;16:697–704.
25. Bassotti G, Germani U, Morelli A. Human colonic motility: physiological aspects. Int J Colorectal Dis. 1995;10:173–80.
26. Kumar D, Williams NS, Waldron D, Wingate DL. Prolonged manometric recording of anorectal motor activity in ambulant human subjects: evidence of periodic activity. Gut. 1989;30:1007–11.
27. Shafik A. Sigmoido-rectal junction reflex: role in the defecation mechanism. Clin Anat. 1996;9:391–4.
28. Ballantyne GH. Rectosigmoid sphincter of O'Beirne. Dis Colon Rectum. 1986;29:525–31.
29. Rao S, Welcher K. Periodic rectal motor activity: the intrinsic colonic gatekeeper? Am J Gastroenterol. 1996;91:890–7.
30. Porter NH. A physiological study of the pelvic floor in rectal prolapse. Ann R Coll Surg Engl. 1962;31:379–404.
31. Snooks SJ, Swash M. The innervation of the muscles of continence. Ann R Coll Surg Engl. 1986;68:45–9.
32. Mahieu P, Pringot J, Bodart P. Defecography: I. Description of a new procedure and results in normal patients. Gastrointest Radiol. 1984;9:247–51.
33. Frenckner B. Function of the anal sphincters in spinal man. Gut. 1975;16:638–44.
34. Lestar B, Penninckx F, Kerremans R. The composition of anal basal pressure. An in vivo and in vitro study in man. Int J Colorectal Dis. 1989;4:118–22.
35. Miller R, Lewis GT, Bartolo DC, Cervero F, Mortensen NJ. Sensory discrimination and dynamic activity in the anorectum: evidence using a new ambulatory technique. Br J Surg. 1988;75(10):1003–7.
36. Duthie HL, Bennett RC. The relation of sensation in the anal canal to the functional anal sphincter: a possible factor in anal continence. Gut. 1963;4:179–82.
37. Haynes WG, Read NW. Ano-rectal activity in man during rectal infusion of saline: a dynamic assessment of the anal continence mechanism. J Physiol. 1982;330:45–56.
38. Duthie HL, Gairns FW. Sensory nerve-endings and sensation in the anal region of man. Br J Surg. 1960;47:585–95.
39. Meunier P, Mollard P, Marechal JM. Physiopathology of megarectum: the association of megarectum with encopresis. Gut. 1976;17:224–7.
40. Sun WM, Read NW, Miner PB. Relation between rectal sensation and anal function in normal subjects and patients with faecal incontinence. Gut. 1990;31:1056–61.
41. Broens PM, Penninckx FM, Lestar B, Kerremans RP. The trigger for rectal filling sensation. Int J Colorectal Dis. 1994;9:1–4.
42. Goligher J, Hughes E. Sensibility of the rectum and colon. Its role in the mechanism of anal continence. Lancet. 1951;1:543–7.
43. Gregersen H, Kassab G. Biomechanics of the gastrointestinal tract. Neurogastroenterol Motil. 1996;8:277–97.
44. Gladman MA, Aziz Q, Scott SM, Williams NS, Lunniss PJ. Rectal hyposensitivity: pathophysiological mechanisms. Neurogastroenterol Motil. 2009;21(5):508–16, e4–5.
45. Petersen P, Gao C, Arendt-Nielsen L, Gregersen H, Drewes AM. Pain intensity and biomechanical responses during ramp-controlled distension of the human rectum. Dig Dis Sci. 2003;48:1310–6.
46. Lynn PA, Olsson C, Zagorodnyuk V, Costa M, Brookes SJ. Rectal intraganglionic laminar endings are transduction sites of extrinsic mechanoreceptors in the guinea pig rectum. Gastroenterology. 2003;125:786–94.
47. Olsson C, Costa M, Brookes SJ. Neurochemical characterization of extrinsic innervation of the guinea pig rectum. J Comp Neurol. 2004;470:357–71.
48. Spencer NJ, Kerrin A, Zagorodnyuk VP, et al. Identification of functional intramuscular rectal mechanoreceptors in aganglionic rectal smooth muscle from piebald lethal mice. Am J Physiol Gastrointest Liver Physiol. 2008;294:G855–67.
49. Frenckner B, Ihre T. Influence of autonomic nerves on the internal anal sphincter in man. Gut. 1976;17:306–12.
50. Gunterberg B, Kewenter J, Petersen I, Stener B. Anorectal function after major resections of the sacrum with bilateral or unilateral sacrifice of sacral nerves. Br J Surg. 1976;63:546–54.
51. Todd Jr LT, Yaszemski MJ, Currier BL, Fuchs B, Kim CW, Sim FH. Bowel and bladder function after major sacral resection. Clin Orthop Relat Res. 2002;397:36–9.
52. Craig AD. A new view of pain as a homeostatic emotion. Trends Neurosci. 2003;26:303–7.
53. Willis WD, Al-Chaer ED, Quast MJ, Westlund KN. A visceral pain pathway in the dorsal column of the spinal cord. Proc Natl Acad Sci U S A. 1999;96:7675–9.
54. Enck P, Vodusek DB. Electromyography of pelvic floor muscles. J Electromyogr Kinesiol. 2006;16:568–77.
55. Petros PE, Swash M. The musculoelastic theory of anorectal function and dysfunction. Pelviperineology. 2008;27:89–93.
56. Lynch AC, Anthony A, Dobbs BR, Frizelle FA. Anorectal physiology following spinal cord injury. Spinal Cord. 2000;38:573–80.
57. Nyam DC. The current understanding of continence and defecation. Singapore Med J. 1998;39:132–6.
58. Lazarescu A, Turnbull GK, Vanner S. Investigating and treating fecal incontinence: when and how. Can J Gastroenterol. 2008;23:301–8.
59. Norton C, Thomas L, Hill J. Management of faecal incontinence in adults: summary of NICE guidance. BMJ: British Medical Journal. 2007;334(7608): 1370–1371
60. Power D, Fitzpatrick M, O'Herlihy C. Obstetric anal sphincter injury: how to avoid, how to repair: a literature review. J Fam Pract. 2006;55:193–200.

61. Fitzpatrick M, O'Herlhy C. Postpartum care of the perineum. Obstet Gynaecol. 2007;9:164–70.
62. Sood AN, Nygaard I, Shahin MS, Sorosky J, et al. Anorectal dysfunction after surgical treatment for cervical cancer. J Am Coll Surg. 2002;195:513–9.
63. Heilbrun ME, Nygaard IE, Lockhart ME, Richter HE, Brown MB, Kenton KS, Rahn DD, Thomas JV, Weidner AC, Nager CW, Delancey JO. Correlation between levator ani muscle injuries on magnetic resonance imaging and fecal incontinence, pelvic organ prolapsed, and urinary incontinence in primiparous women. Am J Obstet Gynecol. 2010;202:488.e1–6.
64. Valsky DV, Lipschuetz M, Bord A, Eldar I, Messing B, Hochner-Celnikier D, Lavy Y, Cohen SM, Yagel S. Fetal head circumference and length of secondary stage of labor are risk for levator ani muscle injury, diagnosed by 3-dimensional transperineal ultrasound in primiparous women. Am J Obstet Gynecol. 2009;201:91–7.
65. Evers EC, Blomquist JL, McDermott KC, Handa VL. Obstetrical anal sphincter laceration and anal incontinence 5–10 years after childbirth. Am J Obstet Gynecol. 2012;29:287–91.
66. Räisänen S, Vehviläinen-Julkunen K, Gissler M, Heinonen S. Hospital-based lateral episiotomy and obstetric anal sphincter injury rates: a retrospective population-based register stud. Am J Obstet Gynecol. 2012;206:347.
67. Stedenfeldt M, Pirhonen J, Blix E, Wilsgaard T, Vonen B, Øian P. Episiotomy characteristics and risks for obstetric anal sphincter injuries: a case–control study. BJOG. 2012;119:724–30.
68. Murphy DJ, Macleod M, Bahl R, Goyder K, Howarth L, Strachan B. A randomised controlled trial of routine versus restrictive use of episiotomy at operative vaginal delivery: a multicentre pilot study. BJOG. 2008;115:1695–702.
69. Wheeler TL, Richter HE. Delivery method, anal sphincter tears and fecal incontinence: new information on a persistent problem. Curr Opin Obstet Gynecol. 2007;19:474–9.
70. Sood AN, Nygaard I, Shahin MS, Sorosky J, et al. Anorectal dysfunction after surgical treatment for cervical cancer. J Am Coll Surg. 2002;195:513–9.
71. Hayden DM, Weiss MD, Eric G. Fecal incontinence: etiology, evaluation, and treatment. Clin Colon Rectal Surg. 2011;24:64–70.
72. Baeten CG, Uludag OO, Rongen MJ. Dynamic graciloplasty for fecal incontinence. Microsurgery. 2001;21:230–4.
73. Miller L, Murray L, Richards L. Comprehensive overview of nursing and interdisciplinary rehabilitation care of the stroke patient: a Scientific Statement from the American Heart Association. J Stroke. 2010;41:2402–48.
74. Feldman HH, Woodward M. The staging and assessment of moderate to severe Alzheimer disease. J Neurol. 2005;27:10–7.
75. Zesiewicz TA, Sullivan KL, Amulf I, Chaudhuri KR, Morgan JC. Practice parameter: treatment of nonmotor symptoms of Parkinson disease. J Neurol. 2010;16:924–31.
76. Verhoef M, Lurvink M, Barf HA, Post MVM, van Asbeck FVA, Gooskens RHJM, Prevo AJH. High prevalence of incontinence among young adults with spina bifida: description, prediction and problem perception. J Spinal Cord. 2005;43:331–40.
77. Krogh K, Mosdal C, Gregersen H, Laurberg S. Rectal wall properties in patients with acute and chronic spinal cord lesions. Dis Colon Rectum. 2002;45:641–9.
78. Russo A, Botten R, Kong M-F, Chapman IM, Fraser RJL, Horowitz M, Sun W-M. Effects of acute hyperglycaemia on anorectal motor and sensory function in diabetes mellitus. Diabet Med. 2004;21:176–82.
79. Munteis E, Andreu M, Martinez-Rodriguez JE, Ois A, Bory F, Roquer J. Manometric correlations of anorectal dysfunction and biofeedback outcome in patients with multiple sclerosis. Mult Scler. 2008;14:237–42.
80. Ricciardi R, Mellgren AF, Madoff RD, Baxter NN, Karulf RE, Parker SC. The utility of pudendal nerve terminal motor latencies in idiopathic incontinence. Dis Colon Rectum. 2006;49:852–8.
81. Petros P, Swash M, Bush M, Fernandez M, Gunnemann A, Zimmer M. Defecation 1: testing a hypothesis for pelvic striated muscle action to open the anorectum. Tech Coloproctol. 2012;16(6):437–43.
82. Thekkinkattil DK, Dunham RJ, O'Herlihy S, Finan PJ, Sagar PM, Burke DA. Measurement of anal cushions in idiopathic faecal incontinence. Br J Surg. 2009;96:680–4.
83. Sultan AH. Obstetric perineal injury and anal incontinence. Clin Risk. 1999;5:193–6.
84. Koelbl H, Igawa T, Salvatore S, Laterza RM, Lowry A, Sievert KD, et al. Pathophysiology of urinary incontinence, faecal incontinence and pelvic organ prolapse. In: Abrams P, Cardozo L, Khoury S, Wein A, editors. Incontinence. 5th ed. [place unknown]: ICUD-EAU; 2013. p. 261–359.

Endoanal Ultrasound

3

Domenico Mascagni, Gianmarco Grimaldi, and Gabriele Naldini

Since its introduction in 1989 [1], endoanal ultrasonography (EAUS) has been widely accepted as a popular technique for evaluating the anal sphincters and pelvic floor in patients with anorectal diseases. Exact knowledge of the normal ultrasonographic anatomy of the anal canal provides an important foundation for identifying abnormalities.

In particular, EAUS is currently the gold standard technique for internal and external anal sphincter evaluation in fecal incontinence (FI). Most studies revealed 80–100% sensitivity in identifying sphincter's defects.

Endosonographic scanning (2D) is performed with a 7 or 10 MHz rotating endoprobe, providing a 360° axial view of the anal canal. The rotating transducers provide images only in the axial direction. Three-dimensional (3D) endosonography allows multiplanar imaging of the anal sphincters, thus enabling more reliable anal sphincter measurements and volumetric description of anal and perianal US morphological alterations. Color or power Doppler imaging technology can also be used with endosonography [2].

For an accurate exam, the rectum should be cleansed thoroughly to avoid artifacts: patients are given a simple cleansing enema, 2 h before the examination.

The examination is usually performed with the patient placed in the left lateral decubitus position, in the knee-chest position (Sims' position). A digital anorectal examination should be performed in advance, trying to identify the lesion's size and location and the clinical status of the internal anal sphincter (IAS) and external anal sphincter (EAS) before the insertion of the probe realized by the operator [3, 4].

To perform endoanal sonography, a hard, sonolucent plastic cone (diameter of 17 mm) covering the transducer is used. Before imaging, the plastic cone is fixed to the tip of the transducer and filled with degassed water for acoustic coupling. Ultrasound (US) gel is applied to the transducer before and after placement of the condom, to allow a better US contact.

When the probe is placed into the anal canal, it is commonly aligned in standard orientation, in which the anterior anatomical structures are at the uppermost or 12 o'clock side of the image, the patient's left side is at 3 o'clock, the patient's posterior side is at 6 o'clock, and the patient's right side is at 9 o'clock.

As the transducer rotates, the probe is carefully introduced. To cover the entire length of

D. Mascagni (✉) • G. Grimaldi
Department of Surgical Sciences, Sapienza University of Rome, Rome, Italy
e-mail: dmascagni@tiscali.it

G. Naldini
Proctological and Perineal Surgery, University Hospital of Pisa, Pisa, Italy

M. Mongardini, M. Giofrè (eds.), *Management of Fecal Incontinence*,
DOI 10.1007/978-3-319-32226-1_3

the anorectal canal, the probe should be introduced up to 8–9 cm, approximately at the level of peritoneal reflection. Then, the probe is slowly retracted, and images are obtained at different levels through the anal canal [5] (Fig. 3.1).

The anatomy of the anal sphincter complex is based on four layers (Figs. 3.2, 3.3, and 3.4):

1. Subepithelial tissues (moderate reflectivity)
2. The internal anal sphincter – IAS – hypoechoic (low reflectivity)
3. The longitudinal muscle layer (variable reflectivity)
4. External anal sphincter – EAS – hyperechoic (variable reflectivity)

The anal canal is usually divided into three different levels during examination:

- The *upper anal canal* which is a hyperechoic horseshoe sling of the puborectalis muscle posteriorly and loss of the EAS in the midline anteriorly (Fig. 3.2).
- The *middle anal canal* level which is the completion of the EAS ring anteriorly in combination with the maximum IAS thickness. The IAS is seen as a hypoechoic ringlike structure. The EAS is echogenic, less well defined, and broader than the IAS (Fig. 3.3).
- The *lower anal canal* level is defined as that immediately caudal to the termination of the IAS and comprises the subcutaneous EAS (Fig. 3.4).

The means of EAS thickness are different between endoanal sonography and MRI; there is a greater variability and a thicker EAS with endoanal sonography and a light spread of measurement between women and men [6] (Table 3.1).

Moreover, the IAS gets slightly thicker, and the EAS gets thinner with increasing age.

It is important to mention a few pitfalls in the interpretation of endoanal sonographic images. The female anatomic characteristics of the anterior EAS below the level of the puborectalis sling may be misinterpreted as an anterior EAS defect. Moreover, posteriorly, the EAS and puborectalis

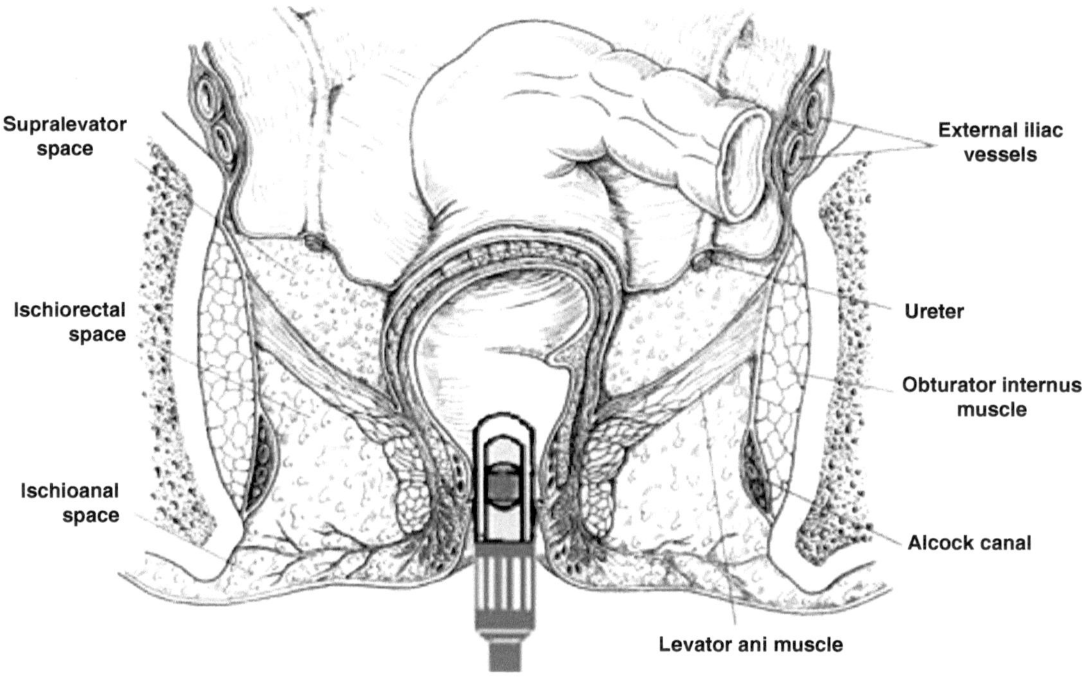

Fig. 3.1 Transanal probe

muscle are attached to the coccyx by means of the anococcygeal ligament. The anococcygeal ligament, which appears as a triangular hypoechoic structure on the axial images posteriorly, should not be confused with a sphincter defect (Fig. 3.5).

Fecal incontinence is due to local, anatomical, or systemic disorders and nontraumatic or traumatic lesions. Not every patient with sphincter injury develops incontinence, and, in addition, patients can have incontinence without sphincter injury.

Sphincter atrophy may occur without sphincter trauma, and although the cause of this remains uncertain, there may be a relationship to neurologic degeneration from denervation and aging [7].

On endoanal sonography, atrophic or degenerative sphincters are seen as thin and poorly defined and often with heterogeneous increased echogenicity. Increased echogenicity on endoanal sonography has been shown histologically to be correlated with replacement of smooth muscle by fibrous tissue (Fig. 3.6). It will be important to distinguish abnormal thinning from physiologic age-related EAS differences. This should be a problem in the EAS; because the EAS muscle is also thinner at older ages, it may be difficult to distinguish sufficiently between atrophy and age-related changes [8].

IAS thickness measurement is indicative of degeneration if less than 2 mm, and generalized EAS atrophy is difficult to evaluate in EAUS. Perineal body measurement improves

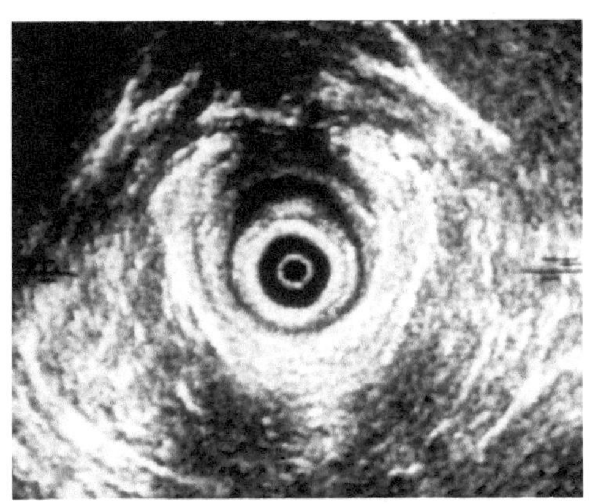

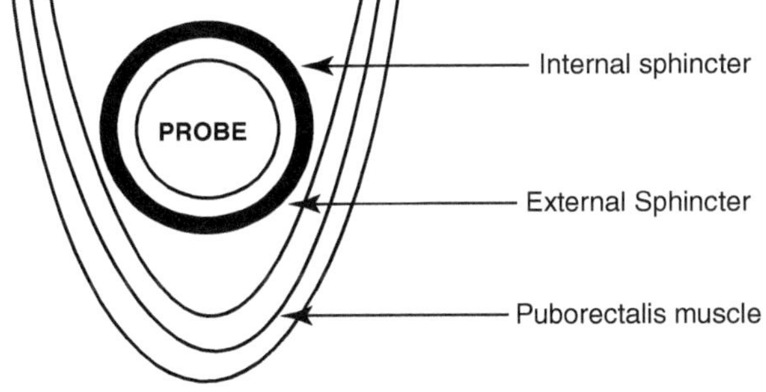

Fig. 3.2 The upper anal canal

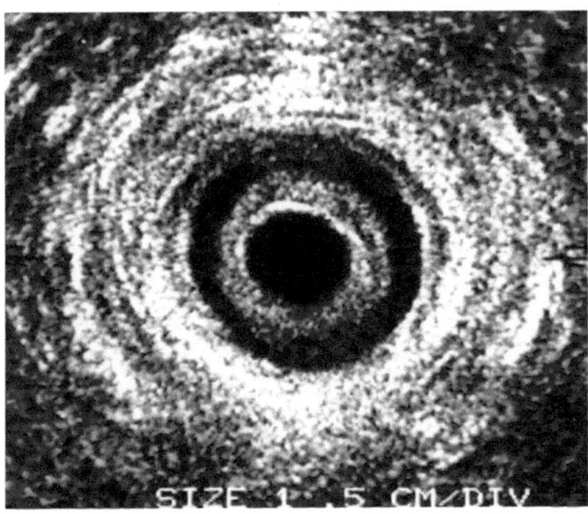

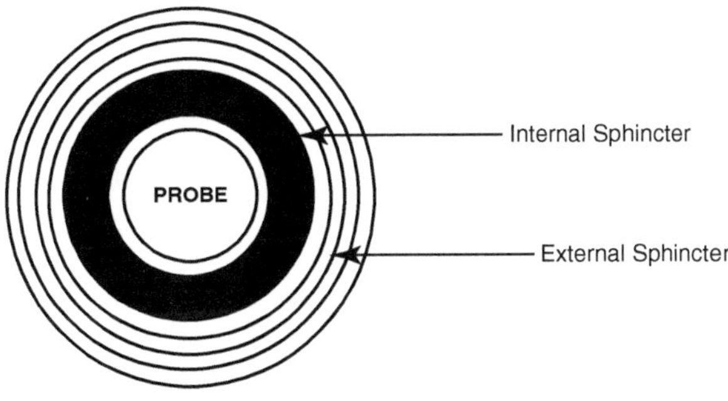

Fig. 3.3 The middle anal canal

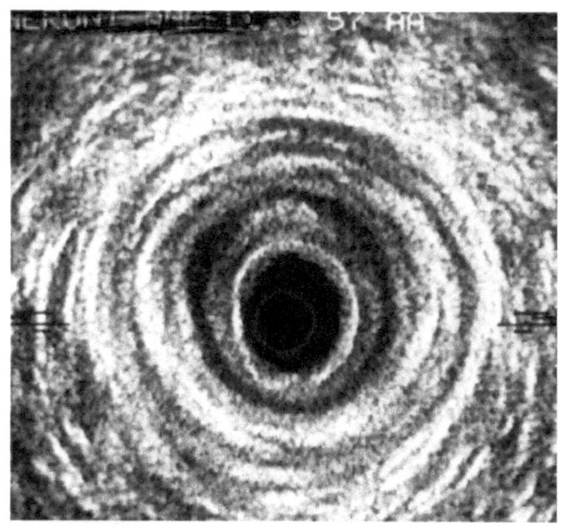
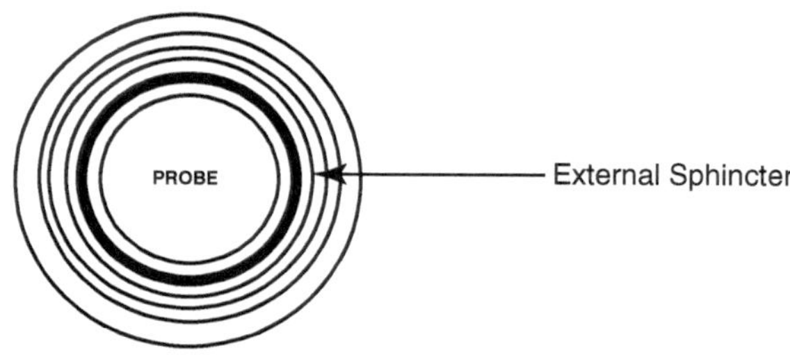

Fig. 3.4 The lower anal canal

Table 3.1 Sphincter muscle thickness measured at endoanal sonography [6]

	Endoanal sonography	
Measurement	Women	Men
Internal sphincter (IAS), mm	3.8 ± 1.2	3.4 ± 1.4
Longitudinal muscle, mm	2.9 ± 1.0	2.3 ± 1.0
External sphincter (EAS), mm	7.2 ± 2.3	6.1 ± 1.7
Total sphincter thickness, mm	18.7 ± 4.1	18.7 ± 5.2

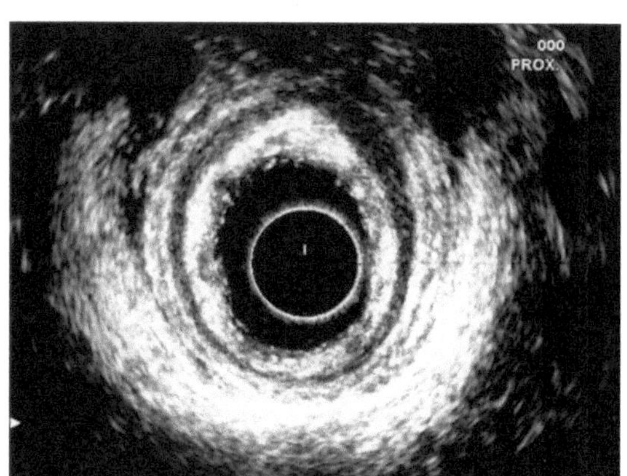

Fig. 3.5 EAUS demonstrating the "U-shape" of the puborectalis muscle

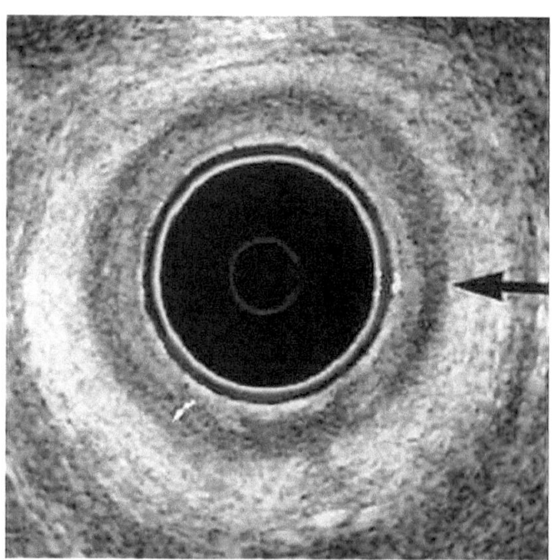

Fig. 3.6 IAS has an increased echogenicity (*Black arrow*)

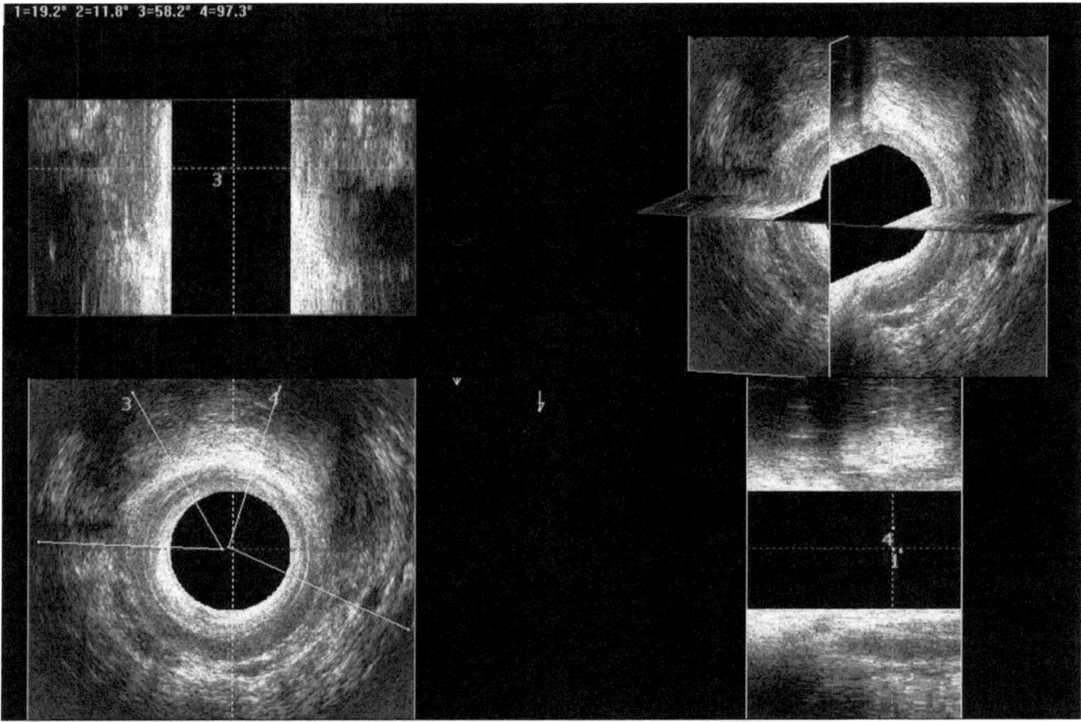

Fig. 3.7 Endoanal US 3D with multiplanar imaging of the anal sphincters: double sphincter defects of the EAS

visualization of anterior sphincter lesions in females. A perineal body thickness of 10 mm or less is considered abnormal, whereas 10 to 12 mm is associated with sphincter defect in one-third of patients and those with 12 mm or more are unlikely to harbor a defect unless they previously have undergone reconstructive perineal surgery [9].

The IAS is very clearly seen on endoanal sonography, and it is easier to appreciate atrophy and small tears of this sphincter. Moreover, 3D endoanal sonography facilitates sagittal and coronal reconstruction of the anal canal, resulting in better delineation of the normal anatomy and defects of the anal sphincter (Fig. 3.7).

EAUS is the gold standard for diagnosing anal sphincters tear and IAS degeneration.

If EAS atrophy is suspected, endoanal MRI should be performed. Needle electromyography of the anal sphincter should be considered in patients with clinically suspected neurogenic sphincter weakness, particularly if there are features suggestive of proximal (i.e., sacral root) involvement [10].

Sphincter injury is the most common cause of fecal incontinence and frequently occurs as the consequence of vaginal delivery, perineal laceration, episiotomy, anorectal surgery, or other accidental injuries [11–13].

Anal sphincter damage can be subdivided into *localized scarring*, *generalized scarring*, *localized defects*, *fragmentation*, *and atrophy*. *Localized or generalized scarring* is often due to the replacement of normal muscle fibers by scar tissue. On endoanal sonography, scar tissue is seen indirectly as an area of mixed echogenicity. A *localized defect* is visible as a discontinuity of the anal sphincters. On endoanal sonography, the localized defect of the IAS appears, usually as hyperechoic break, and

EAS tears appear as relatively hypoechoic areas. *Fragmentation* of the anal sphincter is defined as two or more fragments in the axial plane.

An EAS injury due to vaginal delivery is typically located anteriorly, mostly, in the right anterolateral side. In contrast, an isolated IAS injury almost never follows childbirth and indicates a primary traumatic cause from within the anal canal, most commonly surgery [13].

During the exam, the number, the circumferential extent (radial angle in degrees or in hours of the clock), and the longitudinal extent (proximal, distal, or full length) of the defect should be carefully reported.

The most common cause of fecal incontinence is anal sphincter injury related to vaginal delivery in female, due to direct anal sphincter laceration or indirect damage to sphincter innervation.

The classification of the obstetric tears described by Sultan 1999 [11, 14] has been adopted by the International Consultation on Incontinence and the Royal College of Obstetricians and Gynaecologists (RCOG) 2007 [15]:

Grade 1, injury to the perineal skin
Grade 2, injury to the perineum involving the perineal muscles
Grade 3, injury to perineum involving the anal sphincter complex
  Grade 3a, involving the anal sphincter < 50 % EAS
  Grade 3b, > 50 % EAS
  Grade 3c, involvement of the IAS
Grade 4, involvement of the anal sphincter as well as the anorectal epithelium

Obstetric anal sphincter injuries *(OASIS)* encompass both third- and fourth-degree perineal tears. They are identified in 0.6–9.0 % of vaginal deliveries where mediolateral episiotomy is performed, but the detection in EAUS is much higher.

In 2003, Oberwalder et al. published a meta-analysis of 717 vaginal deliveries and found an incidence of occult anal sphincter injury of 26.9 % in primiparous women and 8.5 % of new defects in multiparous women. In one-third of these women, postpartum sphincter damage was symptomatic [16].

Usually, anal sphincter defects after vaginal delivery are ultrasonically observed as an interruption of the normal U-shaped, upper – or round – middle, and low aspect of the EAS characterized by a “loss” of the right anterolateral arm of the EAS (from 9 o’clock to 11 o’clock), because the episiotomy is usually realized, by a right-hander gynecologist, in this anterolateral area (Fig. 3.8) [17].

In 30 % of these cases, also an IAS defect, in the same area (from 9 o’clock to 12 o’clock), can be associated and US detected (Fig. 3.9).

Usually, only patients with clinical FI were included for endoanal US study.

The current guidelines of the RCOG from 2007 [15], in fact, state that there is no recommendation about screening women after vaginal delivery for occult sphincter defects. However, we think that not only old patients and those at high risk (multiparous) but even young women should be well informed on the risk of the potential, post vaginal delivery, sphincter lesions and submitted to a postpartum survey to identify those patients with a light, not referred, symptomatology that could be submitted to a simple endoanal US to demonstrate the eventual presence of sphincter lesions well balanced at the moment. These women, with subclinical sphincters defect, without an evident FI, can have, in fact, sufficient residual sphincter function or, since several mechanisms contribute to continence, they may compensate for this injury. The peak of incidence of FI in these patients will be evident in the fifth and sixth decades of life, when the cumulative effect of deliveries, aging, menopause, and progression of neuropathy may contribute for sphincter weakness in the long term and FI developing even several years (20 or 30 decades) after delivery. We should consider

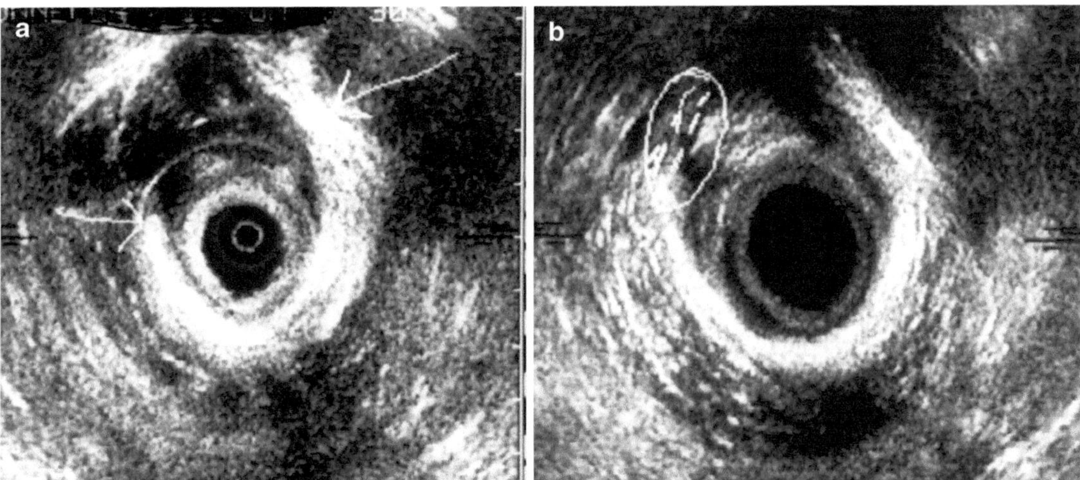

Fig. 3.8 Endoanal US after vaginal delivery: (**a**) "loss" of the right anterolateral side (h 9–11) of the EAS (**b**) with a decreased thickness of the EAS

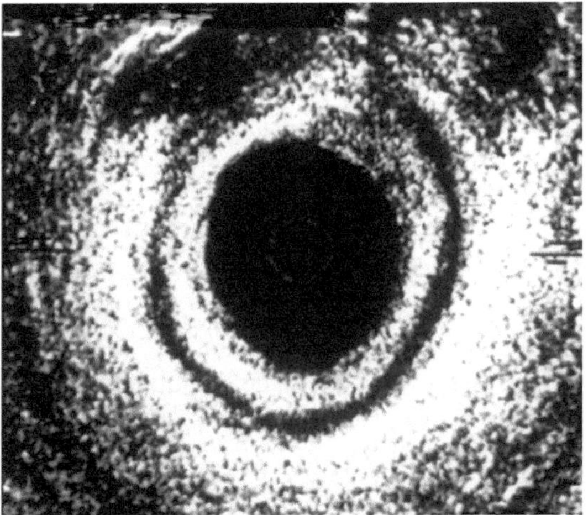

Fig. 3.9 Endoanal US after vaginal delivery: defect (h 9–12) of the IAS

that, in these patients, any future, even innocent trauma, in particular any anorectal surgery, could make manifest a previous, misknown sphincter lesion, due to post vaginal delivery: is evident the correlation of this relief with any subsequent legal event.

If the EAUS after vaginal delivery will detect an important anal sphincter defect – even little symptomatic – it should be immediately repaired to decrease the risk of severe FI [15].

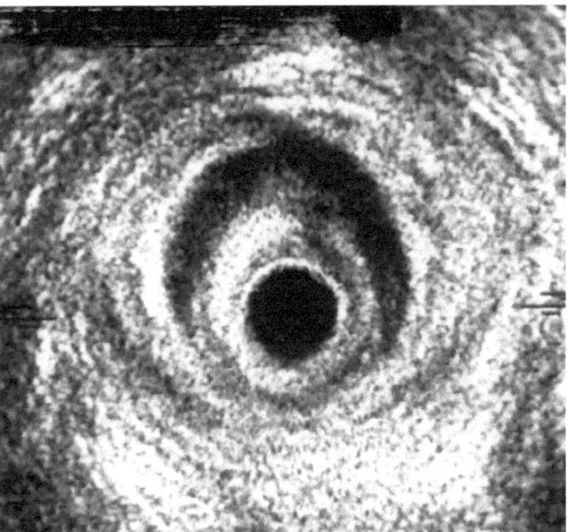

Fig. 3.10 Endoanal US after surgery repair of the EAS: overlapping technique

The RCOG recommends that for repair of the external anal sphincter, either an overlapping technique or end-to-end technique can be used with equivalent outcomes; if the IAS is identified, it is advisable to repair separately using end-to-end technique: a separate repair of the IAS improves the likelihood of subsequent anal continence [15, 18, 19].

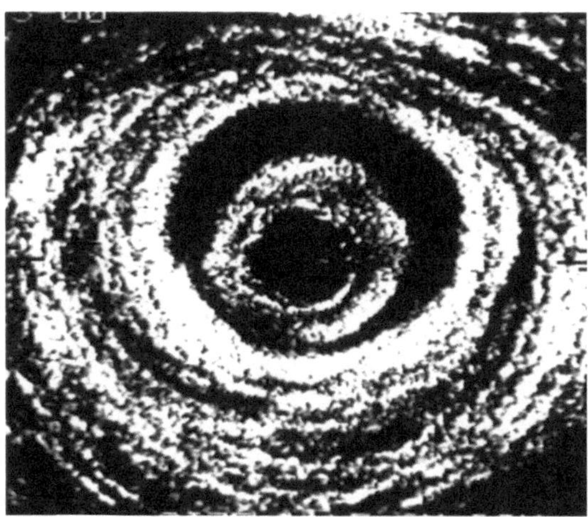

Fig. 3.11 Endoanal US after hemorrhoidectomy: IAS is thinner in the right posterolateral side (h 5–8) with a "compensatory" thickening of the rest of the IAS

Having a persistent sonographic defect after primary repair of OASIS has been shown to be associated with ongoing incontinence symptoms (Fig. 3.10).

Studies show a high frequency of endosonographic sphincter defects after primary repairs, between 54 and 93 % of women, and the extent of the endosonographic defects depend on the surgical experience of the doctor performing the repair and not by the clinical degree of the tear [20].

EAUS can also be important to aid decision for future delivery. According to the RCOG guidelines, "all women who have sustained an OASIS in a previous pregnancy and who are symptomatic or have abnormal EAUS and/or manometry should have the option of elective caesarean birth. Between 17 % and 24 % of these women with previous third degree tear developed worsening fecal symptoms after a second vaginal delivery" [15].

The second most frequent cause of sphincter lesion, after vaginal delivery, is represented by anorectal surgery.

In any case of anorectal surgery, as in the case of a procedure with potential postsurgical sphincter lesion – complex fistula in ano – and even for simple anorectal surgery, as in the case of a patient who is multiparous or with previous perianal surgery or trauma, EAUS should be employed to demonstrate the real status of the sphincters to avoid a simple or complex anorectal procedure that could make manifest a sphincter incontinence in the postoperative period.

When a hemorrhoidectomy or a prolapsectomy is performed, respectively, the removal of hemorrhoidal cushions or the postoperative fecal urgency that can occur after prolapsectomy can improve a light or subclinical fecal incontinence [21] (Fig. 3.11).

Moreover, a simple internal anal sphincterotomy realized for a fissure in ano could became the final act responsible for moving a previous asymptomatic sphincter lesion in a clinical fecal incontinence.

In particular, EAUS in patients surgically treated for a fissure in ano might demonstrate insufficient sphincterotomy and sphincterial thickening because of the persistence of fissure and anal pain or, on the contrary, demonstrate an excessive sphincterotomy with temporary or permanent incontinence (Figs. 3.12 and 3.13).

In case of a surgery for fistula in ano, an endoanal US should be performed in the preoperative diagnostic study not only for mapping the abscess and to identify the fistula, with the internal orifice, but either to exclude the eventual presence of a previous internal, external, or both sphincter lesions. This relief could change the quality of surgery (sphincter sparing should be preferred to a cut surgery) and should be included in the informed consent and well explained to the patient before surgery [22].

The majority of patient candidates for surgery have simple fistulas that can be easily treated successfully. The preoperative EAUS is, however, recommended for every fistula, not only for simple fistulas, because the fistula that was preoperatively judged easy might demonstrate as complex at surgery or at the postoperative follow-up with potential even dramatic sphincter consequences (Fig. 3.14).

On the contrary, an EAUS overstaging can move a fistula from a simple to a complex one, disorientating the patient and obliging to an unmotivated and frustrating surgical exploration, sometimes dangerous for the sphincters' integrity [23, 24].

In recurrent or complex fistula in ano, 3D EAUS (sometimes with hydrogen peroxide) proved to be more accurate than 2D for detecting difficult (hidden) primary or secondary tracks and internal openings [24, 25].

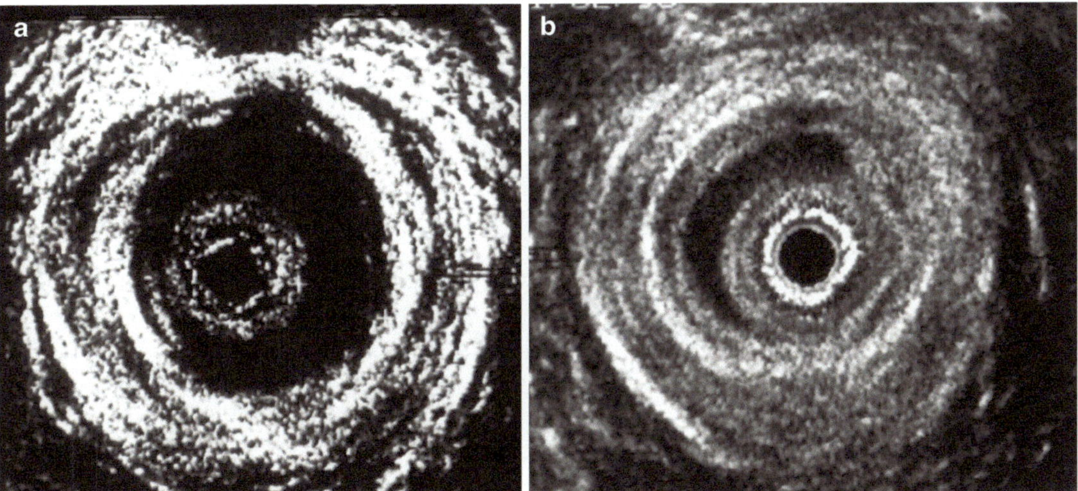

Fig. 3.12 (**a**) Endoanal US after right sphincterotomy: thinning of the IAS (h 7–11) with an important thickening of the rest of the IAS. (**b**) Endoanal US after left sphincterotomy, important "loss" of the IAS (h 1–7)

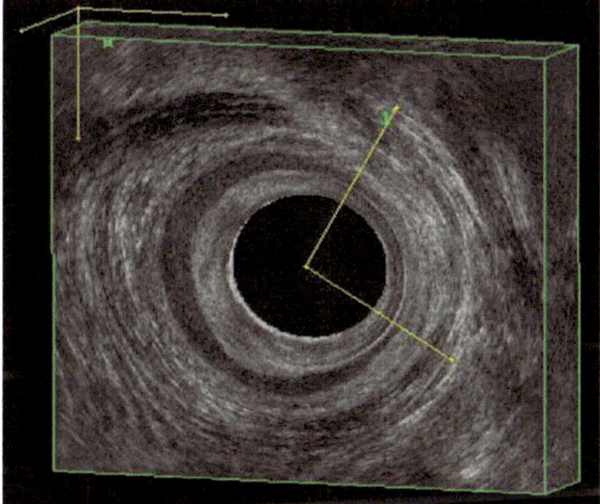

Fig. 3.13 Endoanal US 3D after left sphincterotomy of the IAS

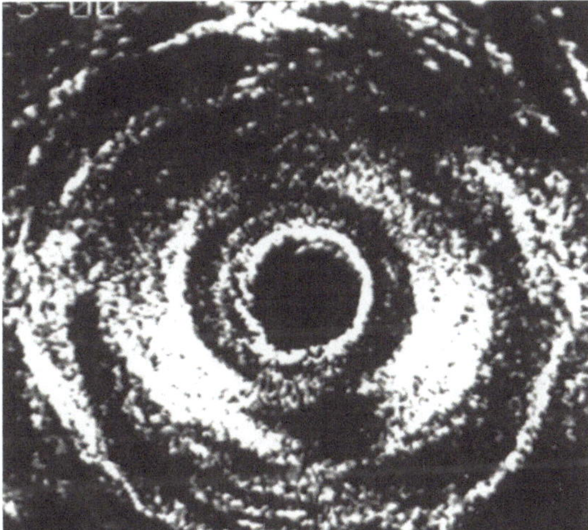

Fig. 3.14 Endoanal US in preoperative fistula in ano: a posterior hypoechoic intersphincteric abscess with an associated ischiorectal "horseshoe" abscess

It should be underlined, however, that an endoanal US realized in an operated patient could offer important difficulties of interpretation of the US images for the presence of fibrosclerotic tissue and/or artifacts.

References

1. Law PJ, Kamm MA, Bartram CI. Anal endosonography in the investigation of fecal incontinence. Br J Surg. 1991;78:312–4.
2. Sudakoff GS, Quiroz F, Foley WD. Sonography of anorectal, rectal, and perirectal abnormalities. AJR Am J Roentgenol. 2002;179:131–6.
3. Frudinger A, Bartram CI, Halligan S, et al. Examination techniques for endosonography of the anal canal. Abdom Imaging. 1998;23:301–3.
4. Thakar R, Sultan AH. Anal endosonography and its role in assessing the incontinent patient. Best Pact Res Clin Obstet Gynaecol. 2004;18:157–73.
5. Abdool Z, Sultan AH, Thakar R. Ultrasound imaging of the anal sphincter complex: a review. Br J Radiol. 2012;85:865–75.

6. Beets-Tan RGH, Morren GL, Beets GL, et al. Measurement of anal sphincter muscles: endoanal US, endoanal MR imaging, or phased-array MR imaging? A study with healthy volunteers. Radiology. 2001;220:81–9.
7. Vaizey CJ, Kamm MA, Bartram CI. Primary degeneration of the internal anal sphincter as a cause of passive faecal incontinence. Lancet. 1997;349:612–5.
8. Frudinger A, Halligan S, Bartram CI. Female anal sphincter: age related differences in asymptomatic volunteers with high-frequency endoanal US. Radiology. 2002;224:417–23.
9. Zetterström JP, Mellgren A, Madoff RD, et al. Perineal body measurement improves evaluation of anterior sphincter lesions during endoanal ultrasonography. Dis Colon Rectum. 1998;41:705–13.
10. Albuquerque A. Endoanal ultrasonography in fecal incontinence: current and future perspectives. World J Gastrointest Endosc. 2015;7:575–81.
11. Sultan AH, Kamm MA, Hudson CN, et al. Anal sphincter disruption during vaginal delivery. N Engl J Med. 1993;329:1905–11.
12. Sultan AH, Kamm MA, Nicholls RJ, et al. Prospective study of the extent of internal anal sphincter division during lateral sphincterotomy. Dis Colon Rectum. 1994;37:1031–3.
13. Felt-Bersma RJ, van Baren R, Koorevaar M, et al. Unsuspected sphincter defects shown by anal endosonography after anorectal surgery: a prospective study. Dis Colon Rectum. 1995;38:249–53.
14. Sultan AH. Editorial: obstetric perineal injury and anal incontinence. Clin Risk. 1999;5:193–6.
15. Royal College of Obstetricians and Gynaecologists (RCOG). The management of third- and fourth-degree perineal tears. RCOG guideline 2007 (revised), vol. 29. London: RCOG Press; 2007. p. 1–11.
16. Oberwalder M, Connor J, Wexner SD. Meta-analysis to determine the incidence of obstetric anal sphincter damage. Br J Surg. 2003;90:1333–7.
17. Baig MK, Wexner SD. Factors predictive of outcome after surgery for faecal incontinence. Br J Surg. 2000;87:1316–30.
18. Sultan AH, Monga AK, Kumar D, et al. Primary repair of obstetric anal sphincter rupture using the overlap technique. Br J Obstet Gynaecol. 1999;106:318–23.
19. Fernando RJ, Sultan AH, Kettle C, et al. Methods of repair for obstetric anal sphincter injury. Cochrane Database Syst Rev. 2013;12, CD002866.
20. Sultan AH, Kamm MA, Hudson CN, et al. Third degree obstetric anal sphincter tears: risk factors and outcome of primary repair. BMJ. 1994;308:887–91.
21. Mascagni D, Naldini G, Stuto A, et al. Recurrence after stapled haemorrhoidopexy. Tech Coloproctol. 2015;19:321–2.
22. Lengyel AJ, Hurst NG, Williams JG. Pre-operative assessment of anal fistulas using endoanal ultrasound. Colorectal Dis. 2002;4:436–40.
23. Pescatori M, Interisano A, Mascagni D, et al. Double flap technique to reconstruct the anal canal after concurrent surgery for fistulae, abscesses and haemorrhoids. Int J Colorectal Dis. 1995;10:19–21.
24. Navarro-Luna A, Garcia-Domingo MI, Rius-Macias JR, et al. Ultrasound study of anal fistulas with hydrogen peroxide enhancement. Dis Colon Rectum. 2004;47:108–14.
25. Ratto C, Gentile E, Merico M, et al. How can the assessment of fistula-in-ano be improved? Dis Colon Rectum. 2000;43:1375–82.

4 Diagnosis and Imaging: MR

Gianfranco Gualdi and Maria Chiara Colaiacomo

4.1 Introduction

Magnetic resonance imaging (MRI) has assumed an important role in the evaluation of patients with fecal incontinence [1, 2]. MRI is a safe technique which provides a detailed multiplanar imaging, producing high-contrast and spatial-resolution images of the sphincter complex and the pelvic floor and accurate dynamic imaging of defecation, without radiation exposure [1–15]. The major advantage of MRI is the ability to detect sphincter integrity, a matter not always exhaustively cleared by physical examination and useful in selecting patient candidates for surgical or conservative treatment [1, 3]. Different MR techniques are available: endoanal MR, with high spatial and contrast resolution on the sphincter complex but limited field of view; external phased-array MR, an alternative to endocoil imaging with more panoramicity; and dynamic imaging, which provides dynamic view of evacuation and dynamic pelvic floor assessment during voiding [1–15].

G. Gualdi (✉)
Department of Anatomical and Histological Sciences, Forensic Medicine and Locomotive System, Sapienza University of Rome, Rome, Italy
e-mail: gianfranco.gualdi@uniroma1.it

M.C. Colaiacomo
Radiology – Department of Emergency and Acceptance, Policlinico Umberto I, Rome, Rome, Italy

4.2 Technique

Conventional closed MR units are suitable for the anorectal imaging, with a magnet field strength up to 3 T; commonly a 1.5 T magnet is used. Any protocol does not require endovenous administration of gadolinium unless inflammatory or neoplastic pathology is suspected [1–15].

4.2.1 Endoanal Imaging

Endoanal imaging is an endoluminal technique which exploits the signal obtained from a dedicated endoanal coil. Due to the small field of view and the strict vicinity to the sphincter complex, this technique provides an optimal visualization of the anatomic structures of the anorectum, but it is limited to the evaluation of such structures only (Figs. 4.1 and 4.2).

Endoanal coil is cylindrical in shape, with a diameter of 15–20 mm and a length of about 10 cm. The coil is covered with a condom and a small amount of lubricant and introduced when the patient lays in lateral position; then the patient turns supine and examination starts. It is important to previously administer intramuscular or endovenous bowel relaxant such as butylscopolamine bromide or glucagon, to reduce patient pain from pelvic floor muscle contraction and artifacts from bowel peristalsis that can affect image quality [1–3].

M. Mongardini, M. Giofrè (eds.), *Management of Fecal Incontinence*,
DOI 10.1007/978-3-319-32226-1_4

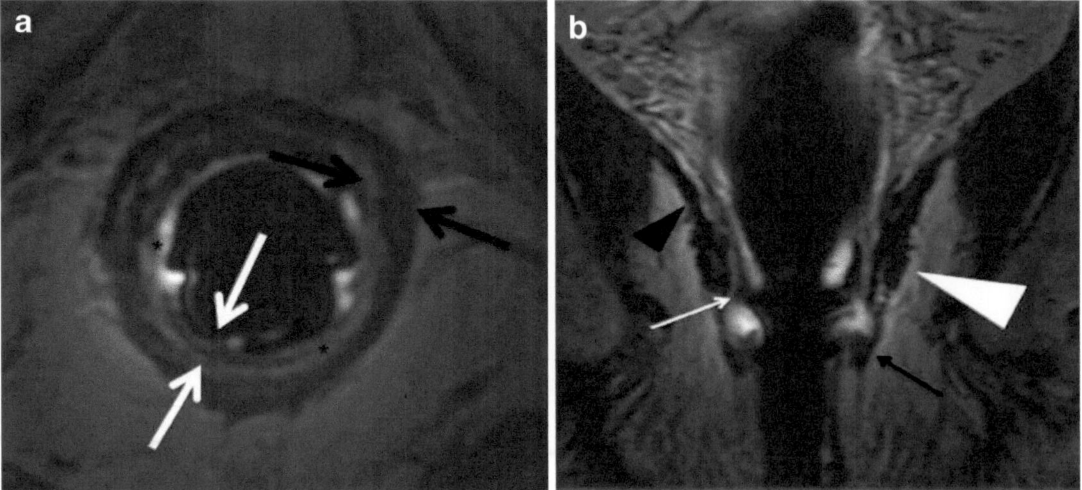

Fig. 4.1 (**a**) Axial T2-weighted image with endoanal coil shows intact external (*black arrows*) and internal (*white arrows*) anal sphincters, and the intersphincteric space (*) (**b**) coronal T2-weighted image with endoanal coil shows intact external (*black arrow*) and internal (*white arrow*) anal sphincters, puborectalis muscle (*white arrowhead*), and levator ani muscle (*black arrowhead*)

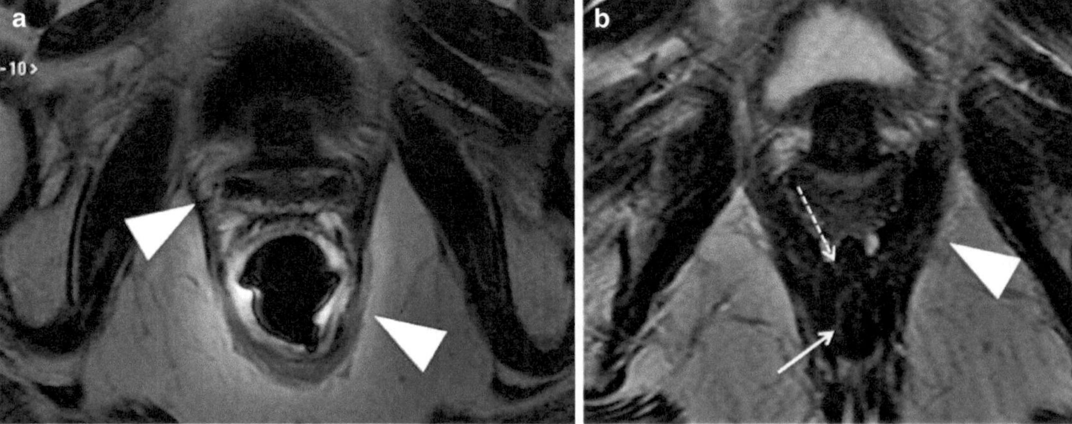

Fig. 4.2 (**a**) Axial T2-weighted image with endoanal coil at an upper level with respect to Fig. 4.1a shows puborectalis muscle (*arrowheads*). (**b**) Corresponding image with phased-array coil shows the puborectalis muscle (*arrowhead*) and external (*dashed white arrow*) and internal sphincters (*white arrow*)

Sequence protocol for endoanal imaging includes high-resolution T2-weighted sequences performed in axial sagittal and coronal planes, oriented along the axis of the anal canal. Sequence parameters are TR/TE, 3240/103, FOV 18×18 cm, thickness 2 mm, matrix 256×224, and gap 0, 1. Time examination is completed in 15 min.

4.2.2 External Pashed-Array Coil Imaging

External phased-array imaging consists in an extensive MR evaluation of the pelvis and the pelvic floor in particular. It is an alternative to endocoil imaging if the introduction of the coil causes too much discomfort to the patient and it is more

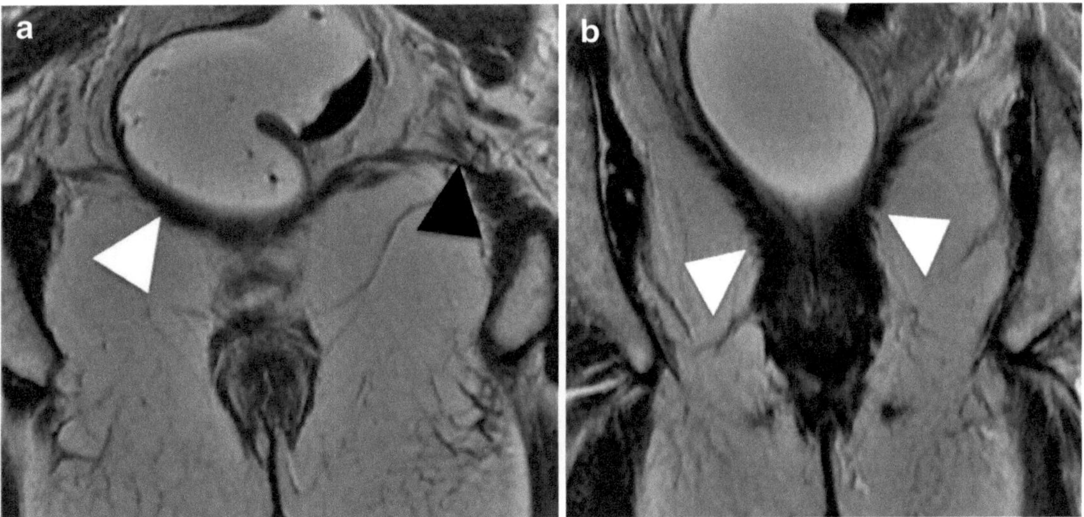

Fig. 4.3 (**a**, **b**) Coronal T2-weighed images nicely show levator ani muscle (*white arrowhead*) and its lateral attachment to the pelvic sidewalls (*black arrowhead*)

widely available [1, 2]. The use of high matrix sequences provides a detailed imaging of the pelvic floor, comparable to that of endocoil imaging [16, 17], with the advantage of a panoramic view of the entire pelvis (Figs. 4.2 and 4.3).

It uses a multicoil array, either pelvic or torso, wrapped around the inferior portion of the pelvis, and the patient is placed in supine position.

Scout images are obtained to identify a midline sagittal section with a rapid T1-weighted large field of view localizer sequence; this image should encompass the symphysis, bladder neck, vagina, rectum, and coccyx.

Examination proceeds acquiring sequences to image pelvic anatomy and any muscle defect, such as thinning and tears. For this aim, T2-weighted high-resolution sequences are acquired (TR 3700; TE 102; FOV 23×23 cm; matrix, 384×224; 5 mm thickness×25 slice; 3–4 min) in axial, sagittal, and coronal planes. The examination is completed in about 15 min.

4.2.3 Dynamic Imaging

Dynamic imaging consists in an evacuation study [4, 18]. It is a helpful study to demonstrate functional laxity of the pelvic floor, to assess if bladder or uterine descent are associated to anal sphincter defect, thus providing useful information if a surgical treatment is planned [10]. A filling media (usually sonographic gel or mashed potatoes) are introduced in the rectum by a short flexible tube with the patient lying lateral decubitus on the scanner table before entering the gantry. Because of the high intrinsic soft tissue contrast of MRI, it is not necessary to opacify bowel loops, the bladder, and the vagina. Covering the gantry with a plastic towel helps to overcome patients' embarrassment, and it helps cleaning after examination.

Dynamic imaging is obtained by using a steady-state sequence (FIESTA, TRUE-FISP, or balanced FFE) (TR 4.8, TE 2.4, FOV 40×40 cm, matrix 224×288, slice thickness 8 mm), acquiring 1 slice every 1 s on the midsagittal plane at rest, at maximal sphincter contraction, at straining, and at defecation. This kind of sequence has the advantage to combine high intrinsic signal and temporal resolution. High-performance magnets and gradients provide an image update every 1 s; 40–50 repetitions are usually enough to cover the time of examination. Images are then analyzed also in the cine loop mode. The dynamic examination is completed in 1–3 min.

4.3 Normal Anatomy

Examinations of MR images start with the evaluation of normal anatomy (Figs. 4.1, 4.2, and 4.3). Muscular structures of the pelvic floor such as the sphincter complex, levator ani, and puborectalis muscle are easily recognized at MRI [19].

In healthy subjects the average internal anal sphincter (IAS) width is approximately 2.8 mm and external anal sphincter (EAS) width is 4 mm without differences from males and females [20]. Intersphincteric space is the space between the internal and external sphincters, and it contains fat and the longitudinal muscle. In the axial plane, both internal and external sphincters show an intact ring shape. Internal and external sphincter can be distinguished by their relative different signal intensity. Striate muscles show lower signal intensity on T2 respect to smooth muscle so external sphincter has a lower intensity compared to the internal one [1].

The levator ani muscle consists of three different muscle groups: the iliococcygeus, the pubococcygeus, and the pubovisceral muscle; the latter is made of the puborectalis and puboanal muscle [1, 19]. The iliococcygeus and the pubococcygeus muscles are horizontal, sheet-like structures, which arise, respectively, from the junction of the arcus tendineus fascia pelvis and the fascia of the internal obturator muscle and from the pubic bone and then fan out to insert at the pelvic sidewall at the tendinous arch [4, 19]. This configuration is nicely assessed on the coronal plane (Fig. 4.3), useful to demonstrate normal thickness and symmetry of the fibers. Posteriorly the fibers fuse anterior to the coccyx to form a midline raphe, the levator plate [14]. The puborectalis muscle arises from the body of the pubic bone and forms a sling around the rectum, aligning to the external anal sphincter [14]. This sling shape is easily imaged on axial plane.

4.4 Findings in Fecal Incontinence and Role of MRI

An imaging assessment is mandatory in evaluating anal incontinence as sphincter tears are overlooked at clinical examination [3]. Loss of ring contiguity and loss of homogeneous signal intensity of the sphincters are pathologic findings due to lesion of muscle fibers [21]. Disruption of the normal shape with hypointense deformation of the muscle fibers is indicative of the presence of scar tissue. Scar tissue is visible as a very hypointense tissue, because of its content in fibrous tissue, more hypointense than the normal external sphincter, distorting the normal multilayered architecture of the sphincter muscle [2]. Endoanal MRI is a valuable tool to identify this finding [22–25]. Atrophy (Fig. 4.4) of the sphincters is shown at MRI as abnormally thinned IAS and/or EAS, with a thickness lower than 2 mm [2]. Fat replacement is also a finding consistent with atrophy even if the sphincter thickness is preserved [2]. Despite in clinical practice no definite criteria are used for the visual diagnosis, EAS atrophy at imaging could be assessed following a useful classification proposed by Terra [1] which considers no atrophy (no thinning and no replacement of sphincter muscle by fat), mild atrophy (<50 % thinning or replacement of muscle by fat), and severe atrophy (>50 % thinning or

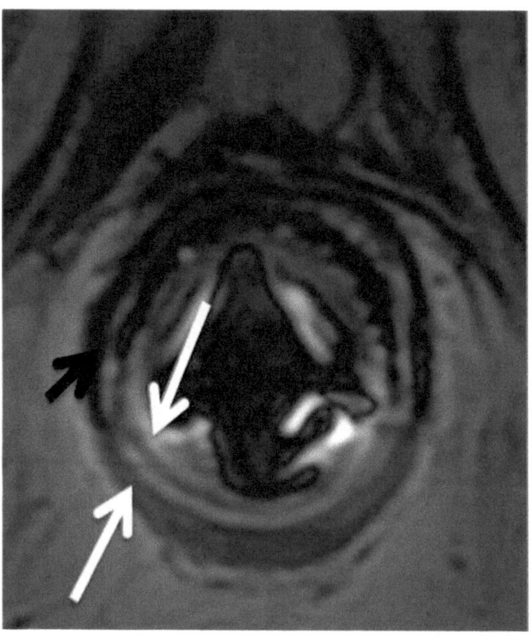

Fig. 4.4 Axial T2-weighted image with endoanal coil shows marked atrophy (*white arrows*) of the posterior internal anal sphincter which is thinned compared to the anterior part (*black arrow*)

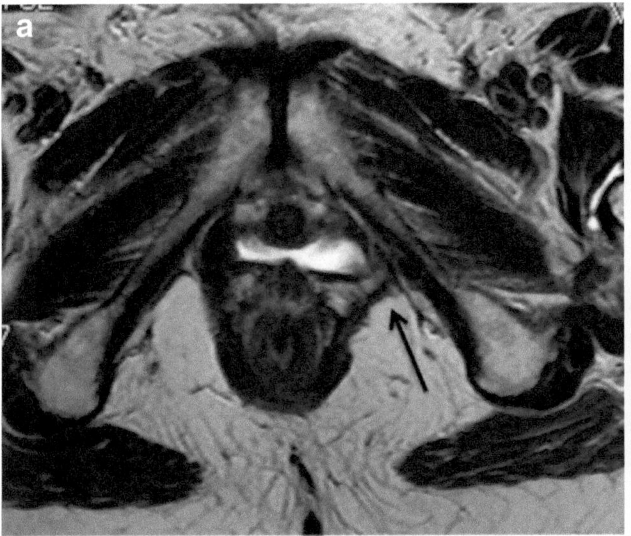

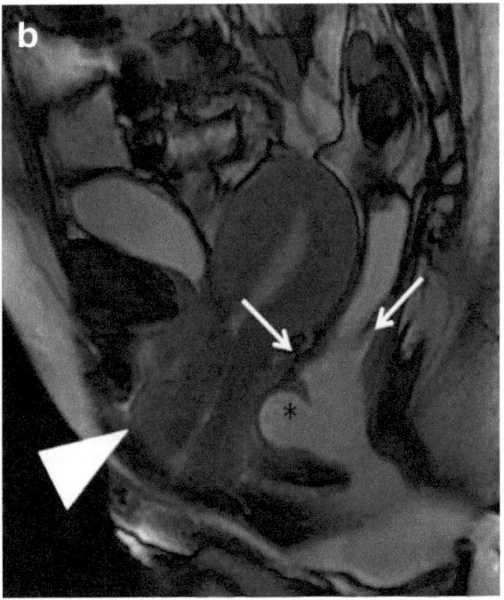

Fig. 4.5 (**a**) Axial T2-weighted image obtained with external phased-array coil shows left lateral detachment of puborectalis muscle from symphyseal insertion (*black arrow*). (**b**) Dynamic MR image obtained during defecation shows an anterior rectocele (*), intrarectal invagination (*white arrows*), and uterine prolapse (*arrowhead*)

replacement of muscle by fat). An evaluation of the relationship between EAS atrophy at endoanal MRI and clinical, functional and anatomical features in patients with fecal incontinence revealed that patients with EAS atrophy were mainly female, older, with lower maximal squeeze pressure and squeeze increment compared with patients without atrophy [26]. Many studies have demonstrated that despite its lower local spatial resolution, external phase-array MR imaging is comparable to endoanal MRI for the depiction of anal sphincter defects and EAS atrophy [16, 17]. Limits of endoanal imaging are discomfort in the introduction of the coil, reduced image quality due to artifacts from motion and interface between the probe surface and the rectum, and possible stretching of the sphincter muscles due to the presence of the probe itself with consequent underestimation of their thickness [16, 17].

External phased-array MRI imaging has demonstrated atrophy of EAS in a large group of women complaining fecal incontinence and an IAS defect in women with previous obstetric trauma [27].

Besides anal sphincter defects, external phased-array MRI can identify defects of other pelvic floor muscles (Figs. 4.5 and 4.6). Puborectalis muscle atrophy, view as an abnormal thinning, has also been found in a considerable number of fecal incontinent patients [28]. Puborectalis and levator ani muscle defects are relatively common in women with severe fecal incontinence, however usually associated to sphincter injury than solitary defects [29]. MRI has demonstrated that levator ani muscle injury is present in a considerable number of women with EAS injuries who delivered vaginally, and those women patients were frequently suffering from fecal incontinence [30]. Hence, an extended evaluation of the entire pelvic floor, in particular in women with obstetric trauma, including puborectalis and levator ani muscle, is important, as it is the evaluation of defecation; this assessment can be achieved by external phased-array MRI and MRI defecography. Anorectal angle (ARA) is defined as the angle between the posterior border of the distal part of the rectum and the central axis of the anal canal [9]. ARA normally measures at rest between 108° and 127° [12, 31] and changes as the puborectalis muscle contracts or relaxes. Normally ARA closes between rest and squeezing and opens between rest and defecation of about 15–20° [6, 31]. ARA change during

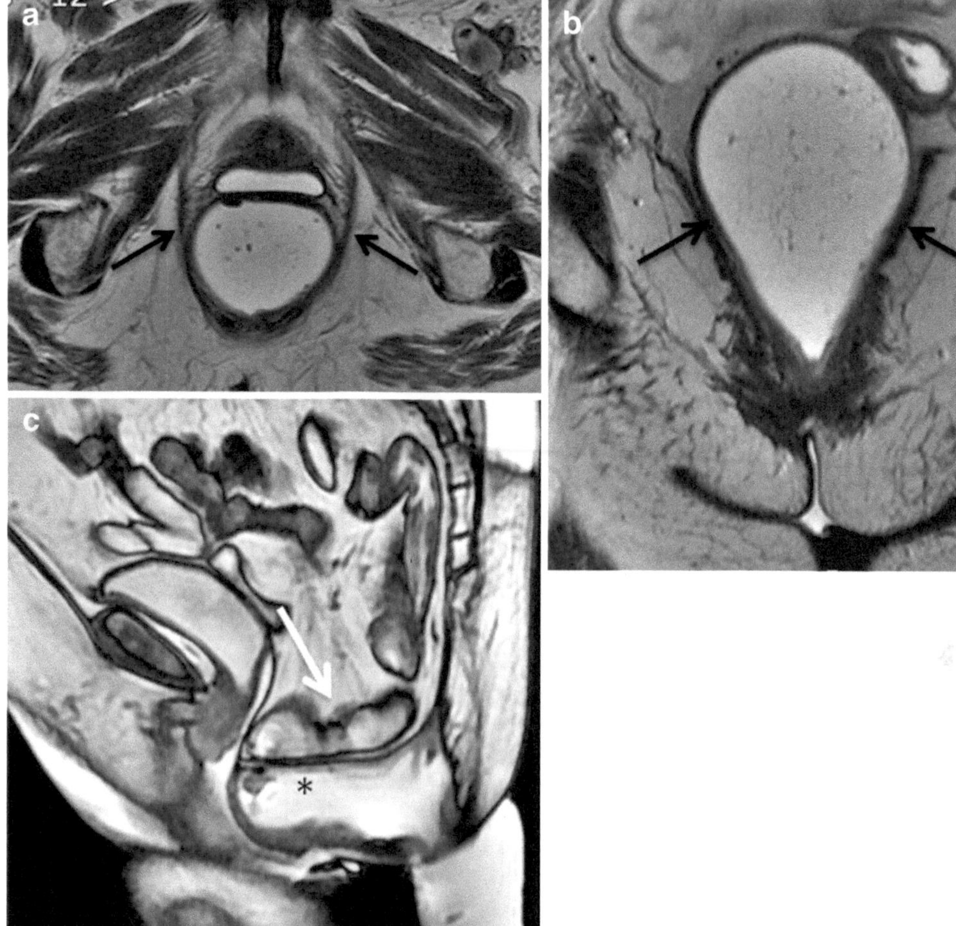

Fig. 4.6 (**a**) Axial T2-weighted image obtained with external phased-array coil shows diffused atrophy of the puborectalis muscle (*black arrows*). (**b**) Coronal T2-weighted image shows thinning (*black arrows*) of levator ani muscles and left lateral detachment (*arrowhead*). (**c**) Dynamic MR image obtained during defecation shows a large anterior rectocele (*) and enterocele (*white arrow*)

squeeze was lower in subjects with fecal incontinence who had a history of a third- or fourth-degree perineal tear, indicating a lower function of the puborectalis muscle [32].

Assessment of sphincter integrity with MR is important because patients with a focal defect may benefit from surgical repair [33], or in the case of incontinence and rectal prolapse, patients may achieve restoration of continence after rectopexy [34]. Conversely EAS atrophy is associated to poor outcome of an anterior anal sphincter repair [35]. In the selection of patients for anal sphincter repair, both endoanal MR and endoanal sonography are sensitive tools for preoperatory assessment, but endoanal MRI is capable of depicting EAS atrophy, with a sensitivity of 81 % and a positive predictive value of 89 % compared to surgical findings, which is associated with a poor outcome of anterior anal sphincter repair [36, 37]. Patients with external sphincter atrophy at a preoperatory assessment have worse outcome after repair [35], while those with normal external thickness show a better postsurgical outcome [38].

MR defecography (dynamic imaging of the pelvic floor) has also been evaluated in selecting surgical options in anal incontinence (Figs. 4.5 and 4.6). MR defecography reveals various pelvic floor abnormalities including rectal descent, cystocele, enterocele, rectocele, and rectal invagination [4–15]. These conditions are hardly assessed at clinical evaluation alone [3]. Cystocele, vaginal vault or cervix descent, enterocele, and rectal prolapse are detected as the vertical lowering of, respectively, the bladder base, the vaginal vault or the cervix, the peritoneal cul-de-sac, and the anorectal junction from the pubococcygeal line, which is a line drawn from the lower border of the pubic symphysis to the last coccygeal joint [4–15]. Rectocele is an abnormal bulging of the rectal wall, usually located at the anterior wall, and it is a cause of incomplete defecation, because of retention of feces into its lumen during evacuation [4–15]. Rectal invagination, or intussusception, is defined as a full-thickness rectal wall prolapse, involving both mucosa and muscular layer; this condition can cause a mechanical obstruction to the passage of stool [4–15]. However, rectocele and internal prolapse are also a cause of fecal incontinence [10]. Evaluation of these findings in a preoperatory assessment has proven to have changed the intended surgical treatment in 68 % [10]. In that series, 36 % was unable to hold the enema and 94 % showed rectal descent, 40 % bladder descent, and 43 % vaginal vault descent, while 34 % showed the presence of anterior rectocele, 32 % the presence of enterocele, and 20 % the presence of rectal invagination. Moreover, 50 % of patients showed ARA changes <10 % between rest and squeezing and rest and defecation, indicating a dysfunction of puborectalis sling mechanism.

Thus, MR imaging in a preoperatory assessment may result in a more accurate selection of patient candidates to surgical treatment. Endoanal MR has showed better evaluation of external sphincter lesions versus sonography compared to surgical results [22]; however, endosonography has reported better results in detecting internal sphincter defect [25]. MR defecography is used to detect previously unknown findings in the pelvic floor, which lead to changes to surgical treatment.

Experience of radiologist is important in evaluating the sphincter complex, being the interobserver agreement stronger if both internal and external sphincters are intact or disrupted [39]. Interobserver agreement for assessing sphincter integrity is moderate for endoanal MRI and poor to fair for external phased-array MRI [17, 39], while the interobserver agreement is fair to very good for both techniques. In assessing EAS atrophy, interobserver agreement has been reported to be moderate for endoanal MRI and moderate to good for external phased-array MRI [26], while intraobserver agreement was moderate to very good for endoanal MRI and fair to very good for external phased-array MRI [26]. Interobserver agreement for MR defecography has been reported to be good to excellent [10].

Conclusions

MRI provides an accurate depiction of anal sphincter complex and pelvic floor anatomy with evaluation of muscle integrity and being a valuable tool to assess functional abnormalities of the pelvic floor as well. Either endoanal or external MRI can be used to evaluate muscle integrity with comparable results. External phased-array MRI provides information on pelvic floor muscle, while dynamic imaging is an additional tool to assess if pelvic floor prolapse (bladder, uterine, or rectal) is associated. These information are of main diagnostic importance in evaluating fecal incontinence and aid treatment decision-making.

References

1. Terra MP, Stoker J. The current role of imaging techniques in faecal incontinence. Eur Radiol. 2006;16:1727–36.
2. Stoker J. Magnetic resonance imaging in fecal incontinence. Semin Ultrasound CT MR. 2008;29:409–13.
3. Stoker J, Halligan S, Bartram CI. Pelvic floor imaging. Radiology. 2001;218:621–41.
4. Colaiacomo MC, Masselli G, Polettini E, Lanciotti S, Casciani E, Bertini L, Gualdi G. Dynamic MR imaging of the pelvic floor: a pictorial review. Radiographics. 2009;29(3):e35.
5. Bertschinger KM, Hetzer FH, Roos JE, Treiber K, Marincek B, Hilfiker PR. Dynamic MR imaging of the pelvic floor performed with a patient sitting in an open-magnet unit versus with patient supine in a closed-magnet unit. Radiology. 2002;223:501–8.

6. Fielding JR, Giffiths DJ, Versi E, Mulkern RV, Lee ML, Jolesz FA. MR imaging of pelvic floor continence mechanism in the supine and sitting positions. AJR Am J Roentgenol. 1998;171:1607–10.
7. Unterweger M, Marincek B, Gottstein-Aalame N, Debatin JF, Seifert B, Ochsenbein-Imhof N, Perucchini D, Kubik-Huch RA. Ultrafast MR imaging of the pelvic floor. AJR Am J Roentgenol. 2001; 176:959–63.
8. Kelvin FM, Maglinte DDT, Hale DS, Benson JT. Female pelvic organs prolapse: a comparison of triphasic dynamic MR imaging and triphasic fluoroscopic cystocoloproctography. AJR Am J Roentgenol. 2000;174:81–8.
9. Goh V, Halligan S, Kaplan G, Healy JC, Bartram CI. Dynamic MR imaging of the pelvic floor in asymptomatic subjects. AJR Am J Roentgenol. 2000;174:661–6.
10. Hetzer FH, Andreisek GA, Tsagari C, Sahrbacher U, Weishaupt D. MR defecography in patients with faecal incontinence: imaging findings and their effects on surgical management. Radiology. 2006;240:449–57.
11. Dvorkin LS, Hetzer F, Scott SM, Williams NS, Gedroyc W, Lunniss PJ. Open-magnet MR defecography compared with evacuation proctography in the diagnosis and management of patients with rectal intussusception. Colorectal Dis. 2004;6:45–53.
12. Mortele KJ, Fairhurst J. Dynamic MR defecography of the posterior compartment: indications, techniques and MRI features. Eur J Radiol. 2007;61(3):462–72.
13. Woodfield CA, Krishnamoorthy S, Hapton BS, Brody JM. Imaging pelvic floor disorders: trend toward comprehensive MRI. AJR Am J Roentgenol. 2010; 194:1640–9.
14. Fielding J. Practical MR imaging of female pelvic floor weakness. Radiographics. 2002;22:295–304.
15. Pannu HK, Kaufman HS, Cundiff GW, Genadry R, Bluemke DA, Fishman EK. Dynamic imaging of pelvic organ prolapse: spectrum of abnormalities. Radiographics. 2000;20:1567–82.
16. Terra MP, Beets-Tan RG, vas der Hulst VPM, et al. MR imaging in evaluating atrophy of the external anal sphincter in patients with fecal incontinence. AJR Am J Roentgenol. 2006;187(4):991–9.
17. Terra MP, Beets-Tan RG, van der Hulst VPM, et al. Anal sphincter defects in patients with fecal incontinence: endoanal versus external phased-array MR imaging. Radiology. 2005;236:886–95.
18. Olson C. Diagnostic testing for fecal incontinence. Clin Colon Rectal Surg. 2014;27:85–90.
19. Bitti G, Argiolas G, Ballicu N, et al. Pelvic floor failure: MR imaging evaluation of anatomic and functional abnormalities. Radiographics. 2014;34:429–48.
20. Rociu E, Stoker J, Eijkemans MJC, Lameris JS. Normal anal sphincter anatomy and age- and sex related variations at high-spatial-resolution endoanal MR imaging. Radiology. 2000;217:396–401.
21. Rociu E, Stoker J, Zwamborn AW, Lameris JS. Endoanal MR imaging of the anal sphincter in fecal incontinence. Radiographics. 1999;19:S171–7.
22. Rociu E, Stoker J, Eijkemans MJ, Schouten WR, Lameris JS. Fecal incontinence: endoanal US versus endoanal MR imaging. Radiology. 1999;212:453–8.
23. de Souza NM, Puni R, Zbar A, Gilderale DJ, Coutts GA, Kraus T. MR imaging of the anal sphincter in multiparous women using an endoanal coil: correlation with in vitro anatomy and appearances in fecal incontinence. AJR Am J Roentgenol. 1996;167:1465–71.
24. de Souza NM, Hall AS, Puni R, Gilderale D, Young IR, Kmiot WA. High resolution magnetic resonance imaging of the anal sphincter using a dedicated endoanal coil. Comparison of magnetic resonance imaging with surgical findings. Dis Colon Rectum. 1996;39:926–34.
25. Malouf AJ, Williams AB, Halligan S, Bartram CI, Dhillon S, Kamm MA. Prospective assessment of accuracy of endoanal MR imaging and endosonography in patients with fecal incontinence. AJR Am J Roentgenol. 2000;175:741–5.
26. Terra MP, Deutekom M, Beets-Tan RG, et al. Relation between external anal sphincter atrophy at endoanal magnetic resonance imaging and clinical, functional, and anatomic characteristics in patients with fecal incontinence. Dis Colon Rectum. 2006;49:668–78.
27. Kessels IMH, Futterer JJ, Sultan AH, Kluivers KB. Clinical symptoms related to anal sphincter defects and atrophy on external phased-array. MR Imaging Int Urogynecol J. 2015;26:1619–27.
28. Bharucha AE, Fletcher JG, Harper CM, et al. Relationship between symptoms and disordered continence mechanisms in women with idiopathic fecal incontinence. Gut. 2005;54:546–55.
29. Terra MP, Beets-Tan RH, Vervoorn I, et al. Pelvic floor muscle lesions at endoanal MR imaging in female patients with faecal incontinence. Eur Radiol. 2008;18:1892–901.
30. Heilbrun ME, Nygaard IE, Lockhart ME, et al. Correlation between levator ani muscle injuries on MRI and fecal incontinence, pelvic organ prolapse, and urinary incontinence in primiparous women. Am J Obstet Gynecol. 2010;202(5):488.e1–6.
31. Healy JC, Halligan S, Reznek RH, et al. Dynamic MR imaging compared with evacuation proctography when evaluating anorectal configuration and pelvic floor movement. AJR Am J Roentgenol. 1997;169:775–9.
32. Bharucha AE, Fletcher JG, Melton III LJ, Zinsmeister R. Obstetric trauma, pelvic floor injury and fecal incontinence: a population based case-control study. Am J Gastroenterol. 2012;107:902–11.
33. Madoff RD. Surgical treatment options for fecal incontinence. Gastroenterology. 2004;126:S48–54.
34. Schiedeck H, Schwandner O, Scheele J, Farke S, Bruch HP. Rectal prolapse: which surgical option is appropriate? Langenbecks Arch Surg. 2005;390:8–14.

35. Briel JW, Stoker J, Rociu E, Lameris JS, Hop WC, Schouten WR. External anal sphincter atrophy on endoanal magnetic resonance imaging adversely affects continence after sphincteroplasty. Br J Surg. 1999;86:1322–7.
36. Dobben AC, Terra MP, Slors JF, et al. External anal sphincter defects in patients with fecal incontinence: comparison of endoanal MR imaging and endoanal US. Radiology. 2007;242:463–71.
37. Cazemier M, Terra MP, Stoker J, et al. Atrophy and defects detection of the external anal sphincter: comparison between three-dimensional anal endosonography and endoanal magnetic resonance imaging. Dis Colon Rectum. 2005;49:20–7.
38. Dobben AC, Terra MP, Deutekom M, et al. The role of endoluminal imaging in clinical outcome of overlapping anterior anal sphincter repair in patients with fecal incontinence. AJR Am J Roentgenol. 2007;189:W70–7.
39. Malouf AJ, Halligan S, Williams AB, et al. Prospective assessment of interobserver agreement for endoanal MRI in fecal incontinence. Abdom Imaging. 2001; 26:76–8.

5 Anorectal Manometry

Danilo Badiali

Several tests are available to evaluate anorectal function as well as gather information about the pathophysiology of disorders that affect continence. Often they complement one another. Anorectal manometry (ARM) is a useful test to categorize anal and/or rectal dysfunction in addition to provide physiological assessment of both anal sphincters and rectum [1–5].

5.1 Procedure

5.1.1 Method

Data concerning ARM in the management of FI are obtained using different methods: conventional water perfusion manometry, solid-state manometry [6], and high-resolution manometry [5, 7].

Solid-state probe with strain gauge transducers or water-perfused probes is currently in use. Solid-state microtransducers are reliable, but too expensive for clinical use. The outer diameter of the probes is between 4 and 6 mm, with at least four recording points (solid-state sensors or perfused side holes) arranged radially and spaced 0.5–1 cm apart longitudinally (Fig. 5.1). A central lumen ends in a 4-cm long, compliant balloon attached to the tip of the catheter, at 4 cm from the distal recording point [6, 8, 9]. The water-perfused manometry systems use pneumohydraulic pumps ensuring a rate of 0.2–0.4 mL/min with a pressure head of 10 psi.

The probe is inserted placing multiple pressure sensors and balloon in the rectum, and a rest period of ~5 min is necessary to allow the anal tone to return to its basal level.

5.1.2 Anal Pressure

The resting anal pressure may be measured with a station pull-through technique withdrawing the probe step-by-step 0.5 cm at the time to record the pressure profile of the anal canal (Fig. 5.2). Anal resting pressure is expressed as the average of the highest recorded values obtained from each transducer [10].

If the patient is not completely relaxed, there is a greater contribution of the striated muscle and higher pressures will be recorded. For this reason, in order to obtain stable values, it would be preferable to place the sensors inside the anal canal and record the pressure at rest for an extended period (5–15 min). The maximal anal pressure is the value obtained during the last period (1–5 min, respectively) in basal condition [6, 9].

D. Badiali, MD
Department of Internal Medicine and Medical Specialties, La Sapienza, Rome University, Rome, Italy
e-mail: danilo.badiali@uniroma1.it

M. Mongardini, M. Giofrè (eds.), *Management of Fecal Incontinence*,
DOI 10.1007/978-3-319-32226-1_5

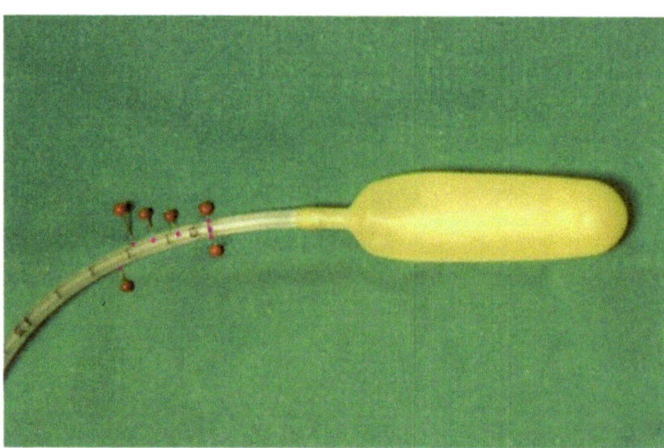

Fig. 5.1 Water-perfused probe with outer diameter of 4 mm and eight side holes (*red points*) radially spaced. Four of them are arranged at the same level, 90° between one another, while the other four are arranged 5 mm apart longitudinally

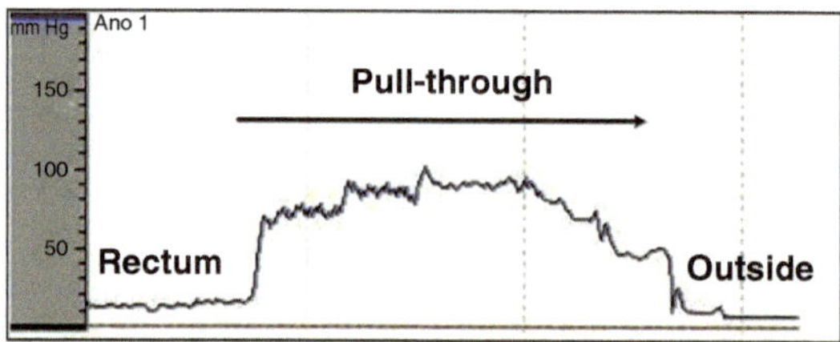

Fig. 5.2 Resting anal pressure assessed by the pull-through technique: the probe is pulled through the anal canal, from the rectum to outward (only one sensor tracing is reported)

In some cases it is possible to observe phasic pressure activities at 1–1.5 cycles per min and with amplitude ±40 mmHg that are named ultra-slow waves. Their pathophysiological and clinical significance is unknown, but they are frequently detected, in subjects affected with a variety of anorectal disorders such as hemorrhoids and dischetia, which can be related to constipation [11, 12]. The detection of ultra slow waves can hinder the measurement of the resting pressure and the interpretation of the tracing [13].

The resting tone is due to the tonic activities of the internal anal sphincter (IAS) and of the external anal sphincter (EAS). Human studies about the effect of the IAS myotomy [14], of the general anesthesia [15], and of the pudendal nerve block [16] on the anal pressures suggest that approximately 75–85 % of the basal pressure derives from the IAS and the remaining part from the EAS.

To evaluate the strength and duration of the voluntary contraction, the manometric probe is positioned in the anal canal with the recording holes in the high-pressure zone and the patient is asked to squeeze (≥2 attempts). The mean of the highest pressures recorded at any site in the anal canal is used to calculate the maximum squeeze pressure [6, 9].

Squeeze duration can be expressed as the period in which squeeze pressure is maintained above the 50 % of the maximal value [6] or as the interval between the onset of pressure increases in the anal canal and the pressure curve returns to baseline values. Some software calculate the area under the squeeze pressure curve [9] providing a reliable assessment of the efficiency of voluntary contraction by combining strength and durability. The squeeze maneuver assesses the function and the voluntary control of the EAS [17].

Pressure asymmetry is present between the proximal and distal segments of the anal canal: proximal pressures of the anterior quadrant are significantly reduced at rest and during maximum voluntary effort [18, 19]. The circumferential asymmetry of this area is due to the "U" shape of the puborectalis muscle, that is, circular in the posterior direction. Recent studies, using manometry and 3D ultrasound of the anal canal [20], reported the association between increased pressure along the entire anal canal and the contraction of both EAS and puborectalis muscle. These data suggest that the puborectalis muscle contributes to the squeezing in the proximal part of the anal canal, while the EAS in the distal part and the maximal values are detected where the puborectalis overlaps EAS.

Involuntary contraction of the EAS occurs during abrupt change in intra-abdominal pressure: this is a multisynaptic sacral reflex that prevents anal incontinence in such conditions and that is voluntarily inhibited during defecation. To test this reflex increase in anal sphincter pressure, the patient is asked to cough: this reflex response causes the anal sphincter pressure to rise above that of the rectum. The cough reflex is rated as the highest positive difference between the increases of the anal pressure in comparison with the increase of the rectal pressure, in two attempts [6].

Scratching the perianal skin is possible to record a contraction of EAS: this is the anocutaneous reflex. It may have potential in the evaluation of the extrinsic innervations of the anus, but there are no data to support its clinical use.

Anal pressures vary by age and sex: they appear higher in men and younger, even though there exists a considerable overlap in values [8, 9, 21, 22]. Measured pressures tend to be higher when you run a quick pull-through [10].

J. Rogers and coworkers [23] reported the reproducibility of the measurement of anal pressures in a small group of patients evaluated blindly by two different investigators in an interval of about 20 days. Recently, the high reproducibility was confirmed measuring the resting and squeeze anal pressures ($r \geq 7$) in the same subject in separate days [24], but both studies evaluated a limited group of healthy subjects.

5.1.3 High-Resolution Manometry

The high-resolution manometry (HRM) uses a probe with 12–36 circumferential sensors. Each sensor is able to detect pressure in each of the radially dispersed sectors and from a 2.5 mm distance. The different values of pressure are identified with different colors, and the space–time pressure data are displayed as isobaric contour plots in topographic form. The technique simultaneously records pressure in the rectum and through the anal canal increasing the accuracy of the interpretation of the findings [5, 7]. The anorectal HRM highly correlates water-perfused manometry [5], and to date there is no evidence that it has clinical, diagnostic, or interventional advantage over conventional manometry [25].

5.1.4 Rectal Properties

The optimal method for assessing the sensorial and viscoelastic characteristics of the rectum is the barostat test, even though it is scarcely use in clinical evaluation because of its cost.

During ARM a balloon is usually inflated in the rectum with increasing volumes of air to get some information over the viscoelastic properties and sensory function. This procedure is certainly less accurate than the detailed barostat test, but it is considered sufficient to get information about clinical rectal properties.

The rectal balloon is intermittently air inflated. Each inflation is realized every 30–60 s and involves a 10 mL volume increase up to 200 mL of air or the onset of pain/discomfort. The rectal balloon is completely air deflated after each step [6, 9].

Rectum responds to filling with visceral relaxation for comfortably storing feces until the voluntary defecation: this adaptability is described by the rectal compliance, which is a volume/pressure curve ($\delta V/\delta P$ ml/mmHg).

The pressure in the balloon during the distension can be considered related to the intrarectal pressure, and its measurement is used to assess the rectal compliance. The balloon inflation causes a rapid increase of the intra balloon pressure, followed by a decline to a steady-state value as the rectum accommodates to the increased volume. The rectal steady state is calculated as the difference between the recorded pressure and the pressure obtained during the inflation of the balloon in ambient with the same volume of distension. The rectal compliance is calculated by plotting the ratio between volume increases and the variations of the stationary state pressures.

High compliance values indicate that the rectum excessively relaxes resulting in poorincreased pressure in its lumen, conversely low compliance values describe a poor adaptation of the rectum to volume increases resulting in high intra-rectal pressures.

The distension of the rectum by increasing volumes is aimed also to evaluate rectal sensibility. The patient is asked to refer the sensations in the rectum. Usually three steps of sensation are identified: (I) sensation of fullness or distention, (II) persistent call to evacuate, and (III) maximum tolerable volume that can be associated with pain [6, 9].

Evaluating the rectal sensibility, it must be appreciated that the rectal size and compliance may affect the threshold and type of perception. Large size and/or high compliant rectum requires large volume to evoke the call to evacuate; in non-compliant rectum, small volume can induce urgency [26].

However, balloon inflections used to assess the rectal compliance and sensibility show some limits: in addition to the fact the rectum is an open-ended cavity, it is also both technique and operator dependent. Recorded data may vary according to the size and the nature of the balloon and the ramp method of inflation and its speed [27, 28]. It is advisable to use a large-volume bag and rectal distension at fixed volumes. The rectal sensibility can also be altered by the discomfort caused by the maneuver and/or by the use of cleansing enema before the test.

5.1.5 Rectoanal Inhibitory Reflex

Distention of the rectum elicits a transient decrease of the resting anal pressure due to the relaxation of the IAS: this characteristic is known as the rectoanal inhibitory reflex. It is an intrinsic reflex that is mediated via the myenteric plexus. It can also last after a pudendal block [29–31], and it is identified as a "sampling mechanism" to discriminate the rectal content: flatus and consistence of feces [32]. Some reports [33, 34] have evaluated the variables of the RAIR (latency, percentage of relaxation, duration, residual pressure) in an attempt to identify discriminating aspects. Even though some differences have been observed between groups of patients affected with incontinence or constipation, those groups overlapped largely showing little clinical significance. The characteristics of the RAIR depend on some technical aspects: the rectum should be free of feces, megarectum needs large volume to reach the proper distension in order to evocate the reflex, the pressure drop can be obscured by the EAS contraction, or it cannot be evident at all when the resting pressure is very low.

The RAIR can be absent after low anterior resection and ileoanal pouch procedures, although there is a tendency for late recovery [35–39]. The absence of RAIR is considered diagnostic for Hirschsprung's disease having sensitivity of 91 % and specificity of 94 % [29, 30, 40].

5.1.6 Defecatory Maneuver

In constipated patients, it is useful to evaluate the defecatory maneuver [1, 3, 5]. The patient is asked to attempt defecation to evaluate sphincter responses during the maneuver, while the rectal balloon can be inflated with air or water. Normal pattern shows increase of the intrarectal pressure, which is synergic with the decrease in the intra-anal pressure. Some constipated patients may exhibit anal pressure increment during straining [41–45] for the paradoxical contraction of the EAS or lack of anal relaxation: in both cases, there is an obstacle to evacuate [6]. In a third pattern of dyssynergic defecation, the intrarectal pressure is lower than anal pressure [6]. The maneuver can be affected by laboratory condition (position of the patient, lack of privacy); actually it is poorly reproducible and altered patterns are recorded also in asymptomatic subjects. The diagnosis of dyssynergic defection should be confirmed with other test (balloon expulsion test, defecography, EMG).

5.2 Clinical Use in Fecal Incontinence

5.2.1 Pressure Alteration

Anorectal manometry is suggested in the work-up for fecal incontinence [1, 3, 46] because it provides objective assessment of the anal sphincter function. The manometric parameters usually considered are resting pressure, squeeze pressure, rectal compliance, and rectal sensibility [6]. The length of the anal canal may seem theoretically important, but there seems to be little evidence to support it. Also the anal vettography is of no apparent benefit for sphincter evaluation because of the scarce correlation with anal ultrasonography [47].

Anal pressures are pathophysiologically important in patients with FI; their assessment can be obtained by digital examination [48–50], but ARM is more accurate than digital examination, especially for minor abnormalities. Several authors [17, 51–53] reported that incontinent patients exhibit lower resting and squeeze pressures than continent patients, regardless of age and gender [51]. Low resting pressure and impairment of voluntary contraction reflect functional deficit of the IAS and EAS, respectively. Impairment in both pressure has been associated with passive incontinence frequency, but not with urge incontinence [17, 54]. Even though there is a large overlapping between incontinent patients and control subjects, the maximum squeeze pressure has been suggested as the best distinctive for FI [52]. This aspect has been confirmed by Raza and Bielefeldt: in order to identify discriminating patterns, they reviewed retrospectively the manometric tracings obtained in incontinent and constipated patients [22]. They reported that a resting pressure of less than 40 mmHg had a good specificity (>90 %), but the sensitivity was low (50 %); reduced squeeze pressures were more often in incontinence, with a sensitivity of 59 % but with a specificity of only 69 %. The low specificity and sensibility can be due to the possible alteration of both sphincters. A recent report [22] performed a retrospective review of anorectal manometry for FI. In 73 % of patients, at least one sphincter dysfunction was recorded and 33 % of tracings showed both IAS and EAS dysfunctions; isolated alteration of IAS or EAS was recorded in 30 % and 11 % of patients, respectively. Note that 26 % of patients did not show any sphincter impairment.

The authors propose classification of FI according to the manometric alteration:

1. IAS dysfunction
2. Isolated EAS dysfunction
3. Combined sphincter dysfunction
4. Normal sphincter function

Some incontinent patients exhibit spontaneous transient anal relaxations, and it is possible that leakage occurs as the anal pressure fell below the rectal pressure [55, 56]; this pattern has been observed in diabetic patients [57].

5.2.2 Alteration of Rectal Properties

It is reported that about 25–40 % of patients affected with FI show a reduced rectal compliance that is often associated with rectal hypersensibility [17, 52, 53]. Even in the absence of sphincter dysfunction, these patterns are associated with symptoms of urgency defecation or passive incontinence [17]. The reduced rectal compliance and urgency can be the result of an enhanced motor response of the rectum to distension (irritable rectum), sometimes associated with a prolonged anal relaxation [55]. R. J. Felt-Bersam and coworkers performed the saline-infusion test in 350 incontinent patients and observed that patients with lower resting and squeeze sphincter pressures and a smaller rectal capacity leaked earlier following saline infusion in the rectum [52].

In one study [53], patients with urgency defecation have been classified according to the presence or absence of hypersensitivity, and all them underwent ARM and prolonged rectosigmoid manometry. The authors reported similar values of the anal pressures in the two groups, but the patients with hypersensitivity demonstrated increased symptoms, enhanced perception, reduced compliance, and exaggerated rectosigmoid motor activity. These data suggest that in the management of urgency defecation, may be useful consider, besides ARC findings, also motor activity of the rectosigmoid.

Reduced rectal compliance is suggested to be useful in discriminating patients with FI [17]; rectal hypersensitivity worsens stool frequency, urgency, and lifestyle in patients with urge fecal incontinence [58].

Rectal compliance is affected by the size and by the tonic contraction of the rectum: patients with megarectum have high values of compliance; conversely patients with rectal fibrosis (Fig. 5.3), such as inflammatory bowel diseases [59] or hypertonic muscle contraction, show a

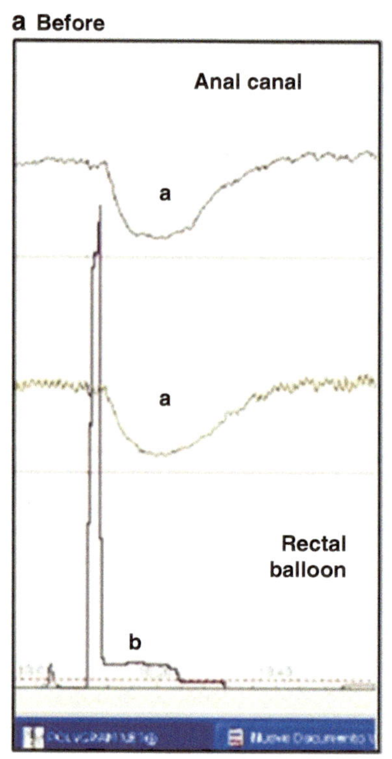

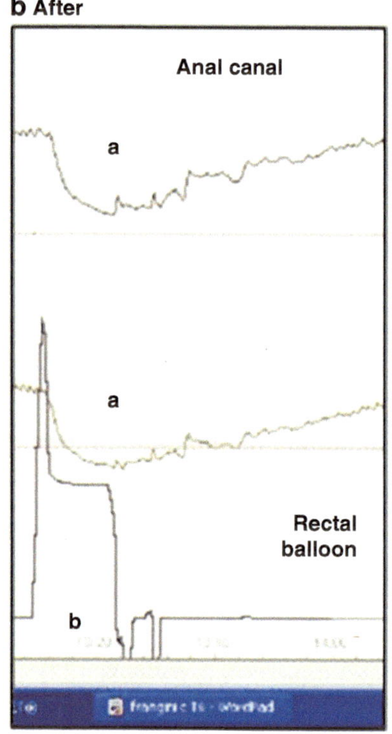

Fig. 5.3 Different rectal adaptability of the rectum before and after radiotherapy: the inflation of the rectal balloon with 100 ml-air elicits the normal rectoanal inhibitory reflex (**a**), but the steady-state pressure (**b**) after radiotherapy is higher than the steady-state pressure before treatment, suggesting a reduce rectal compliance

reduced compliance, due to the rigidity of the rectal wall. Even fibrosis due to other pelvic organs may hinder the expansion of the rectal wall and consequently affect its compliance.

Preserved rectal sensation is necessary for the treatment by biofeedback, and improved sensation after biofeedback therapy predicts improvement of FI [60, 61].

Conclusions

Data of literature do not support the role of discriminating test for ARM in the diagnosis of FI; nevertheless, it is useful to understand the pathophysiology of the symptoms. No prediction can be made about the continence with any single anorectal finding, but the detection of sphincter and/or rectal alteration can facilitate the management of the FI. The accurate assessment of the pathophysiology inducing FI can provide information on the use of new treatments [4, 62], such as α1-adrenoceptor agonists [63] and sacral nerve stimulation [64]; the description of altered EAS efficacy and/or reduce rectal compliance and/or rectal hypersensitivity can guide the rehabilitative protocol with biofeedback [61].

However, FI is a multifactorial disorder resulting from several mechanisms, and the ARM has to be considered complementary to other anorectal tests before formulating a diagnosis.

The procedure must be conducted with appropriate techniques, and the results must be interpreted with caution, in the clinical context of the patient, in relationship with symptoms, clinical features, and other tests.

Since ARM is performed with different equipment and techniques, it is not possible to standardize the procedure, and as a result, different laboratory outcomes cannot be compared. For this reason it is necessary for each laboratory to collect ARM data from its own control group in order to obtain normal values of anal pressures, rectal compliance, and sensitivity.

References

1. Rao SS, Patel RS. How useful are manometric tests of anorectal function in the management of defecation disorders? Am J Gastroenterol. 1997;92(3):469–75.
2. Barnett JL, Hasler WL, Camilleri M. American Gastroenterological Association medical position statement on anorectal testing techniques. American Gastroenterological Association. Gastroenterology. 1999;116(3):732–60. Review.
3. Azpiroz F, Enck P, Whitehead WE. Anorectal functional testing: review of collective experience. Am J Gastroenterol. 2002;97(2):232–40.
4. Bharucha AE. Pro: anorectal testing is useful in fecal incontinence. Am J Gastroenterol. 2006;101(12):2679–81.
5. Rao SS. Advances in diagnostic assessment of fecal incontinence and dyssynergic defecation. Clin Gastroenterol Hepatol. 2010;8(11):910–9. doi:10.1016/j.cgh.2010.06.004.
6. Rao SS, Azpiroz F, Diamant N, et al. Minimum standards of anorectal manometry. Neurogastroenterol Motil. 2002;14(5):553–9.
7. Jones MP, Post J, Crowell MD. High-resolution manometry in the evaluation of anorectal disorders: a simultaneous comparison with water-perfused manometry. Am J Gastroenterol. 2007;102(4):850–5.
8. Rao SS, Hatfield R, Soffer E, et al. Manometric tests of anorectal function in healthy adults. Am J Gastroenterol. 1999;94(3):773–83.
9. Gruppo Lombardo per lo Studio della Motilità Intestinale. Anorectal manometry with water-perfused catheter in healthy adults with no functional bowel disorders. Colorectal Dis. 2010;12:220–5. doi:10.1111/j.1463-1318.2009.01787.x.
10. Diamant NE, Kamm MA, Wald A, Whitehead WE. AGA technical review on anorectal testing techniques. Gastroenterology. 1999;116(3):735–60.
11. Eckardt VF, Schmitt T, Bernhard G. Anal ultra slow waves: a smooth muscle phenomenon associated with dyschezia. Dig Dis Sci. 1997;42(12):2439–45.
12. Yoshino H, Kayaba H, Hebiguchi T, et al. Multiple clinical presentations of anal ultra slow waves and high anal pressure: megacolon, hemorrhoids and constipation. Tohoku J Exp Med. 2007;211(2):127–32.
13. Yoshino H, Kayaba H, Hebiguchi T, et al. Anal ultraslow waves and high anal pressure in childhood: a clinical condition mimicking Hirschsprung disease. J Pediatr Surg. 2007;42(8):1422–8.
14. Duthie L, Watts JM. Contribution of the external anal sphincter to the pressure zone in the anal canal. Gut. 1965;6(1):64–8.
15. Bennett RC, Duthie HL. The functional importance of the internal anal sphincter. Br J Surg. 1964;51(5):355–7.
16. Frenckner B, Euler CV. Influence of pudendal block on the function of the anal sphincters. Gut. 1975;16(6):482–9.
17. Bharucha AE, Fletcher JG, Harper CM, et al. Relationship between symptoms and disordered continence mechanisms in women with idiopathic faecal incontinence. Gut. 2005;54(4):546–55.
18. Taylor BM, Beart Jr RW, Phillips SF. Longitudinal and radial variations of pressure in the human anal sphincter. Gastroenterology. 1984;86(4):693–7.
19. Williams AB, Cheetham MJ, Bartram CI, et al. Gender differences in the longitudinal pressure profile of the anal canal related to anatomical structure as demonstrated on three-dimensional anal endosonography. Br J Surg. 2000;87(12):1674–9.
20. Liu J, Guaderrama N, Nager CW, Pretorius DH, Master S, Mittal RK. Functional correlates of anal canal anatomy: puborectalis muscle and anal canal pressure. Am J Gastroenterol. 2006;101(5):1092–7.
21. Fox JC, Fletcher JG, Zinsmeister AR, et al. Effect of aging on anorectal and pelvic floor functions in females. Dis Colon Rectum. 2006;49(11):1726–35.
22. Raza N, Bielefeldt K. Discriminative value of anorectal manometry in clinical practice. Dig Dis Sci. 2009;54(11):2503–11. doi:10.1007/s10620-008-0631-1.
23. Rogers J, Laurberg S, Misiewicz JJ, et al. Anorectal physiology validated: a repeatability study of the motor and sensory tests of anorectal function. Br J Surg. 1989;76(6):607–9.
24. Bharucha AE, Seide B, Fox JC, Zinsmeister AR. Day-to-day reproducibility of anorectal sensorimotor assessments in healthy subjects. Neurogastroenterol Motil. 2004;16(2):241–50.
25. Dinning PG, Carrington EV, Scott SM. Colonic and anorectal motility testing in the high-resolution era. Curr Opin Gastroenterol. 2016;32(1):44–8. doi:10.1097/MOG.0000000000000229.
26. Felt-Bersma RJ, Sloots CE, Poen AC, et al. Rectal compliance as a routine measurement: extreme volumes have direct clinical impact and normal volumes exclude rectum as a problem. Dis Colon Rectum. 2000;43(12):1732–8.
27. Sloots CE, Felt-Bersma RJ, Cuesta MA, Meuwissen SG. Rectal visceral sensitivity in healthy volunteers: influences of gender, age and methods. Neurogastroenterol Motil. 2000;12(4):361–8.
28. Krogh K, Ryhammer AM, Lundby L, Gregersen H, Laurberg TS, et al. Comparison of methods used for measurement of rectal compliance. Dis Colon Rectum. 2001;44(2):199–206.
29. Howard ER, Nixon HH. Internal anal sphincter: observation on development and mechanism of inhibitory response in premature infants and children with Hirschsprung's disease. Arch Dis Child. 1968;43(231):569–78.
30. Meunier P, Marechal JM, Mollard P. Accuracy of the manometric diagnosis of Hirschsprung's disease. J Pediatr Surg. 1978;13(4):411–5.
31. Lubowski DZ, Nicholls RJ, Swash M, Jordan M. Neural control of internal anal sphincter function. Br J Surg. 1987;74(8):688–90.

32. Duthie HL, Bennett RC. The relation of sensation in the anal canal to the functional anal sphincter: a possible factor in anal continence. Gut. 1963;4(2):179–82.
33. Zbar AP, Aslam M, Gold DM, et al. Parameters of the rectoanal inhibitory reflex in patients with idiopathic fecal incontinence and chronic constipation. Dis Colon Rectum. 1998;41(2):200–8.
34. Kaur G, Gardiner A, Duthie GS. Rectoanal reflex parameters in incontinence and constipation. Dis Colon Rectum. 2002;45(7):928–33.
35. O'Riordain MG, Molloy RG, Gillen P, et al. Rectoanal inhibitory reflex following low stapled anterior resection of the rectum. Dis Colon Rectum. 1992;35(9):874–8.
36. Montesani C, Habib FI, Corazziari E, et al. Continence after restorative proctocolectomy and its correlation to defaecographic and manometric results. Int J Surg Sci. 1995;2(1):111–4.
37. Williamson ME, Lewis WG, Finan PJ, et al. Recovery of physiologic and clinical function after low anterior resection of the rectum for carcinoma: myth or reality? Dis Colon Rectum. 1995;38(4):411–8.
38. Lee SJ, Park YS. Serial evaluation of anorectal function following low anterior resection of the rectum. Int J Colorectal Dis. 1998;13(5–6):241–6.
39. Gross E, Möslein G. Colonic pouch and other procedures to improve the continence after low anterior rectal resection with TME. Zentralbl Chir. 2008;133(2):107–15. doi:10.1055/s-2008-1004735.
40. de Lorijn F, Kremer LC, Reitsma JB, Benninga MA. Diagnostic tests in Hirschsprung disease: a systematic review. J Pediatr Gastroenterol Nutr. 2006;42(5):496–505.
41. Preston DM, Lennard-Jones JE. Anismus in chronic constipation. Dig Dis Sci. 1985;30(5):413–8.
42. Jones PN, Lubowski DZ, Swash M, Henry M. Is paradoxical contraction of puborectalis muscle of functional importance? Dis Colon Rectum. 1987;30(9):667–70.
43. Surrenti E, Rath DM, Pemberton JH, Camilleri M. Audit of constipation in a tertiary referral gastroenterology practice. Am J Gastroenterol. 1995;90(9):1471–5.
44. Bharucha AE, Wald A, Enck P, Rao S. Functional anorectal disorders. Gastroenterology. 2006;130(5):1510–8.
45. Andromanakos N, Skandalakis P, Troupis T, Filippou D. Constipation of anorectal outlet obstruction: pathophysiology, evaluation and management. J Gastroenterol Hepatol. 2006;21(4):638–46.
46. Wald A. Clinical practice. Fecal incontinence in adults. N Engl J Med. 2007;356(16):1648–55. Review.
47. Yang YK, Wexner SD. Anal pressure vectography is of no apparent benefit for sphincter evaluation. Int J Colorectal Dis. 1994;9(2):92–5.
48. Felt-Bersma RJ, Klinkenberg-Knol EC, Meuwissen SG. Investigation of anorectal function. Br J Surg. 1988;75(1):53–5.
49. Hill J, Corson RJ, Brandon H, Redford J, Faragher EB, Kiff ES, et al. History and examination in the assessment of patients with idiopathic fecal incontinence. Dis Colon Rectum. 1994;37(5):473–7.
50. Dobben AC, Terra MP, Deutekom M, et al. Anal inspection and digital rectal examination compared to anorectal physiology tests and endoanal ultrasonography in evaluating fecal incontinence. Int J Colorectal Dis. 2007;22(7):783–90.
51. Enck P, Kuhlbusch R, Lübke H, et al. Age and sex and anorectal manometry in incontinence. Dis Colon Rectum. 1989;32(12):1026–30.
52. Felt-Bersma RJ, Klinkenberg-Knol EC, Meuwissen SG. Anorectal function investigations in incontinent and continent patients. Differences and discriminatory value. Dis Colon Rectum. 1990;33(6):479–85; discussion 485–6.
53. Chan CL, Lunniss PJ, Wang D, et al. Rectal sensorimotor dysfunction in patients with urge faecal incontinence: evidence from prolonged manometric studies. Gut. 2005;54(9):1263–72.
54. Deutekom M, Dobben AC, Terra MP, et al. Clinical presentation of fecal incontinence and anorectal function: what is the relationship? Am J Gastroenterol. 2007;102(2):351–61.
55. Mandaliya R, DiMarino AJ, Moleski S, et al. Survey of anal sphincter dysfunction using anal manometry in patients with fecal incontinence: a possible guide to therapy. Ann Gastroenterol. 2015;28(4):469–74.
56. Sun WM, Read NW, Miner PB, et al. The role of transient internal sphincter relaxation in faecal incontinence? Int J Colorectal Dis. 1990;5(1):31–6.
57. Sun WM, Katsinelos P, Horowitz M, Read NW. Disturbances in anorectal function in patients with diabetes mellitus and faecal incontinence. Eur J Gastroenterol Hepatol. 1996;8(10):1007–12.
58. Chan CL, Scott SM, Williams NS, Lunniss PJ. Rectal hypersensitivity worsens stool frequency, urgency, and lifestyle in patients with urge fecal incontinence. Dis Colon Rectum. 2005;48(1):134–40.
59. Crispino P, Habib FI, Badiali D, et al. Colorectal motor and sensitivity features in patients affected by ulcerative proctitis with constipation: a radiological and manometric controlled study. Inflamm Bowel Dis. 2006;12(8):712–8.
60. Wald A, Tunuguntla AK. Anorectal sensorimotor dysfunction in fecal incontinence and diabetes mellitus. Modification with biofeedback therapy. N Engl J Med. 1984;310(20):1282–7.
61. Chiarioni G, Bassotti G, Stanganini S, Vantini I, Whitehead WE, et al. Sensory retraining is key to biofeedback therapy for formed stool fecal incontinence. Am J Gastroenterol. 2002;97(1):109–17.
62. Prather CM. Physiologic variables that predict the outcome of treatment for fecal incontinence. Gastroenterology. 2004;126(1 Suppl 1):S135–40.
63. Siproudhis L, Jones D, Shing RN, et al. Libertas Study Consortium. Libertas: rationale and study design of a multicentre, Phase II, double-blind, randomised, placebo-controlled investigation to evaluate the efficacy, safety and tolerability of locally applied NRL001 in patients with faecal incontinence. Colorectal Dis. 2014;16 Suppl 1:59–66. doi:10.1111/codi.12546.
64. Thaha MA, Abukar AA, Thin NN, et al. Sacral nerve stimulation for faecal incontinence and constipation in adults. Cochrane Database Syst Rev. 2015;8, CD004464. doi:10.1002/14651858.CD004464.pub3. Review.

6 Electromyography

Maurizio Inghilleri, Maria Cristina Gori, and Emanuela Onesti

6.1 Introduction

Pelvic floor muscles involved in anorectal function, such as in lower urinary tract and sexual functions, share physiological properties with other muscular districts, although with some peculiarities. Neural control of these muscles is complex, working through the pudendal nerve and its terminal branches, the sacral spinal centers, the motor and sensory tracts, and the central brain control centers. The functional integrity of this system can be studied with several electrodiagnostic techniques characterized by partial invasiveness and reliability of results, becoming needful for a correct diagnosis [14, 24]. Moreover, the standard neurophysiological equipment used to test the limbs and trunk might not be appropriate for urogenital-anal studies requiring specific basic knowledge and skills by neurologist. In patients with suspected neurogenic etiology diseases, pelvic floor neurophysiology provides information about the pathogenesis of the disorder (axonal or demyelinating), the anatomical level of lesion, and the extension and kind (acute, chronic) of the lesion.

Evidence-based recommendations for the use of diagnostic tests in clinical practice are needed. To date, several literature reviews on pelvic floor neurophysiology have been published [6, 19, 26]. The most widely accepted diagnostic protocol includes the following tests:

(i) The concentric needle electromyography (CNEMG) of the perineal muscles
(ii) The sacral reflexes: bulbocavernosus reflex (BCR) and pudendal-anal reflex (PAR)
(iii) The pudendal nerve terminal motor latency (PNTML)
(iv) The pudendal somatosensory evoked potentials (SSEP)
(v) The motor evoked potentials (MEPs) of the perineal muscles

6.2 Concentric Needle Electromyography (CNEMG) of the Perineal Muscles

CNEMG is a crucial technique to evaluate the presence of denervation activity (fibrillations, positive slow waves) and to study the characteristics (amplitude, duration, morphology) of the motor unit potentials (PUMs). Previous studies have yet shown that sphincter EMG is useful in the recognition of abnormalities in neurological diseases such as Parkinson's disease and multiple system atrophy and in constipation due to various neurologic anorectal dysfunctions [3, 4, 11, 31]. The usefulness of EMG analysis in patients with

M. Inghilleri (✉) • M.C. Gori • E. Onesti
Department of Neurology and Psychiatry, "Sapienza" University of Rome, Rome, Italy
e-mail: maurizio.inghilleri@uniroma1.it

M. Mongardini, M. Giofrè (eds.), *Management of Fecal Incontinence*,
DOI 10.1007/978-3-319-32226-1_6

idiopathic fecal incontinence (IFI) has been also showed [10, 12]. The analysis of the electrical potentials generated by the depolarization of muscle fiber membranes can be carried out using mono- or bipolar needle electrodes, allowing an accurate qualitative analysis of myoelectric signals. Surface electrodes record the signal less precisely, even if they offer the advantage of non-invasivity [6].

All the muscles of the pelvic floor can be investigated, although the muscles most investigated in clinical routine are represented by the external anal sphincter (EAS) muscle and the bulbocavernosus (BC) muscle (Fig. 6.1).

While the BC muscle has a similar behavior to that of all other skeletal muscles, the EAS presents some peculiarities. Sphincters show continue electrical activity also when they are at rest at low firing rate that disappears only during defecation and urination, consisting of MUP of 150–300 μv at low frequency (4–8 cycles/s) [8, 9, 30]. This activity is essential for the proper function of containment of sphincters, and it is determined by the activation of red muscle fibers (for slow contractions), and by the recruitment of white muscle fibers for the voluntary or reflex rapid activations. When the coaxial needle electrode is inserted, the evaluation of the activity at rest is possible (Fig. 6.2). This muscular activity is enriched during the phase of contraction with the recruitment of MUs. The presence in this phase of denervation is signaled by fibrillation activities or positive slow waves when it is acute, whereas in chronic processes, the presence of potential polyphasic of long duration is detectable. During a voluntary contraction, the definition of morphological characteristics such as width, length, shape, and the firing rate is mandatory (Fig. 6.2). The CNEMG examination ends with the assessment of the recruitment of MUs during a maximum voluntary effort (interferential pattern) or after a reflex contraction (coughing, straining).

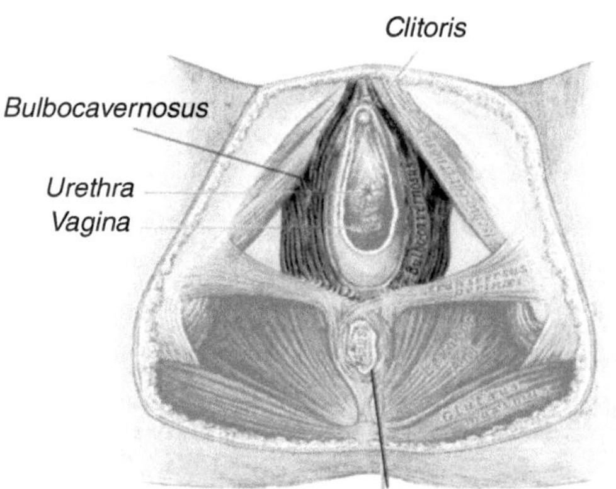

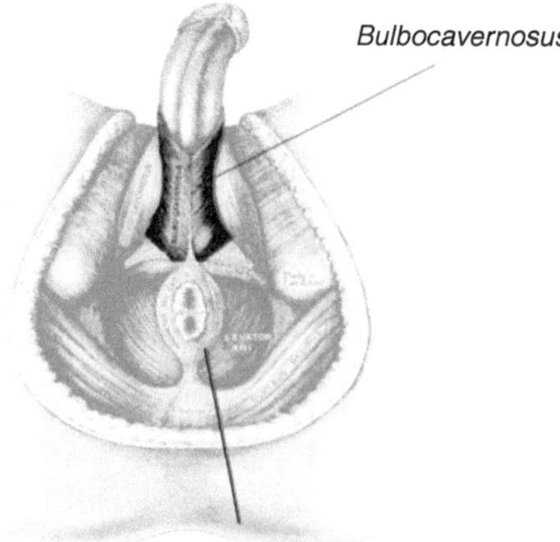

Fig. 6.1 Anatomical representation of the external anal sphincter (EAS) muscle and the bulbocavernosus (BC) muscle

Physiological features of MUs are amplified by an array of amplifiers, converted in digital form and displayed on a screen computer. The contribution of each MUP appears as a sequence of waves on subsequent channels. These waves are progressively time shifted as the source travels underneath the electrode array and generate a typical spatiotemporal pattern [20, 21]. EMG can be performed using a needle electrode or surface electrode [22, 23]. In routine diagnostics, needle electrodes are more commonly used because of its high precision.

According to the placement of needle for the study of the EAS and the BC muscles, the patient lies in the lateral decubitus position; the needle is driven approximately 1 cm lateral to the anal orifice in the case of the EAS and between the anus and the base of the scrotum (or the vaginal orifice) in the case of the BC muscle. Specifically for the EAS study, the concentric needle is usually introduced in different quadrants. In the rear

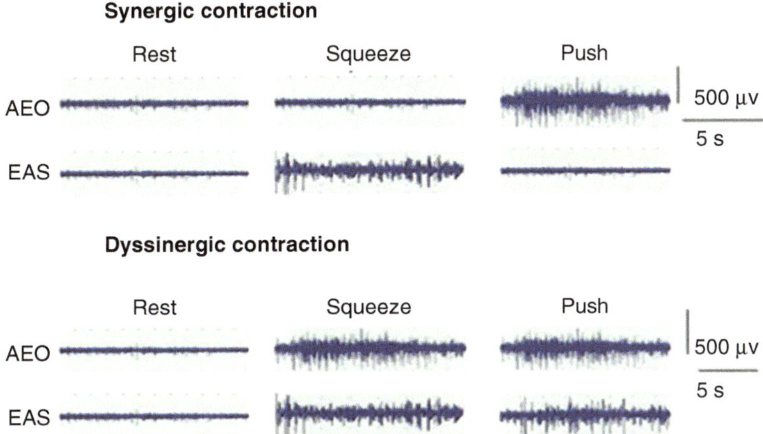

Fig. 6.2 Typical EMG activity at rest and during the phases of voluntary contraction of abdominal external oblique muscle (AEO) and external anal sphincter muscle

quadrant, the needle is inserted at a greater depth in order to study also the activity of the puborectalis muscle. The activity of PUM, both at rest and during voluntary activity, is measured, thus allowing a qualitative and quantitative assessment of innervation of muscle fibers to highlight acute or chronic denervation or total or partial reinnervation. To obtain a maximal voluntary contraction, the examiner asks the patient to imagine holding the urine or feces in the act of urination or defecation. In the normal subject during straining, an interferential pattern with increased number of PUM with the amplitude of 500 μv is detectable until individual potentials are not more evident [15]. Although the amplitude of potential is unquestionably useful into the identification of enlarged MUs, typical of chronic reinnervation processes, the duration is generally more reliable depending much less from the electrode placement. Abnormal EMG activity, such as fibrillation potentials and high-frequency spontaneous discharges, provides evidence of denervation occurring in patients with fecal incontinence, for example, after a pudendal nerve injury or cauda equine syndrome [27]. In patients with anal incontinence, typical frameworks of denervation are characterized by a reduced enrichment of the track base and isolated potentials of denervation (Fig. 6.3).

The single-fiber EMG is a completion of the previous survey, consisting in recording the action potential of a single fiber using a special electrode with a thin diameter (approximately 250 μm). Repeated measurements in the same muscle allow to record the density of the muscle fibers innervated by a single axon; an increased density is indicative of reinnervation, common in the anal incontinence.

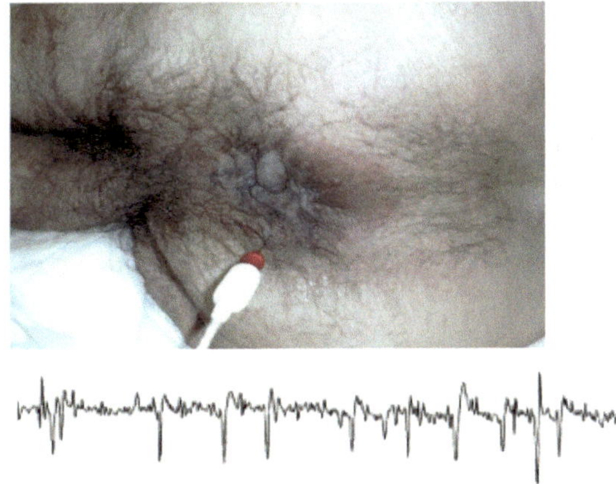

Fig. 6.3 Example of CNEMG in patient with fecal incontinence due to muscle denervation

Therefore, the EMG provides important information regarding the pathogenesis (peripheral, central, or mixed damage) in the case of fecal incontinence [11, 12]. The typical findings in suffering peripheral nervous system are denervation activity (fibrillations, positive slow waves), increase in amplitude and/or duration of PUM, reduction of interferential activity, and enhancement of the percentage of polyphasic potentials in relation to collateral reinnervation phenomena.

6.3 Sacral Reflexes (Bulbocavernosus Reflex, Pudendal-Anal Reflex)

The sacral reflex (SR) is reflex contractions of the striated pelvic floor muscles in response to stimulations of the perineum or the genital region. They provide topographic and pathological information on the sacral somatic pathway controlled by corticospinal system. The recording of stimulus-related responses allows a quantitative analysis of parameters as latency and amplitude.

Clinically, the bulbocavernosus reflex (BCR) is elicited by squeezing the glans or clitoris quickly with fingers, producing a visible and palpable reflex contraction of BC muscle. The presence of this reflex allows to differentiate lesions located above S2–S4 levels, those that interrupt the reflex arc in afferent or efferent (pudendal nerve) branch or in the effector (muscle BC). The neurophysiology allows to obtain a correlated electrophysiological reflex permitting to assess the entire sacral reflex arc, included spinal center located in the Onuf's nucleus (S2–S4) and corticospinal via [7, 28] (Fig. 6.4). This reflex is elicited by electrical stimulation of the clitoris or penis dorsal branches (terminal branches of the sensitive pudendal nerve), and it is recorded using needle electrode in BC muscle. The pudendal-anal reflex (PRA) is elicited with the same technique recording with a needle electrode in EAS muscle [7, 28]. The electrical stimulus consists of a long duration electric square pulse, with an intensity equal to three times the sensory threshold; the electric impulse is given through ring electrodes located at the basis of the penis or clitoris or using an electrical stimulator with electrodes mounted on a plastic assembly positioned on the glans or on the clitoris. The response is recorded with surface electrodes placed on the skin overlying the BC or EAS muscle or with a needle inserted into the same muscle bellies.

The responses to the stimulation of the pudendal nerve are bilateral, and they consist of potentials splitted into two components: an early component with latency between 30 and 40 ms and a delayed response, with variable latency values [18, 28, 33]. The presence of an early and a late component justifies the existence of oligo-polysynaptic circuits [13, 18]. A dysfunction of the pudendal-sacral reflex arc is evident with increased latencies or, in more severe

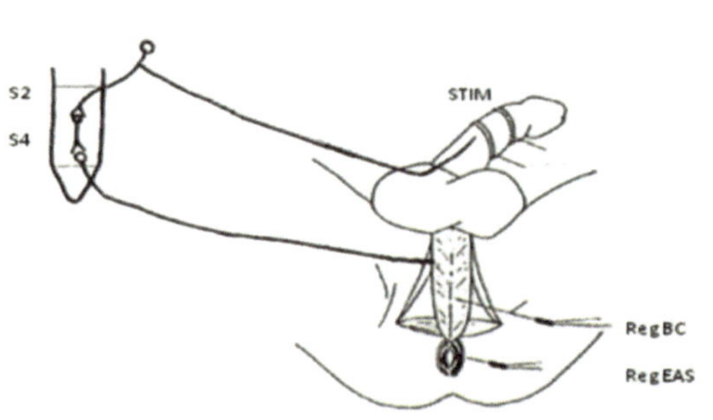

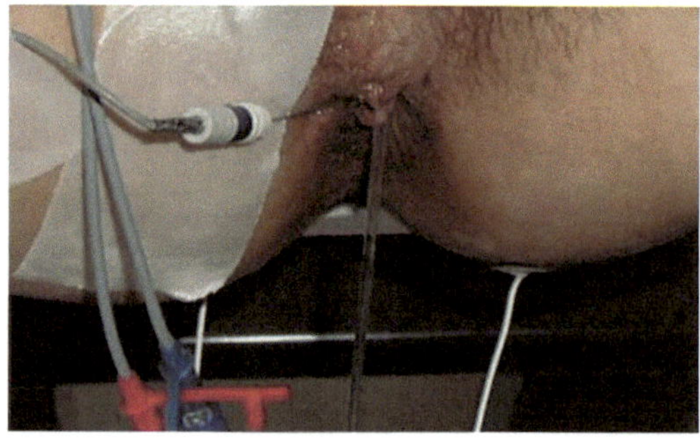

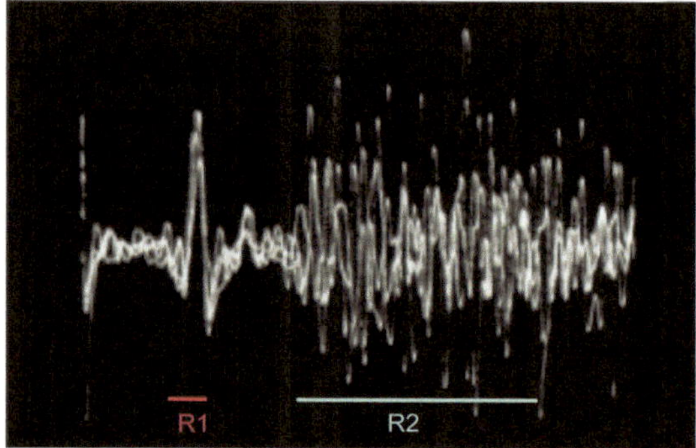

Fig. 6.4 Bulbocavernosus reflex (BCR)

cases, with the complete absence of response. Any deterioration in the latency does not explain clearly the site of the damage that is understandable only with the completion of the entire battery of tests.

6.4 Pudendal Nerve Terminal Motor Latency (PNTML)

The PNTML measures the neuromuscular integrity between the terminal portion of the pudendal nerve and the anal sphincter.

Intrarectal or intravaginal stimulation of the motor branch of pudendal nerve is possible at the ischial spine through the use of the electrode of St. Mark's Hospital, a disposable adhesive plate electrode mounted on the index finger of the glove examiner, recording the needle response by SAE (Fig. 6.5). The normal duration of stimulation is 0.1–0.2 ms, and the maximum amplitude is approximately 15 mv. The latency time is calculated from the stimulus and the onset of contraction, and it is normally about 2 ms.

A lengthening of the PNTML is an expression of suffering of the pudendal nerve on its way. The measurement is to be repeated several times bilaterally to derive the more correct mean value. In some patients with anal incontinence, very long latency is usually detected, while in patients with surgical sequelae or with complete rectal prolapse, a significant difference between the right and the left PNTML can be sometimes evidenced; in other cases any contraction in response to stimuli cannot be detected also after maximal stimuli. The study of PNTML could be significant in the evaluation of anorectal incontinence and chronic pain pelvic syndromes. A literature analysis was conducted to verify the accuracy of PNTML performed according to the St. Mark's technique [16]. Thomas et al. assessed the respective values of PNTML and anal EMG in the diagnosis of fecal incontinence, finding that PNTML has poorer sensitivity and a lack of correlation with manometric parameters compared to EMG examination; authors concluded that PNTML is insufficient alone in the evaluation of patients with suspected neurogenic fecal incontinence and that anal EMG should be performed systematically in all patients [32]. However, its role in constipated patients remains unclear [1, 2, 5, 34].

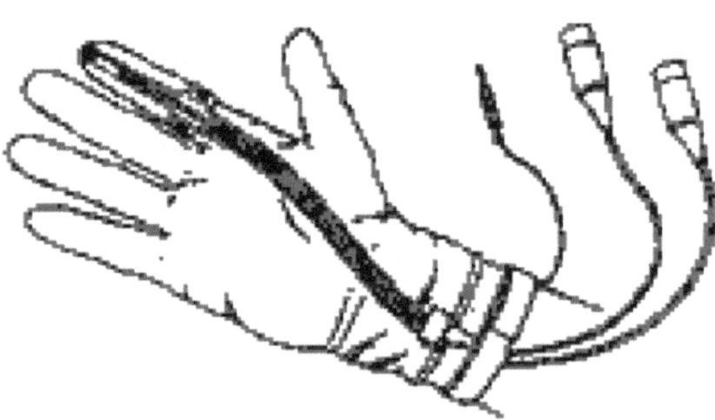

Fig. 6.5 Electrode of the St. Mark's Hospital for the study of the pudendal nerve terminal motor latency (PNTML)

6.5 Pudendal Somatosensory Evoked Potentials (*SSEP*)

The SSEP allows to explore the somatosensory system through the study of the peripheral conduction time from the sensory branch of genital regions. The examination is performed by applying electrical stimuli of low intensity (below the pain threshold) along the branches of the pudendal nerve; the registrant electrode is located on D10–D12 dorsal spinous processes to the sacral cord (N1 latency 17–20 ms) and the referring electrode on the superior anterior iliac spine (or 3–4 cm rostrally) for the spinal potential. Therefore, electrodes are placed on the scalp (Cz), according to the international 10–20 system and the referring electrode in the front median area (Fpz) for the central conduction time (P40 latency 35–40 ms, N50 latency 45–50 ms) [29] (Fig. 6.6). The main component of the cortex response is the P40, considered the expression of the onset of the signal in the parietal cortex. The difference in ms between the spinal and cortical responses constitutes the central conduction time (TCC), an expression of the integrity of the central somatosensory system.

The electrical stimulation of the dorsal clitoral or dorsal penile nerves is made through a low stimulus with an intensity of 2.5 higher than the subjective threshold, a frequency of 3 Hz and a duration of 0.1 ms.

A peripheral or central nervous injury modifies the spinal and/or cortical response leading to a lengthening of conduction time and to a disorganization or abolition of the potential of action.

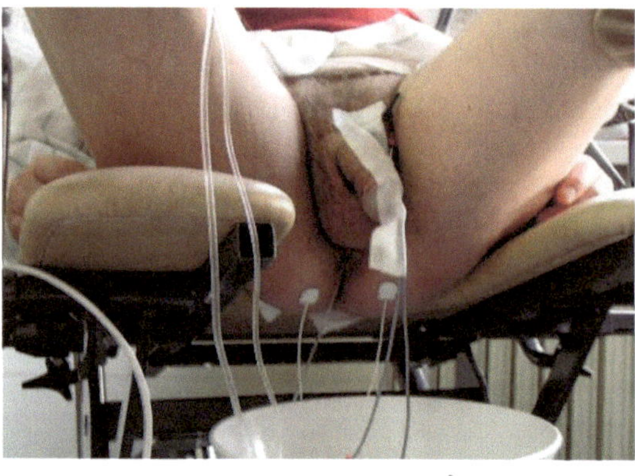

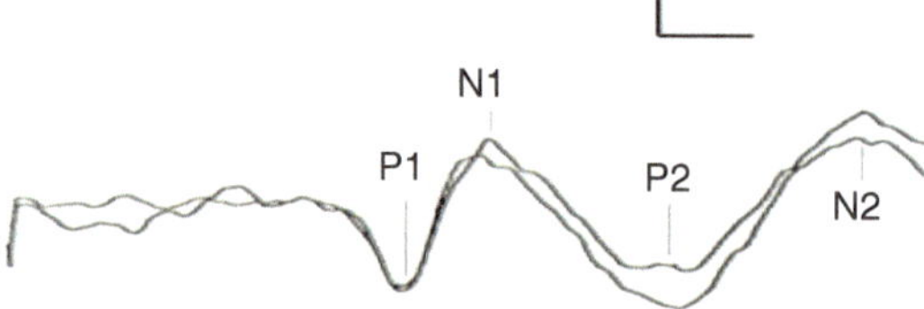

Fig. 6.6 The Pudendal Somatosensory Evoked Potentials (SSEP)

6.6 Motor Evoked Potentials (MEPs) of the Perineal Muscles

The integrity of the spinal anorectal pathway can be assessed through the study of MEPs [17, 25]. The motor cortical representation of urogenital system and pelvic floor corresponds to the primary motor along the mesial surface of the cerebral hemispheres; the corticospinal tract originating from this area runs through the spinal cord and reaches Onuf's nucleus and the motor neurons of pudendal nerve. The MEPs are obtained with transcranial magnetic stimulation (TMS) of motor cortical areas of the pelvic floor. The deeper location along the interhemispheric area of the motor cortex for the target muscles (BC, pelvic floor sphincters) means that the intensity of transcranial stimulation needed results to be higher than the limb muscles. The MEPs are measured centrally by a circular coil placed in Cz and peripherally at the emergence of the sacral roots (Fig. 6.7). When a current is rap-

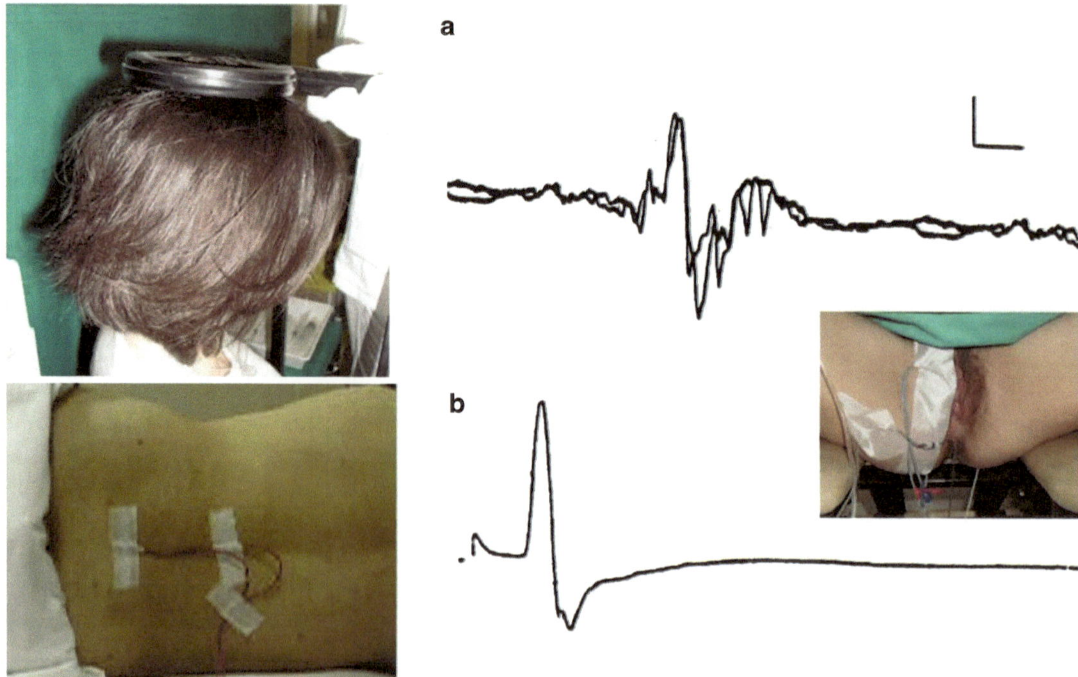

Fig. 6.7 Study of motor evoked potentials (MEPs) of the perineal muscles. (**a**) Transcranial magnetic stimulation; (**b**) root stimulation

idly discharged through a conducting coil, a magnetic flux is produced around the coil, causing stimulation of neural tissue. It can be derived with needle electrodes of the musculature of the pelvic floor permitting the evaluation of the total motor conduction time (TMCT), usually of 30 ms. The considered parameters are usually the latency and the amplitude of motor response. When the stimulation is applied at lumbosacral level, the peripheral motor conduction time (PMCT) can be determined. Therefore, the subtraction of PMCT to TMCT permits to know the central motor conduction time (CMCT). The electrical response is derived by needle electrode from EAS according to the international 10–20 system. The lengthening of latency and amplitude of motor cortical response indicate the site of the damage. Electrical or magnetic stimulation of the lumbosacral nerve roots facilitates diagnosis of sacral motor radiculopathy as a possible cause of fecal incontinence [17]. Normative data are available [25].

Conclusions

In conclusion, the usefulness of pelvic floor neurophysiological tests is widely recognized and supported by evidence. Lower intestinal symptoms such as constipation and fecal incontinence are not uncommon in patients with neurological diseases and they can have a intensely negative impact on quality of life. Understanding their causes can help the planning of effective management strategies. Specifically, the EMG study of the pelvic muscles in combination with measurement of sacral reflex, allows to test the somatic motor innervation in the sacral spinal cord and peripheral components; the pudendal SEP documents the integrity of the afferent pathways from the genital areas to the somatosensory cortex; the application of MEP allows to extend the neurophysiological investigation also to the central motor pathways. Other tests that are not currently supported by high-level evidence could be used in further research settings to corroborate their diagnostic value.

The electrophysiological techniques are becoming essential for a correct diagnosis in the study of fecal incontinence and should come within the store of knowledge not only of specialists in neurology and neurophysiopathology.

References

1. Amarenco G, Kerdraon J. Electromyography and constipation. Pelvi-Perineolog. 2010;5(3):171–7.
2. Azpiroz F, Enck P, Whitehead WE. Anorectal functional testing: review of collective experience. Am J Gastroenterol. 2002;97(2):232–40.
3. Colosimo C, Inghilleri M, Chaudhuri KR. Parkinson's disease misdiagnosed as multiple system atrophy by sphincter electro-myography. J Neurol. 2000; 247(7):559–61.
4. Corazziari E, Badiali D, Inghilleri M. Neurologic disorders affecting the anorectum. Gastroenterol Clin North Am. 2001;30(1):253–68.
5. Diamant NE, Kamm MA, Wald A, Whitehead WE. AGA technical review on anorectal testing techniques. Gastroenterology. 1999;116(3):735–60.
6. Enck P, Hinninghofen H, Merletti R, Azpiroz F. The external anal sphincter and the role of surface electromyography. Neurogastroenterol Motil. 2005;17 Suppl 1:60–7.
7. Ertekin C, Reel F. Bulbocavernosus reflex in normal man and in patients with neurogenic bladder and/or impotence. J Neurol Sci. 1976;28:1.
8. Floyd WF, Wales EW. Electromyography of the sphincter ani externus in man. J Physiol (Lond). 1953;122:599.
9. Giannotti P, Aragona F, Rossi B, Sartucci F. Un caso di incontinenza urinaria da non inibito rilasciamento dello sfintere striato dell'uretra. Rilievi cistometrici ed elettromiografici. Urologia. 1981; XLVIII(IV):1.
10. Gregory WT, Lou J-S, Simmons K, Clark AL. Quantitative anal sphincter electromyography in primiparous women with anal incontinence. Am J Obstet Gynecol. 2008;198(5):550.e1–6.
11. Habib FI, Inghilleri M, Badiali D, Corazziari E. Chronic neurogenic lesions of the external anal sphincter and abdomino-perineal dyssynergia in chronic constipation. Ital J Gastroenterol Hepatol. 1999;31(7):574–9.
12. Infantino A, Melega E, Negrin P, Masin A, Carnio S, Lise M. Striated anal sphincter electromyography in idiopathic fecal incontinence. Dis Colon Rectum. 1995;38(1):27–31.
13. Inghilleri M, Argenta M. Valutazione neurofisiologica del pavimento pelvico nelle lesioni acute del midollo spinale. Neurogastroenterologia. 1997;2(4):133–6.
14. Inghilleri M, Carbone A, Pedace F, Conte A, Frasca V, Berardelli A, Cruccu G, Manfredi M. Bladder filling inhibits somatic spinal motoneurones. Clin Neurophysiol. 2001;112(12):2255–60.

15. Jesel M, Isch-Treussard C, Isch F. Electromyography of striated muscle of anal and urethral sphincters. In: Desmedt JE, editor. New development in electromyography and clinical neurophysiology, vol. 2. Basel: Karger; 1973. p. 406.
16. Kiff ES, Swash M. Slowed conduction in the pudendal nerves in idiopathic (neurogenic) faecal incontinence. Br J Surg. 1984;71(8):614–6.
17. Kimura J. Electrodiagnosis in diseases of the nerve and muscle: principles and practice. 3rd ed. Philadelphia: Davis; 1989.
18. Krane RJ, Siroky MB. Studies on sacral-evoked potentials. J Urol. 1980;124(6):872–6.
19. Lefaucheur JP. Neurophysiological testing in anorectal disorders. Muscle Nerve. 2006;33(3):324–33.
20. Masuda T, Sadoyama T. Skeletal muscles from which the propagation of motor unit action potentials is detectable with a surface electrode array. Electroenceph Clin Neurophysiol. 1987;67:421–7.
21. Merletti R, Rainoldi A, Farina D. Surface EMG for noninvasive muscle characterization. Exerc Sport Sci Rev. 2001;29:20–5.
22. Merletti R, Enck P, Gazzoni M, Hinninghofen H. Surface EMG recording of single motor unit action potentials from the external anal sphincter. Proceedings of the XIV ISEK congress, Vienna; 2002. p. 23–4.
23. Roeleveld K, Stegeman D, Vingerhoets H, Van Oosterom A. Motor unit potential contribution to surface electromyography. Acta Physiol Scand. 1997; 160:1510–7.
24. Olsen AL, Rao SS. Clinical neurophysiology and electrodiagnostic testing of the pelvic floor. Gastroenterol Clin North Am. 2001;30(1):33–54.
25. Opsomer RJ, Caramia MD, Zarola F, Pesce F, Rossini PM. Neurophysiological evaluation of central-peripheral sensory and motor pudendal fibres. Electroenceph Clin Neurophysiol. 1989;74:260.
26. Rao SS. Advances in diagnostic assessment of fecal incontinence and dyssynergic defecation. Clin Gastroenterol Hepatol. 2010;8(11):910–9.
27. Rodi Z, Denislic M, Vodusek DB. External anal sphincter electromyography in the differential diagnosis of parkinsonism. J Neurol Neurosurg Psychiatry. 1996;60(4):460–1.
28. Rushworth G. Diagnostic value of the electromyographic study of reflex activity in man. In: Widen L, editor. Recent advances in clinical neurophysiology. Amsterdam: Elsevier; 1967. p. 65. Suppl 25 to Electroenceph Clin Neurophysiol.
29. Sartucci F, Piaggesi A, Logi F, Bonfiglio L, Bongioanni P, Pellegrinetti A, Baccetti F, Navalesi R, Murri L. Impaired ascendant central pathways conduction in impotent diabetic subjects. Acta Neurol Scand. 1999;99:381–6.
30. Schuster MM. Motor action of rectum and anal sphincters incontinence and defecation. In: Handbook of physiology section 6. Alimentary canal, vol. IV. Washington, DC: American Physiological Soc.; 1968.
31. Stocchi F, Carbone A, Inghilleri M, Monge A, Ruggieri S, Berardelli A, Manfredi M. Urodynamic and neurophysiological evaluation in Parkinson's disease and multiple system atrophy. J Neurol Neurosurg Psychiatry. 1997;62(5):507–11.
32. Thomas C, Lefaucheur JP, Galula G, de Parades V, Bourguignon J, Atienza P. Respective value of pudendal nerve terminal motor latency and anal sphincter electromyography in neurogenic fecal incontinence. Neurophysiol Clin. 2002;32(1):85–90.
33. Trontelj MA, Trontelj JV. Reflex arc of the first component of the human blink reflex: a single motoneuron study. J Neurol Neurosurg Psichiatr. 1978;41:538.
34. Vaccaro CA, Cheong DM, Wexner SD, Nogueras JJ, Salanga VD, Hanson MR, Phillips RC. Pudendal neuropathy in evacuatory disorders. Dis Colon Rectum. 1995;38(2):166–71.

7 Pelvic Floor Rehabilitation

Lucia d'Alba and Margherita Rivera

7.1 Introduction

In the 1950s, the observations of the American surgeon Arnold Kegel led to the recognition of the concept of pelvic floor rehabilitation and to the subsequent use of the muscular portion of the pelvic floor in the treatment of urinary incontinence and genital prolapse. In fact these specific muscular exercises became known as *Kegel exercises*. In the 1970s, this concept of a therapeutic approach to treat the dysfunctions of the pelvic floor was revived and proposed in Europe, above all by French professionals. Today the most distinguished medical organizations recognize the validity of pelvic floor rehabilitation and consider it a first-line therapeutic approach for the treatment of certain pathological conditions: fecal and urinary incontinence, pelvic organ prolapse, syndrome of chronic pelvic pain, sexual dysfunctions, alterations in the sensory control, and evacuation process of defecation.

L. d'Alba, MD (✉)
Gastroenterology Unit, San Giovanni Addolorata Hospital, Rome, Italy
e-mail: luciadalba@tiscali.it

M. Rivera, MD, PhD
Gastroenterology Unit, University of Rome, Sapienza, Italy

The primary goal of all forms of pelvic floor rehabilitation (RT) is to improve pelvic floor and anal sphincter muscle strength, tone, endurance, and coordination to effect a positive change in function with a decrease in symptoms. Additional goals include increasing the patient's awareness of their own muscles, improving rectal sensitivity, and reducing scar burden to allow for improved muscle function. Pelvic floor rehabilitation is performed under the guidance of a pelvic floor physical therapist, although nurses, physicians, and other staff can receive training to perform many of these interventions.

Pelvic floor rehabilitation has been used successfully in the treatment of fecal incontinence (FI) and can produce significant functional and quality of life benefits for patients. Most of the reported literature in this area has been in the form of case reports and nonrandomized prospective trials. In fact, more than 70 such uncontrolled studies have been published with a great range of treatment protocols. Almost all these studies show a significant benefit when using a rehabilitative approach, with the majority reporting a positive response range of 50–80 %. There has only been one published nonrandomized study which reported no benefit to treatment. The patients in that study uniformly had FI due to a neurogenic etiology, which might contribute to the lack of demonstrated benefit from pelvic rehabilitation [1].

M. Mongardini, M. Giofrè (eds.), *Management of Fecal Incontinence*,
DOI 10.1007/978-3-319-32226-1_7

7.2 Conservative Approaches

Conservative approaches are usually first-line therapy, particularly in patients with mild symptoms, and include dietary modifications, medication, muscle-strengthening exercises (*Kegel exercises*), biofeedback, and nonsurgical electrical nerve stimulation. Dietary modification, such as avoiding caffeine, citrus fruits, spicy foods, alcohol, and dairy products (in patients with lactose intolerance) may help, but definitive evidence for these restrictions is lacking. Smoking and sedentary lifestyle are associated with FI [2].

Behavior modification can also be explored with patients, including training on the establishment of a predictable pattern of bowel evacuation, timing of defecation relative to activities to limit incontinent episodes, techniques to reduce straining, proper defecation posture when sitting on the toilet, and fecal urge suppression techniques. Weight reduction is typically encouraged, as obesity is a well-documented risk factor for the development of FI [1].

Opinions differ as to whether the addition of dietary fiber is beneficial or detrimental in the treatment of FI; however, methylcellulose is resistant to fermentation by colonic microflora and may be less likely than some other forms of fiber to exacerbate diarrhea. Several medications are also available to treat FI. Antidiarrheal or antimotility agents, including loperamide or diphenoxylate, may be beneficial in patients with loose stools and urgency. Limited evidence suggests that drugs administered to enhance sphincter tone, such as phenylepinephrine and sodium valproate, may be helpful in patients with passive FI and normal anal sphincter function. In a clinical trial, the tricyclic antidepressant amitriptyline improved FI scores (scale, 1–18) from a median of 16 at baseline to 3 ($P<0.001$) after 4 weeks of treatment. In an open-label uncontrolled study, clonidine, an alpha 2 adrenergic agonist, improved FI after 4 weeks of therapy; however, a randomized, placebo-controlled study showed that clonidine did not significantly improve the number of episodes of FI or quality of life [3].

Pelvic floor rehabilitation is a term which comprises many different therapeutic approaches, including, but not limited to, pelvic floor muscle training (PFMT) and biofeedback-guided electromyography (EMG), which is currently the most widely used rehabilitative treatment modality. The different rehabilitative techniques can be used independently but more frequently are used in conjunction with one another in a multimodal approach to produce the maximum benefit for the patient. Pelvic floor rehabilitation techniques include pelvic floor muscle training PFMT, biofeedback therapy, and the use of electrical stimulation [1].

7.2.1 Pelvic Floor Muscle Training (PFMT)

Kinesitherapy is a rehabilitative method that alleviates symptoms and obtains the greatest possible recovery of lost or altered function, by utilizing therapeutic exercise and movement of the body or part of it to treat disease [4]. Pelviperineal kinesitherapy or PFMT occupies a very important position in rehabilitation in the fields of urogynecology and proctology.

PFMT describes any number of different approaches for increasing strength, endurance, and coordination of the pelvic floor and anal sphincters. Thoracoabdominal pelvic muscle training has also been advocated, as it has been theorized that training all core muscles to work in tandem would be more effective than a narrow focus on the pelvic floor muscles alone. Particular attention is often paid to the transversus abdominis in such expanded approaches. PFMT typically consists of verbally guided instruction in pelvic floor and sphincter contractions (*Kegel contractions*).

Anal sphincter exercises are performed to strengthen the puborectalis muscle, which is continuous with the external anal sphincter (EAS) [3]. Patients can be taught to contract in a variety of ways. Some examples include maximal voluntary sustained sphincter contractions, submaximal sustained contractions, and fast-twitch or "quick-flick" contractions. A commonly reported PFMT technique is to compare the pelvic floor to an elevator, able to stop at different floors as it ascends and descends. Other reported methods include working on coordination of anal sphincter activity and working to isolate a contraction of the anal sphincter. Some practitioners use their hand placed externally, or a digit placed vaginally or rectally to help instruct the patient in the correct exercise techniques, but most would argue that this constitutes a form of low-tech biofeedback training.

The techniques are intended to achieve an improvement of the use of the levator ani muscle that carries out a double function: one as a sphincter and the other as an elevator. The aim of the rehabilitator is to facilitate the education, or the reeducation, of the automatisms of the perineal sphincter, according to the principles of motor development, with which we mean the "system by which humans acquire, modify and conserve movement patterns in their memory, so that they may utilize them whenever they desire to, or whenever it is necessary to do so" [5].

Fundamental to this is the use of feedback: function prevalently correlated to the control of posture and movement; regulated in particular by the cerebellum, the basal nuclei, and the frontal lobe; and finalized to refine specific motor programs [4]. The role of central nervous system (CNS) feedback is to detect errors; this enables consequent modification or interruption of altered motor parameters or patterns. This autocorrection initially leads the patient to achieve a refinement of motor skills and, later, after an adequate training period, to adapt to the new environmental body conditions and acquire the automatization of a new motor skill.

With reference to the general principals of rehabilitation, we consider two types of feedback:

- An intrinsic one that represents all the information that comes from a single patient
- An extrinsic one that registers stimuli and solicitations supplied by an external agent, the rehabilitator

Therefore, the feedback allows the automatization of the motor skills and functions; the rehabilitator specifically guides the patient during the therapy to experience error, thus making him capable of recognizing and then correcting it and in this way determining an actual effective training process.

The reacquisition phases, known as motor training of the competence of the pelvic floor after pelvic dysfunction or disease, are the following:

1. *Acquisition*. This is the phase in which the individual begins to acquire or reacquire a particular movement, through a process of awareness of the different motor skills of the pelvic floor (contraction, relaxation, resting state, action of force of gravity).
2. *Improvement. Improvement* of a given performance and therefore of the altered muscular parameters of the pelvic floor includes hypoactivity, hyperactivity, and impaired coordination of functional activities. The aim here is to improve the quality and efficiency of the performance, reduce the frequency and degree of errors, and increase the safety of the movement. It is necessary for the patient to receive much feedback training, enabling him to adequately elaborate that which he has learned.
3. *Automatization*. The patient transfers what he has learned during the therapy sessions to the actual symptom when it presents itself during various daily life situations.

From this we deduce that it would be simplistic to think that pelviperineal kinesitherapy specifically only serves to reinforce muscle strength. The concept of strength is not solely dependent on the muscular component but is actually the result of three coordinated factors: mechanical, muscular, and neural. The proposed exercises in rehabilitative treatment should take into account types of posture and the use of functional gestures employed in daily life activities.

The electrical activity at the perineal level is influenced by induction, through recall against resistance of various muscle groups, with individual variability. In particular, these groups are comprised of adductors and pelvic trochanter muscles, including both their abductor and external rotator components. Taking these fundamentals into account, it appears correct in the final phases of the therapeutic procedure to introduce combination exercises for the perineal floor and the agonist muscles, with the aim of strengthening a type of synergy that in the early phases is however inhibited in order to encourage an adequate awakening of the sensations of the perineal floor.

The general principles of muscular exercises take into account the following:

1. *Strength*: maximum voluntary contraction defined as the recruitment of the greatest possible number of muscle fibers.
2. *Power*: relationship between maximum strength and the time necessary to obtain it.
3. *Endurance*: the period of time that the contraction is maintained or repeated.
4. *Repetition*: the number of times a contraction is repeated with equal strength.
5. *Fatigue*: exhaustion of the sustainment of the strength required or expected. This is a necessary component for an increase in endurance of muscular exercise [6].

When the muscular deficit is hypoactive, it is then necessary to:

(a) Increase the strength with the use of the maximum voluntary action repeated a few times with the addition of resistance [7]
(b) Increase the endurance and obtain a submaximal contraction [8]
(c) Improve the strength and endurance, with the pause time between contractions lasting double the actual contraction time [9]
(d) Use a maximum voluntary contraction, maintained for a period of 3–10 s, with 8–12 repetitions, performed three times a day; these repetitions are advised to be performed for 5 months. With the aim of obtaining a result [10], it is advised to employ a maximum voluntary contraction for a period of 3–10 s, repeated as many times possible with a rest period of approximately 4 s; this rest period can be reduced when the patient is able to maintain a contraction for 10 s.

Perineal kinesitherapy is organized into progressive sequential phases: a preliminary phase and four specific treatments.

1. *Preliminary phase*. It is indispensible that the patient and rehabilitator establish a trusting collaborative rapport and that the objectives and steps of the treatment are clearly outlined. The issue of discomfort must be considered and discussed with the patient to help in setting up reasonable goals. The rehabilitator needs to attentively and thoroughly illustrate the ano-pelvic anatomy and physiology, with the aid of anatomic models and mirrors, and provide explanations and examples of the correct anal response. The muscular exercises should be explained and verified with positive verbal reinforcement; the rehabilitative treatment plan must be set up and carefully followed.

   The patient must be well informed regarding the preferred strategies chosen to aid in acquiring a satisfactory autonomy while explaining the importance of bowel training and the sharpening of the sensitivity of the evacuation stimulus and the coordination of the action of the muscles of the pelvic floor and abdomen, even during sporadic conditions like the emission of a cough. It is also necessary to evaluate the patient in static equilibrium to correct any eventual postural alterations of the vertebral column and pelvis; these, in fact, constitute an important risk factor to the degree of continence, as relating to the altered distribution of intra-abdominal strength and the involvement of the perineal musculature.
2. *Specific treatment.*

   Gaining awareness of the perineal region, The perineal area has a scant primary motor and sensory representation in the brain cortex, with a consequential reduction in the flow of information between the CNS and the peripheral organs. This results in difficulty in learning automatisms that even more frequently, with the aging process, are lost altogether. The first approach, therefore, is proprioceptive, and all the neuromotor reeducation techniques are applied in order to activate the CNS and to provoke, through reflex, an adequate voluntary muscle activity. The techniques used are the placing under tension of the levator ani muscle and the stretch reflex.

   Elimination of agonist and antagonist synergies. Breathing must be deep and regular. The synergic musculature must not be contracted: the abdominal and pelvic muscles are antagonists.

Training of the levator ani muscle. Isotonic and isometric training exercises. The isometric exercises are used to improve the quality of endurance of the levator ani and/or of the external anal sphincter, while the isotonic exercises increase their strength.

Automatization of the activity of the perineal musculature in conjunction with daily stress. The exercises in this phase require the proper degree of cortical integration to permit rapid association-dissociation activity of different muscle groups. The patient must acquire at least a correct automatism of the perineal contraction in orthostatism and the regaining and reinforcing of the anal closing reflex under pressure.

Kinesitherapy also provides exercises that are to be performed by the patient at home. These exercises are an integral part of the pelvic rehabilitation program and their aim can be outlined in two points:

1. Improvement of the work done with the rehabilitator
2. Maintenance of the acquired results after the termination of the treatment sessions

Only one clinical trial, by Norton et al. in 2003, compared pelvic rehabilitation to a bowel education and retraining program. This study demonstrated comparable benefit in all treatment groups, and the authors concluded that no added benefit was seen with pelvic rehabilitation compared with education alone. However, the education treatment group received instruction in a "bowel urge resistance program" which included training to hold stool in the rectal vault while sitting on the toilet for increasing amounts of time. It is not clear whether such urge suppression techniques are substantially different from pelvic floor muscle strength training with sustained submaximal contractions, and therefore this study's reported conclusions that there is no benefit from PFMT, apart from educational instruction, may not be valid. PFMT without the concurrent use of biofeedback has been well established for use in patients with urinary incontinence. However, there have not been many trials that have looked at PFMT apart from biofeedback training in the treatment of FI. Three studies have shown digitally taught PFMT to be equivalent to PMFT combined with biofeedback. Only one RCT has been done to evaluate the difference between varied types of pelvic floor exercises. Bartlett et al. in 2011 found no difference in outcomes between two separate PFMT techniques, both trained with biofeedback guidance (sustained submaximal anal and pelvic floor exercises versus rapid squeeze plus sustained submaximal exercises). Both groups had significant improvement in FI [1].

7.2.2 Biofeedback Therapy

Biofeedback therapy (BFB) is a term that can be used to describe many different types of training regimens for the pelvic floor. Biofeedback is defined as the process of gaining greater awareness of many physiological functions, primarily using instruments that provide information on the activity of those same systems, with a goal of being able to manipulate them at will. BFB has been used in medicine for more than 30 years and has been used for the treatment of FI since as early as 1974. For pelvic floor rehabilitation purposes, the most common type of biofeedback is EMG biofeedback therapy, which was first introduced in 1979 [1].

Biofeedback is performed using visual, auditory, or verbal feedback techniques with an anorectal manometry or EMG probe inserted into the anorectum to display pressure changes [11].

Data are recorded either through surface electrodes or via the use of intravaginal or intrarectal sensors. Other forms of pelvic floor biofeedback therapy include the use of ultrasound (either intrarectal, intravaginal, or perineal), rectal balloons, digital guidance (the use of an intrarectal/intravaginal finger or hand placed on the perineum), and anorectal manometry [1] (Fig. **7.1**). More recent studies have found a difference between pelvic muscle exercises alone and exercises with biofeedback (the addition of a rectal balloon, electrical stimulation, or EMG), in favor of adding BFB [11].

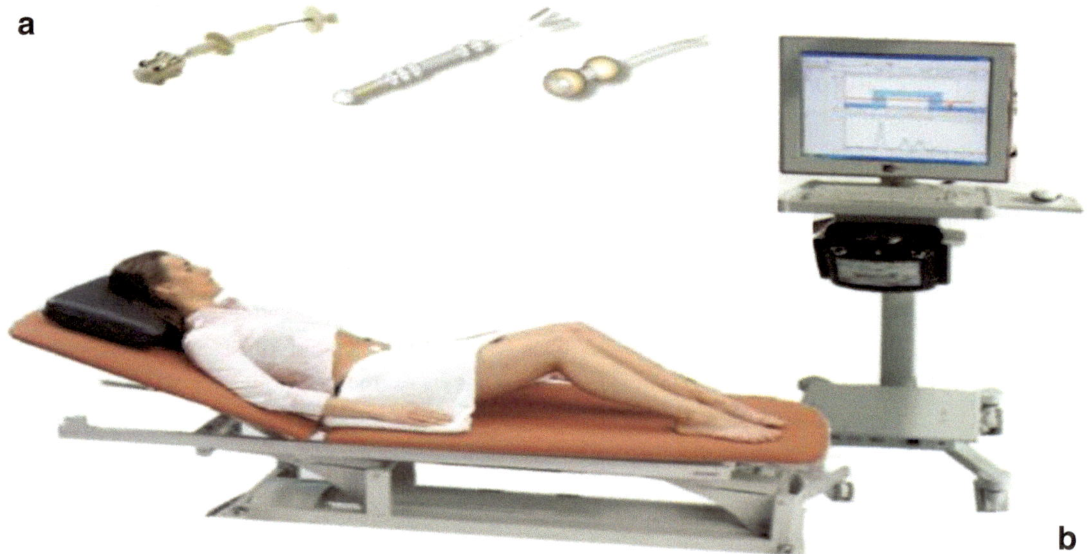

Fig. 7.1 (**a**) Vaginal and anorectal probes. (**b**) Pelvy Tutor System for biofeedback therapy

There are three main methods for the effective use of biofeedback as part of pelvic floor rehabilitation for FI. The most common type is for strength and endurance training for the pelvic floor and/or anal sphincter. The biofeedback apparatus gives information about how strong the muscles are being contracted, and the patient can use that information to learn how to do the pelvic floor exercises more effectively. It is also thought that biofeedback motivates the patient to improve by giving information on performance and progress. The theory behind strength and endurance training is that if the sphincter muscles are stronger, the patient will be able to hold in the stool for a longer period of time and enable them to make it to the restroom with fewer accidents. The second treatment modality is to use biofeedback therapy to improve rectal sensitivity or compliance. This type of treatment has also been termed volumetric rehabilitation or discrimination training and is typically done with rectal balloons. The balloon is inflated with air or water to determine the first sensation of rectal filling. It is then gradually inflated with decreasing amounts of air or water to teach the patient to appreciate stool in the rectal vault at progressively lower volumes. The rationale behind sensory retraining is to allow the patient to detect smaller volumes of stool at an earlier moment, again making it possible for them to reach the restroom before an accident occurs. It also allows for the patient to have more time to perform a voluntary anal sphincter contraction before the volume of stool in the rectal vault overwhelms the patient's ability to hold it.

Rectal balloons can also be used on patients with fecal urgency and rectal hypersensitivity. The balloons are in these cases simply inflated to progressively larger volumes, which the patient is then coached on how to tolerate without feeling the need to expel the rectal contents.

The third biofeedback therapy approach deals with coordination training for the anal sphincter. Multiple balloons are again inserted, a large one in the rectum itself and one or two smaller ones in the anal canal. These are typically connected to a manometric pressure-recording device. When the larger balloon is inflated, the rectal–anal inhibitory reflex is triggered, and the patient is taught to appreciate the momentary internal anal sphincter relaxation that results. The patient can then be taught to do a voluntary external sphincter contraction to counteract the involuntary relaxation of the internal sphincter.

This type of coordination training is not as commonly studied today as it was in the past. More recent studies have referred to "coordination training" instead as a combination between motor skills training and sensory discrimination training [1].

7.2.3 Electrical Stimulation

Electrical stimulation is another modality that has been proposed for the rehabilitative treatment of FI. The goal of electrical stimulation is to enhance the strength and/or endurance of striated muscle contraction with the target being typically the external anal sphincter in the case of patients with FI. Another goal can be to allow patients with decreased kinesthetic awareness to become more cognizant of where their pelvic floor muscles are in space and what it feels like when the muscles and sphincter are contracting. Electrical stimulation has been shown to transform fast-twitch muscle fibers to slow-twitch muscle fibers, which is thought to help with improving endurance. It also increases capillary density, allowing more blood flow to the oxidative slow-twitch fibers. Electrical stimulation can be delivered to the pelvic floor and anal sphincter in many different forms, including via surface electrodes or intrarectal probes and with many different stimulation parameters and treatment protocols. Low-frequency stimulation (LFS) has typically been the norm, although a new form of amplitude-modulated medium-frequency (AM-MF) stimulation has recently been proposed. All forms of electrical stimulation are often used in conjunction with PFMT or biofeedback training, although stimulation can be used without any other concurrent rehabilitative treatment. Electrical stimulation can also be used to augment a volitional contraction once the contraction threshold reaches a predefined level, and such a strategy has also been employed in trials [1].

7.2.4 Comparison Among Rehabilitative Procedures

There is no universally accepted therapeutic algorithm and no specific criteria for evaluating the efficacy of RT. The techniques used, such as biofeedback therapy, kinesitherapy, anal-electrostimulation, and volumetric rehabilitation, can vary greatly in rehabilitation programs among centers. For this reason, the results of studies are not comparable.

Eighteen randomized trials sustain the use of biofeedback therapy in FI. Biofeedback therapy is aimed at improving voluntary EAS contraction. Another effect is training of synchrony for anal sphincter responses during rectal distention. Finally, biofeedback therapy may be used to improve rectal sensation and sphincter responsiveness to balloon distention with the use of instruments that simultaneously monitor sphincter contractions. Some authors have combined biofeedback therapy with kinesitherapy for the pelvic and perineal muscles as supported by two randomized controlled trials. Nevertheless, when used alone, one randomized controlled trial shows that biofeedback therapy is superior to pelvic floor exercises. RT could improve rectal sensations. Such RT may be performed through biofeedback therapy ("sensory retraining") or volumetric rehabilitation, using an inflated balloon, or water enemas of decreasing volume. Neither biofeedback therapy nor volumetric rehabilitation is supported by randomized controlled trials.

Anal-electrostimulation can be used to treat FI. The assumption is that anal-electrostimulation can induce muscle contraction by direct stimulation or indirectly via peripheral nerve stimulation. A Cochrane Library review on four randomized trials raised concerns on the utility of anal-electrostimulation in FI because:

(a) In clinical practice anal-electrostimulation would seldom be given in isolation without exercises and other advice
(b) There is no sufficient evidence for assessing the effectiveness of anal-electrostimulation
(c) There is not enough evidence on how to select patients suitable for anal-electrostimulation nor on which modality of electrical stimulation is optimal

Anal sphincter exercises (pelvic floor muscle training) and biofeedback therapy have been used alone and in combination for the treatment of FI.

A single-center randomized controlled study indicated that a regimen of pelvic floor exercises with biofeedback was nearly twice as effective as pelvic floor exercises alone, with 44 % versus 21 % of patients achieving complete continence at 3 months, respectively ($P=0.008$). In addition,

Table 7.1 Controlled Trials on comparison among rehabilitative procedures

	KT+BFB	ES+BFB	KT	ES	ES+KT
Norton C, Cody JD. *Cochrane Database Syst Rev*. 2012;7.	+	/	–	/	/
	+	/	–	/	+
Bartlett L et al. *Dis Colon Rectum*. 2011;54:846–56.	No differences	/	No differences	/	/
Schwandner T et al. *Dis Colon Rectum*. 2010;53:1007–16.	/	+	/	–	/

KT Kinesitherapy, *BFB* biofeedback, *ES* electrical stimulation

symptom relief was reported for 76% of patients using biofeedback and pelvic floor exercises compared with 41% of patients performing pelvic floor exercises alone ($P<0.01$), and patients adjunctively using biofeedback had greater reductions in Fecal Incontinence Severity Index (FISI) scores.

In a more recent randomized study comparing 2 different pelvic floor exercise regimens, both with biofeedback, 59 of the 69 patients (86%) had improved continence with 20% fully continent, with no statistically significant differences between exercise regimens.

A 2012 systematic review of randomized or quasi randomized controlled trials of patients performing anal sphincter exercises and/or receiving biofeedback and/or surface electrical stimulation of the anal sphincter concluded that the addition of biofeedback or electrical stimulation was superior to exercise alone in patients who had previously failed to respond to other conservative treatments. As indicated above, nonsurgical (surface) electrical stimulation, alone or in combination with biofeedback, has also proven useful. One study found the combination of electrical stimulation 20 min twice daily, and biofeedback was superior to electrical stimulation alone: 53.8% of 39 patients receiving the combination were continent at the end of treatment versus none of 41 patients in the electrical stimulation-alone group [3] (Table 7.1).

7.3 Transcutaneous and Percutaneous Posterior Tibial Nerve Stimulation

Transcutaneous and percutaneous posterior tibial nerve stimulations have been tried in patients with FI. In a randomized, double-blind, sham-controlled trial, 144 patients were randomly assigned to receive either active or sham stimulations for 3 months. No statistically significant difference was seen between active and sham transcutaneous electrical nerve stimulation (TENS) in terms of an improvement in the median number of FI/urgency episodes per week. Thirty-four patients (47%) who received the active TENS treatment exhibited a >30% decrease in the FI severity score compared with 19 patients (27%) who received the sham treatment. No differences in delay to postpone defecation, patient self-assessment of treatment efficacy, or anorectal manometry were seen between the two groups [12]. A recent double-blind, randomized controlled trial compared the short-term efficacy of percutaneous tibial nerve stimulation (PTNS) against sham electrical stimulation in adults with fecal incontinence in 227 patients. In this study PTNS given for 12 weeks did not confer significant clinical benefit over sham electrical stimulation in the treatment of adults with fecal incontinence. Further studies are warranted to determine its efficacy in the long term and in patient subgroups (i.e., those with urgency) [13].

7.4 Rehabilitation Versus Other Therapeutic Techniques

There are no suitable trials testing drug treatment versus another conservative treatment including RT. There are no studies on the usefulness of RT before surgery. Only one randomized trial has studied adjuvant biofeedback therapy following sphincter repair: there was no difference between the groups as regards continence scores, but adjuvant biofeedback therapy improved the patient's QoL. This report confirmed data from previous studies showing partial improvement with bio-

Table 7.2 Expert panel recommendations

After drugs, rehabilitation is the treatment of choice in incontinent subjects (2a-B)
Several randomized trials sustain the use of biofeedback therapy in FI (1a-A)
The combination of biofeedback and kinesitherapy can be useful in FI (1b-B)
There is no sufficient evidence to recommend anal-electrostimulation (4-C)
A partial improvement of continence can be achieved with biofeedback after sphincteroplasty (2b-B)
Rehabilitation improves anorectal function after anorectal surgery (3a-B)
RT can identify patient nonresponders for whom more invasive therapies are needed (3b-C)
RT can maintain medium and long-term effects (1b-A)

feedback therapy used after sphincteroplasty. A review on functional disorders after rectal cancer resection examined the effects of rehabilitative treatment on FI taken from 15 papers, including 11 nonrandomized prospective studies. The methodological quality of the studies was evaluated according to the methodological index for nonrandomized studies (MINORS) scale. The review concluded that RT improves postsurgical anorectal function.

Management of Patients Who Do Not Respond to RT It is not clear how nonresponsive patients should be managed. In one study reported, a mini-irrigation system was used in 50 patients with passive FI and/or evacuation difficulty who had not responded to biofeedback therapy. Two-thirds of the patients believed their symptoms were improved and wanted to continue using the system. Rehabilitation can identify those "nonresponders" who should be next in line for more invasive therapeutic procedures [14].

Medium- and Long-Term Effects of RT Lasting improvement has been observed in patients with FI up to 1 year after rehabilitative treatment. In a randomized study comparing biofeedback therapy versus kinesitherapy, 53 % of biofeedback therapy patients reported adequate relief at a 12-month follow-up compared with 35 % of patients in the kinesitherapy group. Improvement in fecal urgency and subjective rating of bowel control was also maintained at 2 years of follow-up in incontinent patients who had undergone biofeedback therapy with different exercise regimens [14] (Table 7.2).

References

1. Scott KM. Pelvic floor rehabilitation in the treatment of fecal incontinence. Clin Colon Rectal Surg. 2014;27:99–105.
2. Townsend MK, Mattews CA, Whithehead WE, Grodstein F. Risk factors for fecal incontinence in older women. Am J Gastroenterol. 2013;108:113–9.
3. Rao SSC. Current and emerging treatment options for fecal incontinence. J Clin Gastroenterol. 2014;48:752–64.
4. Umphred D. Neurological rehabilitation. Mosby Elsevier: St. Louis; 2007.
5. Shumway-Cook A, Woollacott M. Motor control: theory and practical applications. Baltimore: Lippincott, Williams and Wilkins; 1995.
6. Haslam J, Laycock J. Biofeedback. In: Haslam J, Laycock J, editors. Therapeutic management of incontinence and pelvic pain pelvic organ disorders. Springer-Verlag London Limited; 2008.
7. Giruaudo D, Lamberti G. Esercizio terapeutico nel rinforzo muscolare del pavimento pelvico. In: Giraudo-Lamberti, editor. Incontinenza urinaria femminile. Ed. Ermes Bologna, Italy; 2007.
8. Dorey G, Speakman M, Feneley R, et al. Randomised controlled trial of pelvic floor muscle exercises and manometric biofeedback for erectile dysfunction. Br J Gen Pract. 2004;54:819–25.
9. Di Benedetto P. Riabilitazione uro-ginecologica. Ed. Minerva Medica, Torino, Italy; 2004.
10. Bø K, Mørkved S, Frawley H, Sherburn M. Evidence for benefit of transversus abdominis training alone or in combination with pelvic floor muscle training to treat female urinary incontinence: a systematic review. NeurourolUrodyn. 2009;28:368–73.
11. Meyer I, Richter HE. An evidence-based approach to the evaluation, diagnostic assessment and treatment of fecal incontinence in women. Curr Obstet Gynecol Rep. 2014;3:155–64.
12. Leroi AM, Siproudhis L, Etienney I, et al. Transcutaneous electrical tibial nerve stimulation in the treatment of fecal incontinence: a randomized trial (CONSORT 1a). Am J Gastroenterol. 2012;107:1888–96.

13. Knowles CH, Horrocks EJ, Bremner SA et al. CONFIDeNT Study Group. Percutaneous tibial nerve stimulation versus sham electrical stimulation for the treatment of faecal incontinence in adults (CONFIDeNT): a double-blind, multicentre, pragmatic, parallel-group, randomised controlled trial. Lancet. 2015;386(10004):1640–8.
14. Italian Society of Colorectal Surgery (SICCR), Italian Association of Hospital Gastroenterologists (AIGO). Diagnosis and treatment of faecal incontinence: Consensus statement of the Italian Society of Colorectal Surgery and the Italian Association of Hospital Gastroenterologists. Dig Liv Dis. 2015; 47:628–45.

8 Radiofrequency (SECCA® Procedure)

Marco Frascio and Francesca Mandolfino

8.1 Background

The SECCA® procedure, which involves the administration of temperature-controlled radiofrequency energy to the anal canal, was first used for the treatment of fecal incontinence in Mexico in 1999 [1].

This procedure evidenced a therapeutic effect in the treatment of gastroesophageal reflux [2]. In 2002, the Food and Drug Administration of the United States approved the SECCA® system for use specifically in the treatment of fecal incontinence in those patients with solid or liquid incontinence occurring at least once per week and who already had unsuccessfully tried more conservative therapies [3].

After this initial report, a few studies assessed the results of the SECCA® procedure as a treatment for fecal incontinence, and the results of these studies suggested its safety and efficacy.

M. Frascio (✉)
Department of Surgical Sciences (DISC), University of Genoa, IRCCS Azienda Ospedaliera Universitaria San Martino - IST Istituto Nazionale per la Ricerca sul Cancro, Largo R. Benzi 10, Genoa, Italy
e-mail: mfrascio@unige.it

F. Mandolfino
Department of Surgical Sciences (DISC), University of Genoa, Largo R. Benzi 10, Genoa, Italy
e-mail: fcmandolfino@gmail.com

8.2 Procedure

The SECCA® procedure is performed delivering temperature-controlled RF to the anorectal junction to treat fecal incontinence.

The radiofrequency generator uses heat generated by a high-frequency alternating current that flows from four electrodes causing frictional movements of ions and tissue heating (Fig. 8.1).

The patient is placed in the lithotomic position.

After induction of general anesthesia, the SECCA® device is inserted into the anal canal, and submucosal RF energy is circumferentially delivered to the anorectal junction.

Four temperature-controlled needle electrodes are deployed after the device is correctly positioned in the anal canal. Each needle is monitored by the generator, which measures tissue resistance, surface mucosal temperature, and deep submucosal temperature. Tissue impedance should be kept below 250 ohms. The goal with delivery of the RF energy is to generate a submucosal temperature of 85 °C while maintaining mucosal temperature below 42 °C.

To maintain a surface temperature of less than 42 °C, the needles and mucosa are irrigated with cold sterile water at a rate of 42 mL/min. The device has a separate suction port, which allows removal of the irrigant and liquid stool. The energy is delivered for a total of 1 min at each level.

The anus is divided into four quadrants, and the RF energy is delivered at five different levels

M. Mongardini, M. Giofrè (eds.), *Management of Fecal Incontinence*,
DOI 10.1007/978-3-319-32226-1_8

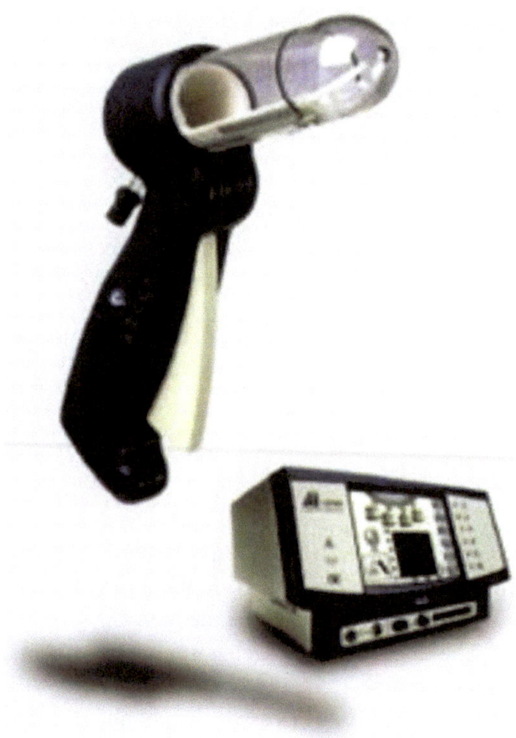

Fig. 8.1 SECCA®®® manipulo and RF generator

in each quadrant. After initial RF delivery 5 mm below the dentate line, the device is advanced proximally into the anus and lower rectum deploying the needles electrodes and delivering energy at 5 mm increments until a total of 5 level of energy have been delivered. The device is rotated 90°, and the next anal quadrant is treated. Extreme care is taken in the anterior quadrant of the anus to prevent penetration of the needles through the rectovaginal septum or perineal body to prevent the possible formation of a rectovaginal fistula. Delivery of the energy to the four quadrant of the anus takes between 25 and 35 min.

Anoscopy was routinely performed upon completion of the procedure to verify hemostasis and absence of thermal injury.

The therapeutic effects of the procedure have been related to the improvement of sphincter function and restored anorectal sensitivity and rectoanal coordination, but the real mechanism of action has only been hypothesized. In particular four actions have been imagined: an improvement in anorectal sensation and coordination through C and A delta afferent fiber neuromodulation, a collagen and a smooth muscle remodeling, and then a modulation of interstitial Cajal cell function.

It had been also been hypothesized that radiofrequency could alter the muscular and connective tissues inducing a fibrosis so determining an improvement in clinical manifestation of incontinence. A double-blind randomized crossover study about radiofrequency utilization at the gastroesophageal junction (GEJ) seemed to exclude fibrosis as the primary mechanism. The study was conducted in a tertiary care center. Patients underwent two upper gastrointestinal endoscopies 3 months apart, during which active or sham Stretta treatment was performed in a randomized double-blind manner. Symptom assessment, endoscopy, manometry, 24-h esophageal pH monitoring, and a distensibility test of the GEJ were done before the start of the study and after 3 months.

A barostat distensibility test of the GEJ before and after administration of sildenafil, a smooth muscle relaxant, was the main outcome measure. Three months after the initial Stretta procedure, no changes were observed in esophageal acid exposure and lower esophageal sphincter (LES) pressure. In contrast, the symptom score was significantly improved, and GEJ compliance was significantly decreased. Administration of sildenafil normalized GEJ compliance again to pre-Stretta level, arguing against GEJ fibrosis as the underlying mechanism. Similar studies regarding Stretta are currently underway [2].

8.3 Costs and Diffusion of SECCA®

Every SECCA® procedure needs a disposable manipulo using device and the RF generator to be performed.

In Italy every SECCA® procedure costs about 2500 euros, but it can depend on the chance to keep the RF generator or to book it for every patient so the cot can vary from 1500 to 3000 euros each.

The technique is diffused especially in the United States, in Europe, and also in the Emirates.

The centers that perform SECCA® routinely are Cleveland Clinic Weston, FL, USA; Previty Clinic for Surgical Care Beaumont, TX, USA;

East Texas Medical Center Jacksonville, TX, USA; Towson, MD, USA, Jagiellonian University School of Medicine Krakow, Poland; and Cleveland Clinic Abu Dhabi, UAE.

8.4 Our Experience

After Institutional Review Board (IRB) approval, 19 patients with FI were recruited into this prospective, single center, observational study.

Patients were eligible for this study if they had experienced fecal incontinence for at least six months and had attempted, but not effectively, one or more of the more common conservative treatments (lifestyle and diet modification, pharmacological therapy, or electrostimulation).

Exclusion criteria were constipation or chronic diarrhea, inflammatory bowel diseases, pregnancy, psychiatric disorder, anal abscess or fistula, prior pelvic irradiation, or prior sphincter repair or artificial bowel sphincter implantation.

Actually 11 patients completed the one-year follow-up.

All patients were female, with an average age of 68 (range 59–77) years and a mean duration of FI of 21.5 (range 12–31) months. Six patients (67 %) had prior vaginal delivery, five of which included an episiotomy. After informed consent, the RF procedure was performed delivering temperature-controlled RF to the anorectal junction.

The mean operative time was 45 (range, 37–53) min.

All patients completed the CCF-FI score and Fecal Incontinence Quality of life (FIQoL) scales at 1, 3, 6, and 12 months after the procedure; similarly all patients underwent anorectal manometry and endoanal ultrasound.

8.4.1 CCF-FI Score Evaluation

The mean CCF-FI score significantly improved at 3 months follow-up from 14 (+3.8) to 12.8 (+3.7). Improvement was maintained at 6 months follow-up ($p<0.05$), although a slight decrease was observed at 12 months to 13 (+3.1) (Fig. 8.2).

8.4.2 Fecal Incontinence Quality of Life Score

The mean FIQoL score was significantly improved in only the embarrassment category (one of four categories) ($p<0.05$) (Table 8.1). A positive trend was noted for the other domains.

8.4.3 Anorectal Manometry

Anorectal manometry showed significant improvement in basal anal pressure (BAP) and in rectal compliance (RC), although not in squeeze anal pressure (SAP) at 6 months follow-up ($p<0.05$). These changes were transient since

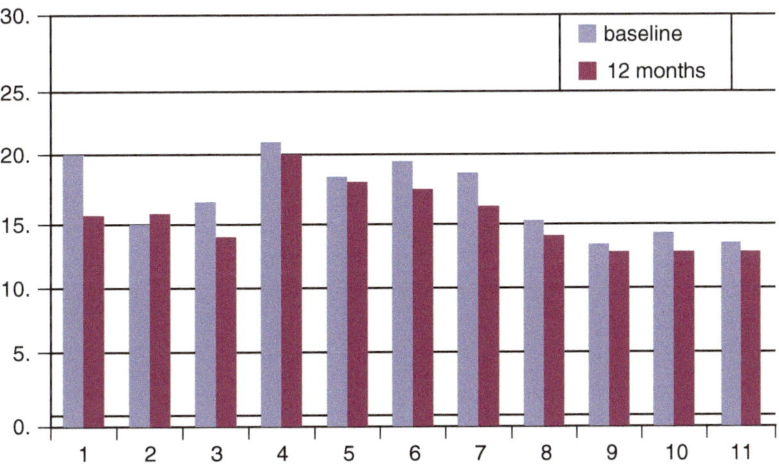

Fig. 8.2 CCF-FI score evaluation

Table 8.1 Fecal Incontinence Quality of Life score

FIQL category	Mean at baseline	Mean at 12 months
Lifestyle	3.14 ± 0.7	2.99 ± 0.8
Coping	2.03 ± 1	1.86 ± 0.86
Depression	2.16 ± 0.78	2.11 ± 0.67
Embarrassment	2.89 ± 0.9	1.78 ± 0.6

Table 8.2 Anorectal manometry results

Manometric parameters	Mean at baseline	Mean at 6 months	Mean at 12 months
BAS (mmHg)	25.63 ± 5.61	31.6 ± 6.2	26.47 ± 7.8
SAP (mmHg)	67.9 ± 11.24	82.4 ± 14.8	69.3 ± 12.4
RC (H_2O cc)	> 200 ± 25	174 ± 18	186 ± 19.1

they were not sustained at 12 months follow-up (Table 8.2).

8.4.4 Endoanal Ultrasound

Preoperative ultrasound did not reveal any sphincter defect prior to the procedure and any significative modification at the 6- and 12-month follow up.

8.4.5 Morbidity

No intraoperative complications were noted; however, at 1 month after surgery one intra-anal submucosal abscess was successfully treated by surgical drainage and intravenous antibiotics with complete resolution.

8.5 Discussion and Conclusion

Fecal incontinence is not a life-threatening disease; however, it can seriously affect quality of life and cause significant disability.

A variety of treatment modalities for FI currently exist, including medical and pharmacologic treatments, biofeedback, and surgical approaches [4–8].

Patients with FI are generally initially managed with noninvasive low-risk treatments, including diet modification, antimotility agents, Kegel exercises, biofeedback, and/or controlled evacuation. However, data obtained in randomized controlled trials are limited [9, 10].

Since the RF procedure was introduced into clinical practice in 2000, several studies have endeavored to determine its efficacy. The authors have recently published a complete review of RF including results in 220 patients from 11 studies [11]. In several clinical studies, RF was clearly shown to effectively treat mild-to-moderate FI. When patient selection is appropriate, this treatment has demonstrated clinically significant improvements in symptoms, as demonstrated by statistically significant reductions in the CCF-FI scores as well as significant improvements in quality of life scores [9, 10, 12–16].

The mechanism of action of non-ablative radiofrequency application to the internal anal sphincter has recently been clarified. Specifically, a pathologist blinded porcine model study has shown that RF induces the structural rearrangement of internal anal sphincter smooth muscle and interstitial cell of Cajal distribution with an increase in internal anal sphincter smooth muscle actin and reactive myofibroblast contents [17].

Our experience, not yet published, seems to confirm good results of improvements in FI at 6 months sustained at 12 months follow-up with a morbidity of only 5 % (1 case).

RFE for fecal incontinence seems to be encouraging.

Ideally, a prospective randomized trial with a larger number of patients would be necessary to explore what improvement does mean and how RFE does relate to quality of life.

Finally, another crucial concept to stress is that radiofrequency option does not preclude further surgery so it can be considered as a bridge to a more invasine surgery in selected and non responsice patients.

References

1. Takahashi T, Garcia-Osogobio S, et al. Radiofrequency energy delivery to the anal canal for the treatment of fecal incontinence. Dis Colon Rectum. 2002;45:915–22.

2. Triadafilopoulos G, DiBaise JK, et al. Radiofrequency energy delivery to the gastroesophageal junction for the treatment of GERD. Gastrointest Endosc. 2001;53:407–15.
3. Takahashi T, Garcia-Osogobio S, et al. Extended Two-year results of radio-frequency energy delivery for the treatment of fecal incontinence (the SECCA® procedure). Dis Colon Rectum. 2003;46:711–5.
4. Takahashi-Monroy T, Morales M, et al. SECCA® procedure for the treatment of fecal incontinence: results of a five-year follow-up. Dis Colon Rectum. 2008;51(3):355–9. Epub 2008 Jan 19.
5. Efron JE, Corman ML, et al. Safety and effectiveness of temperature-controlled radiofrequency energy delivery to the anal canal (SECCA® procedure) for the treatment of fecal incontinence. Dis Colon Rectum. 2003;46(12):1606–16. discussion 1616–8.
6. Efron JE. The SECCA® procedure: a new therapy for treatment of fecal incontinence. Surg Tech Intl. 2004;XIII:107–10.
7. Parisien CJ, Corman ML. The SECCA® procedure for the treatment of fecal incontinence: definitive therapy or short-term solution. Clin Colon Rectal Surg 2005;18(1):42–5.
8. Felt-Bersma RF, Mulder CJ. Temperature controlled radiofrequency energy (SECCA®Æ) to the anal canal for the treatment of fecal incontinence: pilot seems promising. Presented at DDW. 2006.
9. Walega P, Jasko K, Kenig J, Herman RM, Nowak W. Radiofrequency waves in the treatment of faecal incontinence. Preliminary report. Proktologia. 2009;10(2):134–43.
10. Ruiz D, Pinto RA, et al. Does the radiofrequency procedure for fecal incontinence improve quality of life and incontinence at 1-year follow-up? Dis Colon Rectum. 2010;53:1041–6.
11. Frascio M, Mandolfino F, Imperatore M, et al. The SECCA® procedure for faecal incontinence: a review. Colorectal Dis. 2014;16:167–72.
12. Felt-Bersma RJ, Szojda MM, Mulder CJ. Temperature-controlled radiofrequency energy (SECCA®) to the anal canal for the treatment of faecal incontinence offers moderate improvement. Eur J Gastroenterol Hepatol. 2007;19:575–80.
13. Kim DW, Yoon HM, Park JS, et al. Radiofrequency energy delivery to the anal canal: is it a promising new approach to the treatment of fecal incontinence? Am J Surg. 2009;197:14–8.
14. Lefebure B, Tuech J, Bridoux V, et al. Temperature-controlled radio frequency energy delivery (SECCA®® procedure) for the treatment of fecal incontinence: results of a prospective study. Int J Colorectal Dis. 2008;23:993–7.
15. Parisien C, Corman M. The SECCA® procedure for the treatment of fecal incontinence: definitive therapy or short-term solution. Clin Colon Rectal Surg. 2005;18:42–5.
16. McHorney CA, Ware JE, Lu JF, Sherbourne CD. The MOS 36-item health survey (SF-36): tests of data quality, scaling assumptions, and reliability across diverse patient groups. Med Care. 1994;32:40–66.
17. Herman R, Wojtysiak D, Rys J, et al. Interstitial cells of Cajal and smooth muscle actin activity after non-ablative radiofrequency energy application to the internal anal sphincter: an animal study. Poster presented at DDW. 2013.

9 Sacral Nerve Stimulation in Fecal Incontinence

Marileda Indinnimeo, Cosima Maria Moschella, Gloria Bernardi, and Paolo Gozzo

Sacral nerve stimulation (SNS) has been used to treat urinary dysfunction by Tanagho EA and Schmidt RA since 1988. In 1995, Matzel et al. treated patients with functional bowel disorders with SNS, and this therapy was later proved to be also effective for fecal incontinence (FI) secondary to various functional or morphological causes, including large sphincter lesions (up to 180°). SNS delivers mild, non-painful, electrical pulses to the sacral nerves, ultimately improving or restoring function. Validated questionnaires should be administered to FI patients proposed for SNS, in order to assess the severity of FI and its impact on quality of life (QoL). Moreover, anorectal manometry, endoanal ultrasound, pelvic floor electromyography, pudendal nerve assessment, and also MRI should be performed, because every exam analyzes a specific aspect related to FI. Limited information is available to explain the mechanism of action of SNS, and the neurologic mechanism behind this procedure is still unclear. However, SNS is an easy surgical technique that can be performed under local anesthesia and totally reversible. InterStim® Therapy (Medtronic) is the only implantable system currently approved for SNS. As recommended by most of the authors, the optimal implantation site for the electrode is the third sacral foramen. SNS is usually performed with a two-stage procedure, where the first phase consists in a test stimulation period allowing the patient to evaluate the effectiveness of therapy, while at the second stage, the implantable pulse generator (IPG) is connected to the previously placed quadripolar wire. Device can be programmed in monopolar or bipolar configuration, with variable amplitude, frequency, and pulse width. The complications are sporadic and mainly consisting in sepsis and wire displacement. Patients are followed up regularly, 1 month, 6 months after the implant, and yearly thereafter. Long-term results are positive and prove SNS as significantly more effective than medical treatment on clinical outcomes and QoL. The cost of SNS, including diagnostic studies, implant, medication, and outpatient visits, amounts approximately to €14.973 per patient; however, the therapy is demonstrated to significantly reduce direct and indirect costs associated with FI, with respect to standard medical treatment.

9.1 Introduction

Fecal incontinence (FI), defined as the complaint of involuntary loss of liquid/solid stool, is a physically and psychosocially debilitating condition which negatively impacts quality of

M. Indinnimeo (✉) • C.M. Moschella • G. Bernardi
P. Gozzo
Department of Surgery "P. Valdoni",
Sapienza – University of Rome, Rome, Italy
e-mail: marileda.indinnimeo@uniroma1.it

M. Mongardini, M. Giofrè (eds.), *Management of Fecal Incontinence*,
DOI 10.1007/978-3-319-32226-1_9

life (QOL). Anal incontinence (AI) and FI are often used interchangeably; however, the terms are not synonymous. According to the terminology by the International Urogynecology Association (IUGA) and the International Continence Society (ICS), AI is the involuntary loss of feces and/or flatus, whereas FI pertains to involuntary loss of feces [1]. Both conditions cause social or hygienic problems. FI can lead to social isolation, embarrassment, loss of employment, as well as self-esteem. In addition, the impact of FI is influenced not only by severity, but by multiple other individual factors, such as age, lifestyle, occupation, cultural issues, and personal values. Fecal incontinence affects up to 15 % of the adult population. Its prevalence is probably underestimated due to reluctance of most people to discuss the problem. Brown HW and Manchio JV reported that women discussed their FI symptoms with a family physician (56 %), an internist (19 %), and a gastroenterologist (27 %) and were less likely to talk to surgical specialists, such as a colorectal surgeon (7 %) or gynecologist/urogynecologist (7 %) [2, 3]. Many clinical studies have shown a higher prevalence of FI in women (28.4 %). However, recent epidemiologic studies tend to show an equal gender distribution [4, 5]. FI depends on impairment of some mechanisms such as anal sphincter morphology and function, rectal sensation, rectoanal reflex, rectal compliance, stool consistency, colonic transit time, and cognitive and neurologic factors. Incontinence occurs when any one or more of these factors are impaired. A correct treatment requires a careful understanding of the complex pelvic floor musculature and innervation, as well as compensatory mechanisms. The etiology of incontinence is multifactorial and may depend on anal causes (injury, surgery for fistula, hemorrhoids, carcinoma, infection, congenital malformations), rectal causes (proctitis, previous surgery, radiotherapy), central and peripheral neurological causes (stroke, dementia, spinal cord injury, tumor, multiple sclerosis, cauda equina, pudendal neuropathy, diabetes mellitus), and functional causes (fecal impaction, chronic diarrhea, irritable bowel syndrome).

9.2 History of Sacral Nerve Stimulation

Electrical stimulation was first used to treat urinary dysfunctions. The first report was published in 1878 by Saxtorph who described direct vesical stimulation in urinary retention patients [6]. The technique has been developed, and the first implantations were performed by Tanagho and Schmidt in 1988 [7]. SNS has been used for over 20 years to successfully treat patients with urinary urge incontinence, urgency-frequency, and urinary retention. In 1995 Matzel employed SNS in patients with functional bowel disorders [8], and later, SNS proved to be an effective and safe treatment for fecal incontinence in the short and long terms [9–14]. It delivers mild, non-painful electrical pulses to the sacral nerves, to improve or restore function. Initially it was confined to patients with a functionally deficient but morphologically intact anal sphincter complex. Subsequently, the indications for SNS have extended to patients with various functional and morphological causes of fecal incontinence, including large sphincter lesions (180°). SNS has therefore been employed in FI due to obstetric trauma, anorectal surgery, and postradiation therapy to treat anorectal or prostatic cancer and in patients affected by neurological disorders secondary to trauma, infections, long-standing diabetes, or degenerative neurological disease. The concept was to enhance residual function of the anal sphincter and pelvic floor muscles by electrical stimulation of the peripheral nerve supply. Many authors have demonstrated the beneficial effect of SNS in other diseases such as severe constipation, obstructive defecation syndrome, irritable bowel syndrome, urinary and bladder dysfunction, and chronic pelvic pain, sometimes in association with FI [15–17].

9.3 Clinical Assessment of Patients with FI

The assessment of the severity of FI is important in order to choose a treatment modality as well as to evaluate the treatment outcomes. The patients with FI who can benefit from SNS should be selected by a careful history and by validated questionnaires to assess the severity of the FI and its effect on QOL. Continence diaries to document bowel habits and episodes of incontinence are a very useful tool in measuring the severity of symptoms. It is interesting to note that total FI severity scores based on recall (from patient history) compared to daily report (from bowel diary) are significantly lower [18, 19].

The Fecal Incontinence Severity Index (FISI) for assessment of severity was developed by surgeons with patient input [19]. The importance of qualitative research on the impact of FI on QOL gained support in the 1990s. Current data indicate that disease-specific health-related QOL (HRQOL) questionnaires, instead of general questionnaires, have been shown to best quantify the impact of FI [20, 21].

The Fecal Incontinence Quality of Life index (FIQOL) is a validated quality outcome measure consisting of 29 questions divided into 4 individual scales of lifestyle, coping/behavior, depression/self-perception, and embarrassment [22].

The Manchester Health Questionnaire (MHQ) comprises 31 items with subscales of role limitations, physical/social limitations, personal relationships, emotions, and sleep/energy to measure HRQOL in women with AI [23].

The International Consultation on Incontinence Questionnaire – Bowel Symptoms (ICIQ-B) was most recently developed to evaluate symptoms of AI and impact on HRQOL in a single scale for a general adult population [24]. This tool has been shown to have all three factors (validity, reliability, and responsiveness), making it one of the most valid tools for assessing the impact of FI [25]. It was traditionally believed that the more severe the condition, the higher the impact of the condition on a patient's QOL; thus, the two measures (severity and QOL) should correlate. However, more recent data demonstrate a weak correlation between severity and some QOL measures [26–31]. We believe that, even for the choice of treatment, it is vital to take into account not only the severity of incontinence but above all the impact of this on social and emotional aspects of life and in the relational sphere. One must also consider that filling out the QOL questionnaires may not always prove easy for all patients. In this regard, a tool that can quantify the perception of the severity of incontinence by the patients and the impact of the disease on their quality of life is represented by a simple analog scale graded 0–10. The use of this simple measuring system has proved effective both for the selection of patients to be treated with SNS and for the evaluation of the results.

9.4 Diagnostics

Although multiple diagnostic tests are available to assess FI, few guidelines exist to delineate when specific testing should be performed [32]. We consider it essential to always perform anorectal manometry, endoanal ultrasound (EAU), pelvic floor electromyography (EMG), pudendal nerve assessment, and sometimes magnetic resonance imaging (MRI). Only from an analysis of these tests can a correct indication for SNS be achieved, because each of them analyzes a specific component responsible for FI. Digital examination provides a preliminary assessment of the anal resting tone and squeeze pressure, anal sphincter defects, the anorectal angle, pelvic floor descent, rectal masses, and other pathologic conditions. The accuracy of digital examination is operator dependent. Any correlation between physical examination and manometric measures has been controversial [33–37]. Even if the positive predictive value of digital examinations in identifying resting and squeeze pressure was reported to be 67 % by Hill [38] and 81 % by Rao [39], we believe that it is always necessary to perform anorectal manometry with rectal sensory testing, for defining the functional weakness of the anal sphincters and detecting abnormal rectal sensation [40, 41].

EAU provides an accurate assessment of the morphology of the anal sphincters, and it is useful in ruling out other anorectal and pelvic floor disorders. A traditional probe has a 7 mHz rotating transducer with a focal length of 1–4 cm. Higher-frequency transducers (10–15 mHz) can provide better delineation of the sphincter complex [33,

42, 43]. Both 2D and 3D ultrasound approaches are currently available. For accurate diagnosis, a sphincter defect must be viewed in the upper, middle, and distal anal canal. EAU also permits accurate assessment of the thickness of the anal sphincters and the size of the defect. Muscular thinning is indicative of altered nervous support, and it may represent an indication for SNS, while a sphincter defect higher than 180° represents a contraindication. With improvements in sonographic technology, there is no significant difference between endoanal MRI and ultrasound in detecting external anal sphincter (EAS) defects in patients with FI [44]. The sensitivity for detecting EAS defects by MRI and ultrasound was 81 and 90 %, respectively, and the positive predictive value (PPV) was 89 % for MRI and 85 % for EAU [45]. The cost and availability are often contraindications to the use of MRI.

EMG assesses anal sphincter activity using a surface electrode or a concentric needle and can be helpful in distinguishing neurogenic from myogenic damage. Studies comparing EMG with EAU showed a high concordance rate for identifying sphincter defects [33]. Patients who show signs of complete denervation cannot be treated with SNS. Pudendal nerve terminal motor latency (PNTML) measures the time required after stimulating the pudendal nerve with an electrode to induce an EAS contraction. Prolongation of PNTML suggests pudendal neuropathy. However, one may have normal fast-twitch muscle function demonstrated but abnormal slow-twitch which would not be measured by PNTML. Bilateral, not unilateral, neuropathy has been associated with diminished sphincter function and higher incontinence scores [46]. Some studies have reported that PNTML is useful in predicting the outcome of sphincteroplasty in conjunction with other modalities [40]. However, PNTML is operator dependent and has a poor correlation with clinical symptoms and histologic findings. The American Gastroenterological Association (AGA) does not recommend PNTML for routine evaluation [40, 47, 48]. Emerging neurophysiological tests have been recently introduced. The neural circuitry of afferent and efferent pathways can be evaluated using cortical evoked potentials (CEP) and motor evoked potentials (MEP) of the rectum and anal sphincter response to magnetic stimulation of the motor cortex (transcranial magnetic stimulation [TMS]). CEP, MEP, and TMS are largely used in research and clinical trials, currently not available for clinical use [49–53].

9.5 Mechanism of Action

Anorectal and pelvic floor innervation is derived from both the autonomic and the somatic nervous systems. Motor innervation of the levator ani muscle and puborectalis sling originates in the sacral nerve roots (S2-S5) [54–56]. The external anal sphincter muscle is mainly innervated by a branch of the pudendal nerve, the inferior rectal nerve [54]. Autonomic innervation is both sympathetic and parasympathetic. Parasympathetic innervation is through the pelvic plexus, derived from the sacral nerves (S2-S4) [54]. Anal and distal rectal sensory innervation is mainly through the pudendal nerve [57]. Electrical stimulation of this dual innervation seems to excite both systems and cause both direct and reflex-mediated responses in the fecal continence mechanism [58, 59]. The exact mechanism of action of SNS in the treatment of bowel and urinary dysfunctions is not completely understood. Most of the studies were conducted in patients affected by urinary dysfunctions. For infants, who have not yet achieved voluntary control, a critical level of bladder distention is required to stimulate the voiding reflex. This sensory input, on reaching the pontine micturition center, simultaneously allows for a coordinated detrusor contraction and concomitant urethral relaxation. Gaining voluntary control, the voiding reflex becomes a complex process mediated at a higher level in the cerebral cortex. Voluntary voiding is a result of inhibition of the sympathetic system and activation of the sacral parasympathetic system [60]. For patients with urinary retention, SNS is believed to activate the pudendal nerve afferents originating from the pelvic organs into the spinal cord. At the level of the spinal cord, pudendal afferents may turn on voiding reflexes by suppressing exaggerated guarding reflexes, thus relieving the symptoms of patients with urinary retention. Research with positron emission tomography (PET) scans in urge-incontinent individuals suggests that SNS influences brain areas involved in bladder alertness and awareness [61]. In patients with fecal incontinence, limited information is available to explain the mechanism of action. A small study demonstrated that SNS was associated with higher tolerance of rectal distention, but the neurologic mechanism behind this is unclear [62]. Probably, the pudendal afferent somatic fibers work by inhibiting colonic propulsive activity and activating the internal anal sphincter [63]. The action on colonic motility may explain why patients with significant anal sphincter defects may benefit from SNS. Nevertheless, chronic constipation is also an approved indication for SNS in Europe. Dinning et al. have demonstrated increased colonic peristalsis and frequency of bowel movements in slow-transit constipation patients with SNS stimulation [64, 65]. As with the bladder, it is difficult to understand how SNS may be effective in both bowel storage and emptying disorders.

9.6 Procedure

SNS involves the insertion of an electrode into a sacral foramen for the stimulation of the sacral nerve roots. The ideal implantation site of the electrode was considered to be the third sacral foramen as recommended in the literature [66] and by all participants in the consensus statement from the Italian Group [67]. Benson [68] demonstrated that the third sacral nerve root provides the majority of innervation to the pelvic organs. However, the sacral anatomy is extremely variable, and thus, occasionally the S4 or S2 nerve roots are stimulated.

It is a simple surgical technique that can be performed under local anesthesia, completely reversible. Preoperative antibiotic prophylaxis was recommended by all the experts; although bacteria have been found in about 50% of explanted electrodes, modest levels of clinical infections have been recorded. By contrast, local antibiotic therapy was not considered useful.

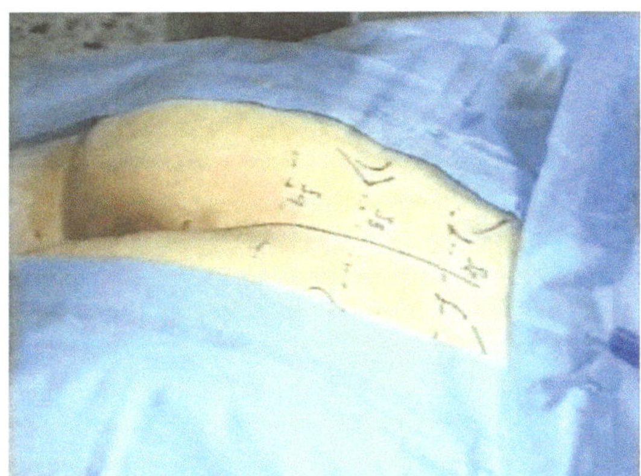

Fig. 9.1 Reference points for the identification of the sacral foramen

SNS is performed in two stages using insertion kits, electrodes, and pacemakers manufactured by Medtronic (InterStim System Medtronic Inc Minneapolis, MN). The first phase is the test stimulation period where the patient can evaluate the effectiveness of therapy. A positive test phase was shown to be highly predictive of a good outcome with implantation. The patient is positioned prone on the operating table, with a cushion under the abdomen, taking care to expose the anal region, the sacral region, and feet. The identification of the sacral foramina is done with some landmarks, namely, the posterior-superior iliac spine, the sciatic notch, and the spinous processes of the sacral vertebrae. The second sacral foramen is identified approximately at the level of the posterior-superior iliac spine, 1.5 cm from the midline, the third sacral foramen approximately 1 cm below S2, and the fourth at the upper edge of the sciatic notch, about 1.5 cm under the third foramen (Fig. 9.1).

There are two techniques to perform test stimulation. The first is termed percutaneous nerve evaluation (PNE) and consists of placing a temporary monopolar wire through the sacral foramen under local anesthesia. The wire is connected to an external generator for a short period of 3–7 days. The disadvantages of this method lie in the impossibility of varying the programming, given that the electrode is monopolar, by the shortness of the test period which cannot allow correct evaluation of the stimulation and by displacement

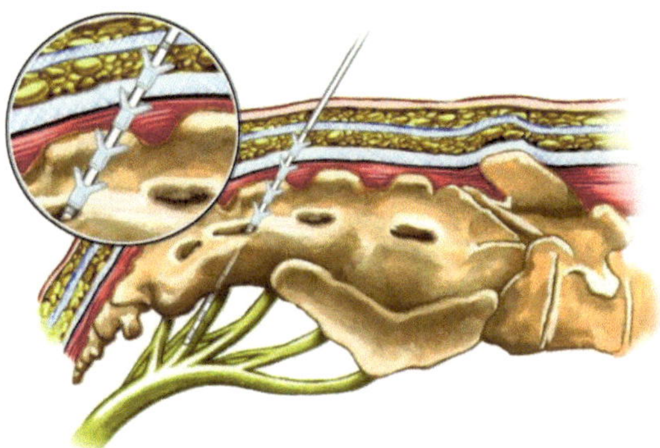

Fig. 9.2 Introduction of the quadripolar electrode with self-anchoring tines in the third sacral foramen

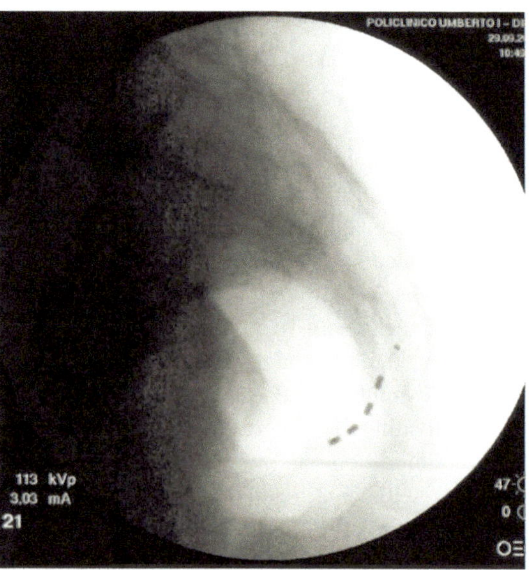

Fig. 9.3 Radiological monitoring of the correct positioning of the quadripolar electrode

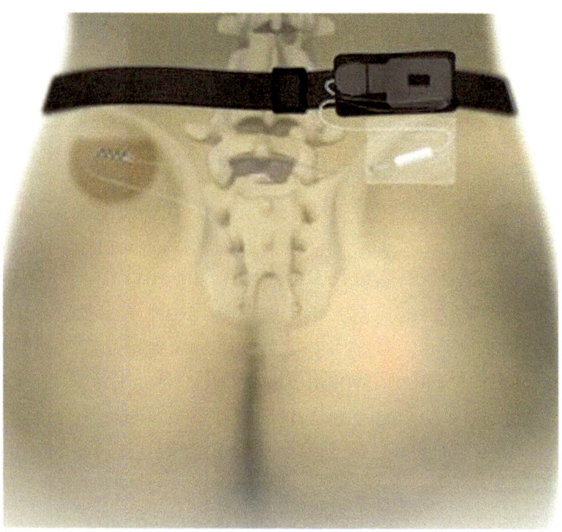

Fig. 9.4 Electrode in the third sacral foramen; connection capsule in the subcutaneous pouch, output cable; external electrostimulator

of the wire, not securely anchored in place. The second option is the staged implant introduced by Spinelli in 2003 [69, 70] that is typically performed as an outpatient procedure using local anesthesia. This procedure involves placement of a quadripolar lead wire adjacent to a sacral nerve root (typically S3) (Fig. 9.2). In order to evaluate correct positioning in the sacral foramen and depth of the wire, intraoperative fluoroscopy is considered necessary by most authors, during the implantation phase [66, 71] (Fig. 9.3). The lead is self-anchoring and therefore reduces the risk of migration. The quadripolar wire is transferred subcutaneously on the opposite side and connected to an external electrostimulator by means of a connecting cable. The connection is placed in a subcutaneous pouch in the supragluteal region (Fig. 9.4). Using this electrode, the test phase can continue for 60 days, reducing the percentage of false-positive results due to a transient efficacy of the treatment, avoiding an unnecessary pacemaker implantation. It also reduces the rate of false-negative results due to a shorter stimulation period. The quadripolar wire is provided with 4 electrodes, offering a wide range of programming in the test phase. During the trial test, the electrical pulse parameters can be varied, i.e., the polarity, the amplitude, the frequency, and the duration up to a threshold value that does not cause discomfort to the patient. During the second stage, the previously placed quadripolar wire remains in place; under local anesthesia, a new incision is made at the site of the previous scar, in the supragluteal region, in correspondence with the subcutaneous pouch, which is expanded in order to position the implantable pulse generator (IPG). The connection cable between electrode and external electrical stimulator is removed, and the electrode is connected to the IPG (Figs. 9.5, 9.6, 9.7, and 9.8). In 2006, the second-generation

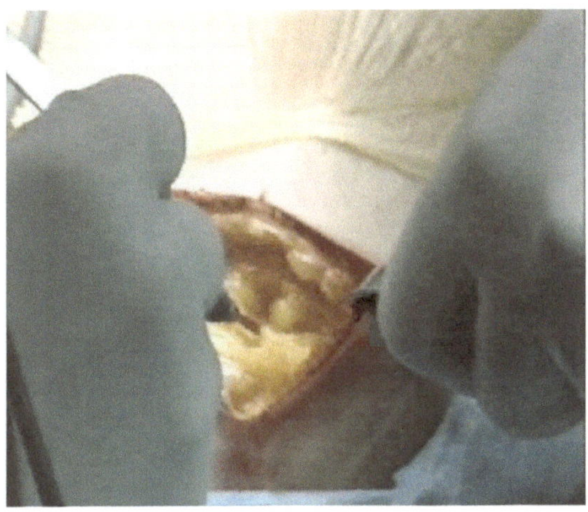

Fig. 9.5 Packaging of the subcutaneous pouch

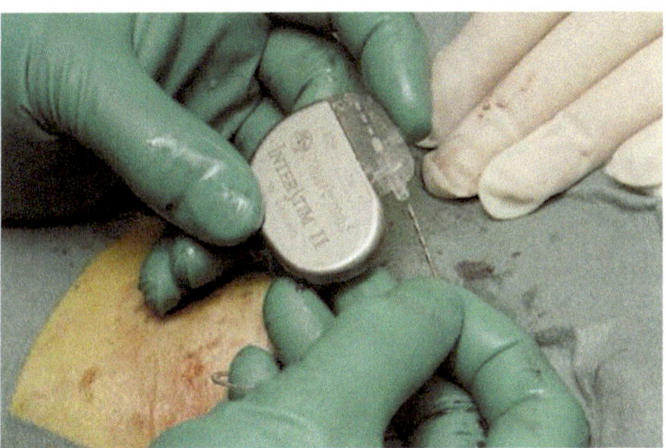

Fig. 9.6 Connection between definitive quadripolar electrode and sacral pacemaker

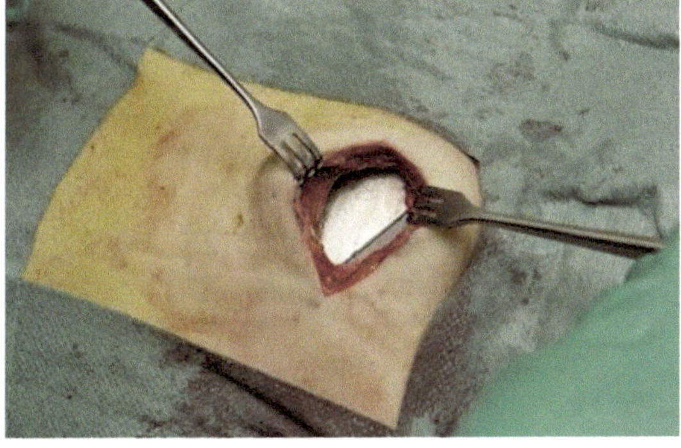

Fig. 9.7 The pacemaker is positioned in the subcutaneous pouch

IPG was introduced, which is one-third the volume of the original. In a prospective study comparing the PNE with the staged implant, there

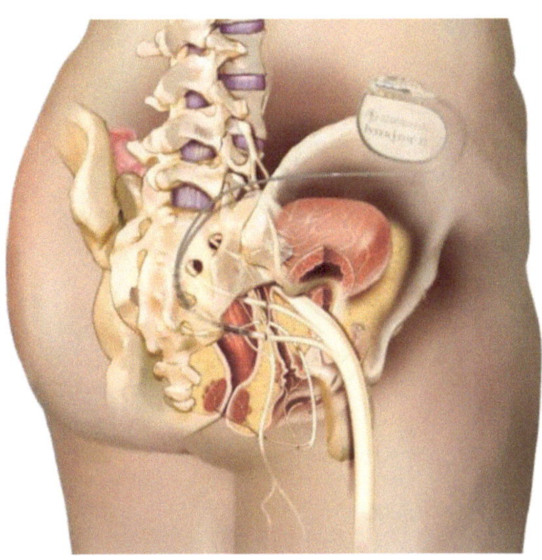

Fig. 9.8 Definitive implantation with IPG in the subcutaneous pouch in the supragluteal region and electrode positioned in the third sacral foramen

was a significantly higher rate of conversion to definitive implant with the stage procedure vs. the PNE (88 % vs. 46 %) [72]. To determine optimal lead placement, both motor and sensory responses are desirable. The sensory responses are formication, vibration, paresthesia, or even pain at the level of the vagina, rectum, and/or perineum. Motor responses vary according to the foramen stimulated. S2 stimulation causes contraction of the external anal sphincter and the levator complex. There is associated external rotation of the leg and foot flexion. S3 stimulation causes bellows contraction of the anus and hallux flexion. S4 stimulation, finally, leads to clamp contraction of the anus without lower limb response (Fig. 9.9). There has been no definitive study to determine which factor is more predictive of success. One small, prospective study, in a urological setting, did report that a positive motor response was more predictive than a sensory response in achieving a successful trial stimulation [73]. A larger retrospective analysis reported both to be highly predictive [74]. Although these findings may suggest that motor response alone may be adequate, the best predictor of a successful response is still not known, and many surgeons prefer to have both motor and sensory responses

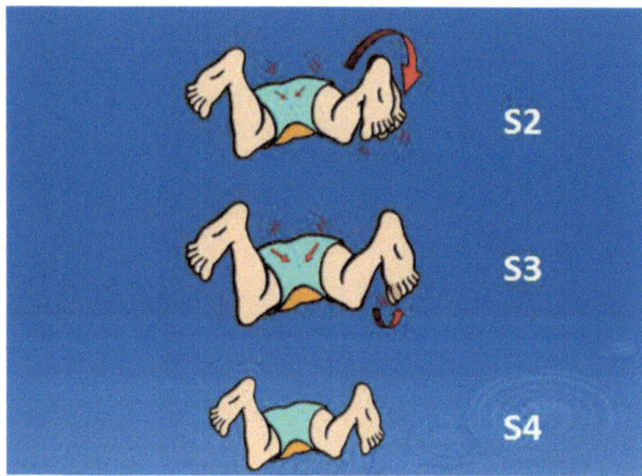

Fig. 9.9 Motor responses during the trial test. *S2* stimulation, contraction of the anal sphincter and external rotation of the leg and/or foot flexion; *S3* stimulation, bellows contraction of the anus and hallux flexion; and *S4* stimulation, clamp contraction of the anus

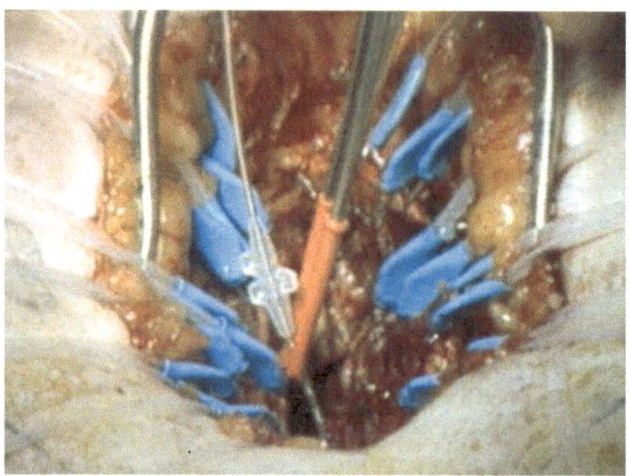

Fig. 9.10 Wide incision at the sacral foramen and fixing of the electrode to the periosteum

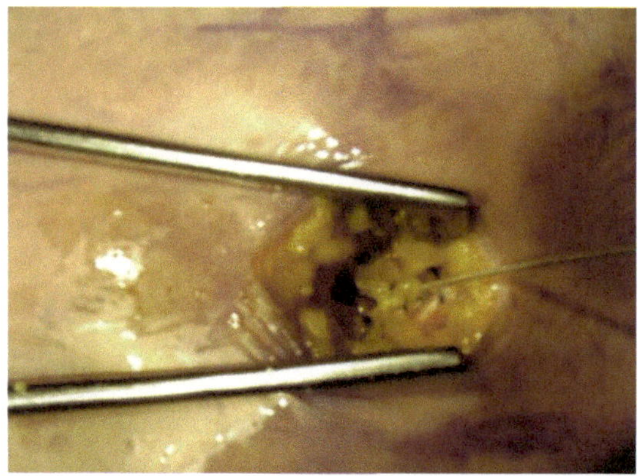

Fig. 9.11 Skin and fascial incision: electrode fixed to the fascia

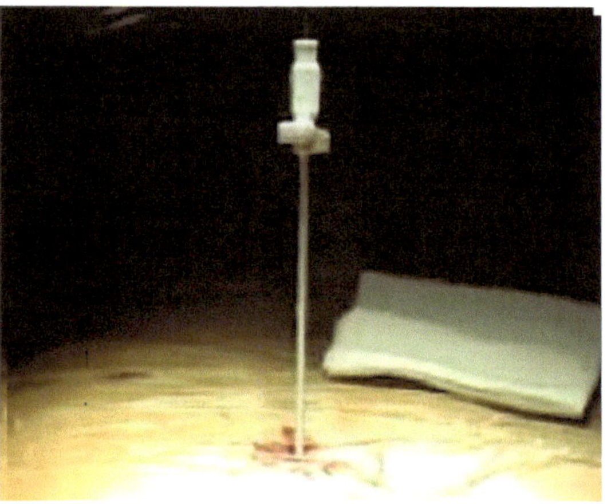

Fig. 9.12 Introduction of the self-anchoring electrode percutaneously

and therefore advise the routine use of local anesthesia. A greater probability of success has been demonstrated in patients who require lower induction values of the motor responses [75]. Since its introduction, SNS has undergone significant improvements in design and application. The initial implantation technique required general anesthesia and a 5–7 cm incision over the sacrum that was taken down to the periosteum, where the electrode was fixed (Fig. 9.10). Subsequently, a less extensive incision was made, and the fixing was performed at the fascia (Fig. 9.11). The current technique involves the percutaneous insertion, on an introducer guide, in accordance with the Seldinger technique, of a quadripolar electrode, fitted with self-anchoring tines. This procedure has allowed the skin incision to be reduced up to a few millimeters, decreasing the intervention time and the need for general anesthesia (Figs. 9.12, 9.13, and 9.14). More recently, a curved stylet was added to the tined lead kit. The curved stylet has been postulated to facilitate an advantageous placement of the lead proximal to the nerve root. A recent randomized crossover trial demonstrated the superiority of the curved over straight stylet in achieving motor response at lower amplitudes, thus increasing programming options and potentially extending battery life [76].

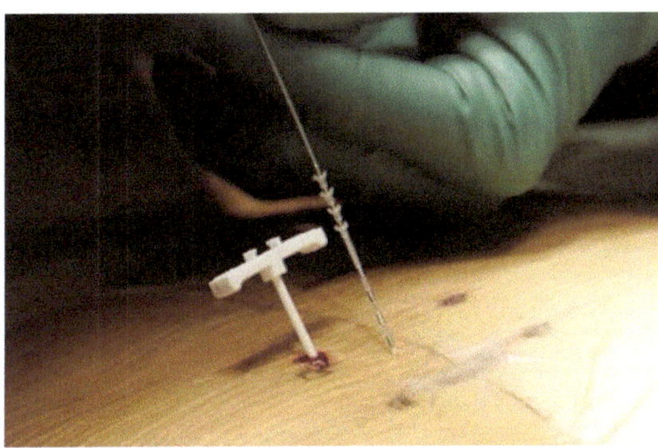

Fig. 9.13 Introducer placed percutaneously and definitive quadripolar electrode

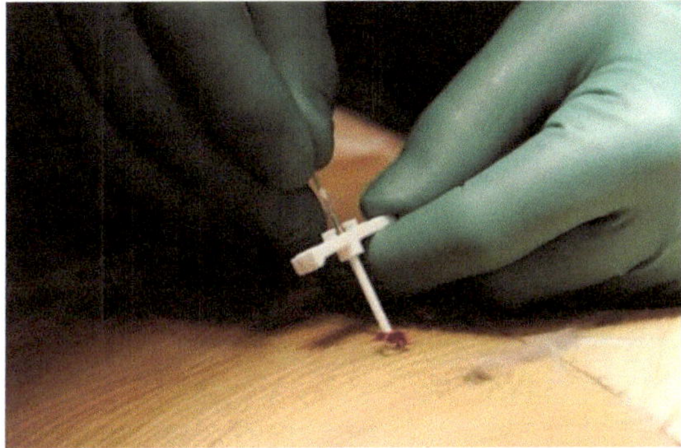

Fig. 9.14 Positioning of the electrode onto the introducer guide

9.7 Stage I Efficacy Assessment

The evaluation of the results during the trial period does not consider instrumental tests, because, often, they are not changed. The most reliable parameters are patient satisfaction, improved defecation diary, improved Wexner score, and improved QOL. In the past an improvement of more than 50 % of clinical parameters was necessary to proceed to definitive implant [66]. Currently, based on the experience of the Italian authors, an improvement of at least 70 % in clinical parameters alone or a 50 % improvement in clinical parameters together with a significant improvement in QOL should be considered satisfactory [67]. According to our experience, patients are definitive implant candidates when they have an improvement higher than 70 % in Wexner score and improvement higher than 50 % in incontinence and quality of life on the basis of the analogical scales. In the event of an unsatisfactory result, the Italian experts suggest changing the stimulation parameters at least once after 15 days and trying different program settings on the basis of polarity, frequency (Hz), amplitude (V), and duration (μs). In the event of suboptimal result with unilateral SNS, it has been described in urology that bilateral stimulation was superior to unilateral stimulation [77, 78]. Leroi reported that contralateral testing has been deemed unhelpful in fecal incontinence [66]. After the definitive implant, the same programming that provided the best results during testing is mostly maintained. Programming aims to ensure optimal relief of symptoms, minimize patient discomfort, and preserve the battery life of the neurostimulator. A stimulation program consists of programming electrical parameters, active electrode settings, and modality of stimulation. The electrical pulse output from the neurostimulator may vary based on three different parameters: amplitude, frequency, and duration of the stimulus. The amplitude or intensity of the stimulus is measured in volts, and the optimum setting is based on the patient's comfort. The second parameter is the pulse rate and is measured in pulses per second (pps) or in Hertz (Hz). At high frequencies, the patient perceives a vibration sensation and at low frequencies a pulsation. Optimal values range between 10 and 30 Hz. The third parameter is pulse duration or width which is measured in microseconds and oscillates between 180 and 240 μs. The smaller the pulse width, the more targeted the stimulation. The larger the pulse width, the wider the spread of stimulation. By increasing amplitude or pulse duration, therefore, the patient perceives a sensation of pulsation or vibration that involves a wider and wider area. As these parameters are increased, INS battery longevity decreases. It is possible to select a unipolar or bipolar mode of stimulation. In the unipolar configuration, the IPG is positive, and one of the four electrode contacts is negative. In the bipolar configuration the IPG is in the off position, and two of the four electrodes have opposite polarities (Fig. 9.15). The unipolar configuration determines a very

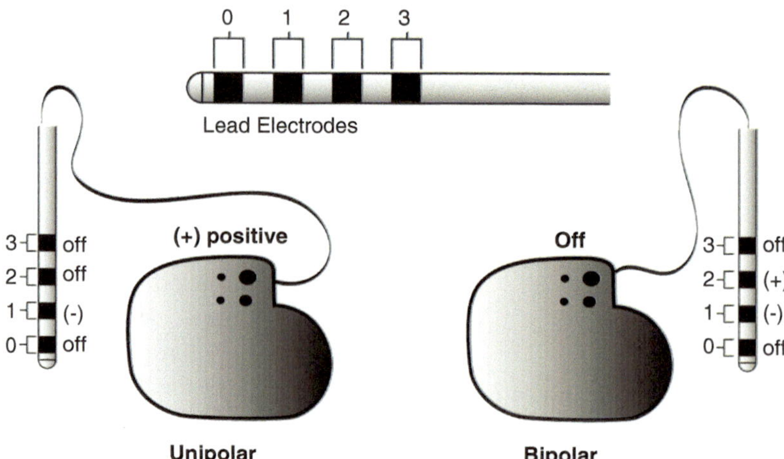

Fig. 9.15 Unipolar or bipolar configuration. The action potential is generated near the cathode

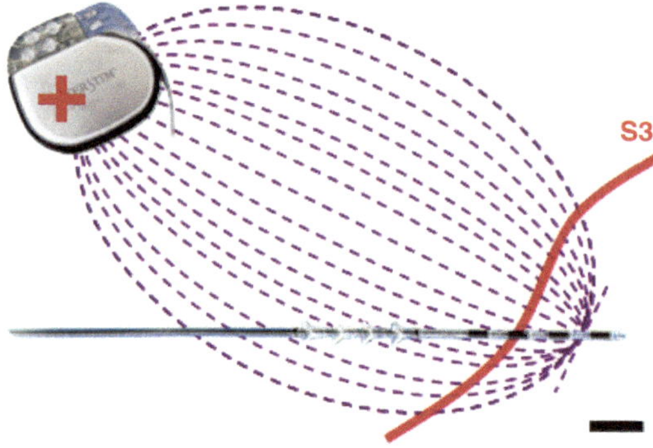

Fig. 9.16 Unipolar configuration: The negative pole is at the level of the electrode, and the positive pole is at the level of the case

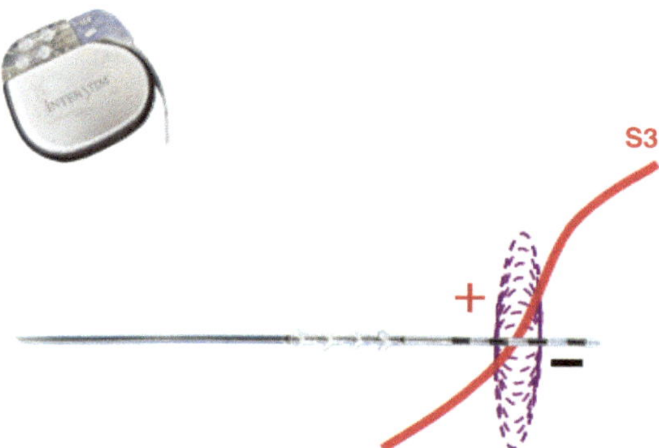

Fig. 9.17 Bipolar configuration: both poles are positioned on the electrode

large electrical stimulation field, while in the bipolar configuration the electrical field is more restricted (Figs. 9.16 and 9.17). However, more than two active electrodes can be selected. The more active electrodes that are selected, the faster the INS battery is depleted. The stimulation mode may be continuous or cyclic. The cyclic mode consists of periods of stimulation alternating with periods of pulse interruption. The start/stop soft cyclic variant is characterized by a progressive increase and decrease of amplitude during the on phase. The Medtronic InterStim System is generally programmed within 1 week after operation. Programming is done by the doctor with an N'Vision programmer, which communicates externally telemetrically with the IPG. The patient is also given a programmer "InterStim iCon Patient Programmer," of the size of a mobile phone, provided with an interactive display. Its function can be limited to basic operations (on, off, amplitude increase and decrease) but can offer up to four clinician-set therapy programs, if programmed on and downloaded from the N'Vision® Clinician programmer.

9.8 Follow-Up and Evaluation of Results

According to most authors, the first follow-up examination should be carried out 1 month after definitive implantation and subsequently at 6 months and 1 year. Subsequent controls are scheduled once a year or, where necessary, at the patient's request. Each control evaluates the stimulation parameters and the remaining life of the IPG battery, and the clinical outcome is noted on the basis of the Wexner score and QoL. A decrease in effectiveness of the stimulation may be due to a low bat-

Table 9.1 Studies of outcomes of sacral nerve stimulation

Ref.	Year	Patients (*n*)	Significant reduction in incontinence scores and incontinent episodes	Significant increase in quality of life
Leroi et al. [91]	2005	27	Y	Y
Boyle et al. [92]	2009	15	Y	NR
Brouwer et al. [93]	2010	55	Y	Y
Wexner et al. [86]	2010	120	Y	Y
Hollingshead et al. [83]	2011	18	Y	NR
Lim et al. [85]	2011	41	Y	Y
Mellgren et al. [79]	2011	83	Y	Y
George et al. [84]	2012	23	Y	Y
Devroede et al. [88]	2012	78	Y	Y
Hull et al. [14]	2013	76	Y	Y
Damon et al. [87]	2013	92	Y	Y

Y yes, *NR* not reported

tery; the dislocation of the electrode, detectable with an X-ray of the sacral region; a rupture of a system component, detectable with the N'Vision programmer; or, lastly, a fibrotic reaction around the electrodes. In such cases it is recommended to proceed with a change in the programming parameters and only later with the implantation of a new wire in a contralateral position. The most frequent complications after SNS include lead displacement, pain at the surgical site, and paresthesias. Infection of the permanent device on surgical site occurs in 10 % of patients requiring surgical management in 5 % [79, 80]. Hull et al. reported that about one-third of patients required surgical revision of the site of the device in long-term follow-up [14]. Duelund-Jacobsen et al. [81], in a case study of 164 patients with fecal incontinence, reported a percentage of infections in the surgical site of 3 % that led to the explantation of the pacemaker. Pain or dislocation was present in 12.1 % with the need for repositioning of the pacemaker. During follow-up, it was necessary to undertake a surgical revision in 19.5 % of cases. The SNS results at a distance also use the evaluation of patient satisfaction, the defecation diary, the Wexner score, and QOL. Long-term results are available.

In fecal incontinence sacral nerve stimulation is significantly more effective than medical treatment [82]. A recent report showed that after 5 years after SNS, 89 % of patients have significant reduction in fecal incontinence, and 36 % have a complete response [14]. Numerous other studies have demonstrated significant long-term reduction in fecal incontinence scores [14, 83–86] and improvement in QoL scores [79, 86–89]. Furthermore, women treated with sacral nerve stimulation for fecal incontinence showed improvement in sexual and urinary symptoms, demonstrating also a beneficial effect of SNS on the pelvic floor [90]. Long-term results are reported in Table 9.1 in a review of the literature after sacral nerve stimulation [94].

9.9 Personal Experience

Our experience is based on the observation of 97 patients with medium-to-severe fecal incontinence undergoing trial tests between 2004 and 2014. Patient selection was made through the clinical diary, the Wexner score, diagnostic tests (manometry, EAU, and EMG of the pelvic floor), and the analogical scales to assess subjective perception of disease severity and QoL. The trial test was performed with the quadripolar electrode system, positioned in the operating room, under local anesthesia, after antibiotic prophylaxis and using intraoperative fluoroscopy. The test lasted on average 42 days (min 27–max 50). Completely unsatisfactory results were observed in patients with resection of the rectum with coloanal anastomosis, often associated with stenosis and fibrosis secondary to the surgery and to radiation therapy, such as to constitute, in our opinion, an absolute contraindication to SNS. Eighty patients were deemed suitable for permanent implantation, due to having presented an improvement higher than 70 % in Wexner score and improvement higher than 50 % in incontinence and quality of life on the basis of the analogical scales. Particularly with the analogical scales, patients had a significantly reduced perception of the seriousness of the disease (from an average of 8.7 to 2.8) and a much improved quality of life (from 1.5 to 8). Of the patients subjected to IPG implantation, 23 were males and 57 females with a mean age of 59 years (range 30–77); 56.3 % were suffering from urge fecal incontinence, 6.3 % from passive fecal incontinence, and 37.4 % from mixed (urge + passive) incontinence. In 31.6 % of cases, patients had previously been submitted to anterior resection of the rectum with colorectal anastomosis also associated with radiochemotherapy, and in 26.3 % of cases, other proctological interventions were performed. In 42.1 % there was degenerative, postinfectious, post-traumatic, and diabetic-based neurological disorder present. The mean follow-up was 4 years. Eighty-five percent of all implanted patients showed a stable and significant improvement for the Wexner score (p value <0.001) and for QoL, especially for the role limitations due to physical health and emotional state. The benefits obtained regarding the perception of the general state of health conditioned by the presence of the pacemaker, perceived as a foreign body, were more limited. Only 5 % of implanted patients had complications that required surgical revision; in 2 cases the pacemaker was explanted due to a reaction to the implanted material after 60 days, and in further 2 cases, it was necessary to reposition the pacemaker.

9.10 Costs

The costs of SNS cannot be separated from the evaluation of the direct costs of fecal incontinence represented by the costs of clinical visits, hospitalization, drugs, and consumables (absorbent diapers, ointments, sanitizing products). There are also considerable indirect costs due to absence from work, reduced work efficiency, the need to change the type of work, avoiding jobs requiring contact with the public, and those that take place in locations devoid of toilets. An American study calculated that patients with major incontinence (leakage of over 400 g of feces per day) are absent from work for about 50 days a year versus 5 days in the general population [95]. Among the indirect costs, we must also consider working days lost or even loss by relatives who have to assist patients with fecal incontinence. A significant social cost is also the payment of disability benefits. The average annual cost per person in American people, including direct medical and nonmedical costs, as well as lost productivity, was 4,110.00 US dollars. Of these costs, direct medical and nonmedical costs averaged 2,353 and 209 USD, respectively, whereas the indirect costs associated with productivity loss averaged 1,549 USD per patient annually [96]. FI severity was significantly associated with higher annual direct costs. A Dutch study estimated an annual total cost of € 2.169 for FI patients, of which € 714 was for direct medical costs, € 337 for direct nonmedical costs, and € 1.118 for indirect costs [97]. Regarding costs related to treatment with SNS, in addition to implantation, even outpatient visits, diagnostic procedures, and medications need to be considered. Spending per patient in the first 2 years after implantation was calculated by Leroi to be € 14.973 [98]; similar costs were found by Hetzer et al. [99] who reported a cost of € 15.345 per patient for the first year and € 997 for each subsequent year, including surgical treatment failures, complications, and follow-up. Since SNS is also indicated in the treatment of urinary incontinence, it is likely that the cost-benefit ratio is even more favorable in patients with mixed incontinence.

References

1. Haylen BT, de Ridder D, Freeman RM, et al. An International Urogynecological Association (IUGA)/ International Continence Society (ICS) joint report on the terminology for female pelvic floor dysfunction. NeurourolUrodyn. 2010;29(1):4–20.

2. Brown HW, Wexner SD, Segall MM, Brezoczky KL, Lukacz ES. Quality of life impact in women with accidental bowel leakage. Int J Clin Pract. 2012;66(11):1109–16.
3. Manchio JV, Sanders BM. Fecal incontinence: help for patients who suffer silently. J Fam Pract. 2013;62(11):640–50.
4. Kang HW, Jung HK, Kwon KJ, et al. Prevalence and predictive factors of fecal incontinence. J Neurogastroenterol Motil. 2012;18(1):86–93.
5. Landefeld CS, Bowers BJ, Feld AD, et al. National Institutes of Health state-of-the-science conference statement: prevention of fecal and urinary incontinence in adults. Ann Intern Med. 2008;148(6):449–58.
6. Saxtorph M. Stricture urethrae – Fistula perinee – Retentio urinae. Clinisk Chirurgi, Gyldendalske Forlag, Copenhagen. 1878:265–280.
7. Tanagho EA, Schmidt RA. Electrical stimulation in the clinical management of the neurogenic bladder. J Urol. 1988;140:1331–4.
8. Matzel KE, Stadelmaier U, Hohenfeller M, Gall FP. Electrical stimulation of sacral spinal nerves for treatment of faecal incontinence. Lancet. 1995;346:1124–7.
9. Makol A, Grover M, Witehead WE. Fecal incontinence in women: causes and treatment. Womens Health. 2008;4(5):517–28.
10. Uludag O, Koch SM, van Gemert WG, Dejong CH, Baeten CG. Sacral neuromodulation in patients with fecal incontinence: a single-center study. Dis Colon Rectum. 2004;47(8):1350–7.
11. Altomare DF, Ratto C, Ganio E, Lolli P, Masin A, Villani RD. Long-term outcome of sacral nerve stimulation for fecal incontinence. Dis Colon Rectum. 2009;52(1):11–7.
12. Melenhorst J, Koch SM, Uludag O, van Gemert WG, Baeten CG. Sacral neuromodulation in patients with faecal incontinence: results of the first 100 permanent implantations. Colorectal Dis. 2007;9(8):725–30.
13. Michelsen HB, Thompson-Fawcett M, Lundby L, Krogh K, Laurberg S, Buntzen S. Six years of experience with sacral nerve stimulation for fecal incontinence. Dis Colon Rectum. 2010;53(4):414–21.
14. Hull T, Giese C, Wexner SD, Mellgren A, Devroede G, Madoff RD, et al. Long-term durability of sacral nerve stimulation therapy for chronic fecal incontinence. Dis Colon Rectum. 2013;56(2):234–45.
15. Brazzelli M, Murray A, Fraser C. Efficacy and safety of sacral nerve stimulation for urinary urge incontinence: a systematic review. J Urol. 2006;175:835–41.
16. Gajewski JB, Al-Zahrani AA. The long-term efficacy of sacral neuromodulation in the management of intractable cases of bladder pain syndrome: 14 years of experience in one centre. BJU Int. 2011;107: 1258–64.
17. Herbison GP, Arnold EP. Sacral neuromodulation with implanted devices for urinary storage and voiding dysfunction in adults. Cochrane database Syst Rev. 2009;(2):CD004202.
18. Wang JY, Abbas MA. Current management of fecal incontinence. Perm J. 2013;17(3):65–73.
19. Fisher K, Bliss DZ, Savik K. Comparison of recall and daily self-report of fecal incontinence severity. J Wound Ostomy Continence Nurs. 2008;35(5): 515–20.
20. Alas AN, Bergman J, Dunivan GC, et al. Readability of common health-related quality-of-life instruments in female pelvic medicine. Female Pelvic Med Reconstr Surg. 2013;19(5):293–7.
21. Wiebe S, Guyatt G, Weaver B, Matijevic S, Sidwell C. Comparative responsiveness of generic and specific quality-of-life instruments. J Clin Epidemiol. 2003;56(1):52–60.
22. Meyer I, Richter IE. Impact of fecal incontinence and its treatment on quality of life in women. Womens Health. 2015;11(2):225–38.
23. Abrams P, Andersson KE, Birder L, et al. Fourth International Consultation on Incontinence Recommendations of the International Scientific Committee: evaluation and treatment of urinary incontinence, pelvic organ prolapse, and fecal incontinence. NeurourolUrodyn. 2010;29(1):213–40.
24. Cotterill N, Norton C, Avery KN, Abrams P, Donovan JL. A patient-centered approach to developing a comprehensive symptom and quality of life assessment of anal incontinence. Dis Colon Rectum. 2008;51(1): 82–7.
25. Cotterill N, Norton C, Avery KN, Abrams P, Donovan JL. Psychometric evaluation of a new patient-completed questionnaire for evaluating anal incontinence symptoms and impact on quality of life: the ICIQ-B. Dis Colon Rectum. 2011;54(10):1235–50.
26. Smith TM, Menees SB, Xu X, Saad RJ, Chey WD, Fenner DE. Factors associated with quality of life among women with fecal incontinence. Int Urogynecol J. 2013;24(3):493–9.
27. Markland AD, Greer WJ, Vogt A, et al. Factors impacting quality of life in women with fecal incontinence. Dis Colon Rectum. 2010;53(8):1148–54.
28. Rockwood TH, Church JM, Fleshman JW, et al. Patient and surgeon ranking of the severity of symptoms associated with fecal incontinence: the fecal incontinence severity index. Dis Colon Rectum. 1999;42(12):1525–32.
29. Bartlett L, Nowak M, Ho YH. Impact of fecal incontinence on quality of life. World J Gastroenterol. 2009;15(26):3276–82.
30. Bordeianou L, Rockwood T, Baxter N, Lowry A, Mellgren A, Parker S. Does incontinence severity correlate with quality of life? Prospective analysis of 502 consecutive patients. Colorectal Dis. 2008;10(3):273–9.
31. Glasgow SC, Lowry AC. Long-term outcomes of anal sphincter repair for fecal incontinence: a systematic review. Dis Colon Rectum. 2012;55(4):482–90.
32. Costilla VC, Foxx-Orenstein AE, Mayer AP, et al. Office-based management of fecal incontinence. Gastroenterol Hepatol. 2013;9(7):423–33.
33. Rao SSC, American College of Gastroenterology Practice Parameters Committee. Diagnosis and management of fecal incontinence. Am J Gastroenterol. 2004;99:1585–604.

34. Coller JA. Clinical application of anorectal manometry. Gastroenterol Clin North Am. 1987;16:17.
35. Orkin BA, Sinykin SB, Lloyd PC. The digital rectal examination scoring system (DRESS). Dis Colon Rectum. 2010;53:1656.
36. Felt-Bersma RJ, Klinkenberg-Knol EC, Meuwissen SGM. Investigation of anorectal function. Br J Surg. 1988;75:53–5.
37. Eckhardt VF, Kanzler G. How reliable is digital examination for the evaluation of anal sphincter tone? Int J Colorectal Dis. 1993;8:95–7.
38. Hill J, Corson RJ, Brandon H, et al. History and examination in the assessment of patients with idiopathic fecal incontinence. Dis Colon Rectum. 1994;37(5):473–7.
39. Rao SSC. Advances in diagnostic assessment of fecal incontinence and dyssynergic defecation. Gastroenterol Hepatol. 2008;2:323–5.
40. Remes-Troche JM, Rao SSC. Neurophysiological testing in anorectal disorders. Gastroenterol Hepatol. 2008;2:323–35.
41. Gurland B, Hull T. Transrectal ultrasound, manometry, and pudendal nerve terminal latency studies in the evaluation of sphincter injuries. Clin Colon Rectal Surg. 2008;21(3):157–66.
42. Law PJ, Kamm MA, Bartram CI. Anal endosonography in the investigation of faecal incontinence. Br J Surg. 1991;78:312–4.
43. Bartrum C. Rao SCC. Disorders of anorectum. Gastroenterol Clin North Am. W.B. Saunders. 1. Vol. 30. 2001. Radiological evaluation of anorectal disorders; p. 55–76.
44. Dobben AC, Terra MP, Deutekom M, et al. Anal inspection and digital rectal examination compared to anorectal physiology tests and endoanal ultrasonography in evaluating fecal incontinence. Int J Colorectal Dis. 2007;22(7):783–90.
45. Abdool Z, Sultan AH, Thakar R. Ultrasound imaging of the anal sphincter complex: a review. Br J Radiol. 2012;85(1015):865–75.
46. Jones MP, Post J, Crowell MD. High-resolution manometry in the evaluation of anorectal disorders: a simultaneous comparison with water-perfused manometry. Am J Gastroenterol. 2007;102:850–5.
47. Barnett JL, Hasler WL, Camilleri M. American Gastroenterological Association medical position statement on anorectal testing techniques. American Gastroenterological Association. Gastroenterology. 1999;116:732.
48. Remes-Troche JM, Paulson J, Attaluri A, et al. A comprehensive assessment of the efferent motor pathways to the anorectum in humans. Neuorgastroenterol Motil. 2007;19:330.
49. Hayden DM, Weiss EG. Fecal incontinence: etiology, evaluation, and treatment. Clin Colon Rectal Surg. 2011;24(1):64–70.
50. Hobson AR, Aziz Q. Brain imaging and functional gastrointestinal disorders: has it helped our understanding? Gut. 2004;53:1198–206.
51. Hobday DI, Hobson AR, Sarkar S, et al. Cortical processing of human gut sensation: an evoked potential study. Am J Physiol Gastrointest Liver Physiol. 2002;283:335–9.
52. Chan YK, Herkes GK, Badcock C, et al. Alterations in cerebral potentials evoked by rectal distension in irritable bowel syndrome. Am J Gastroenterol. 2001;96:2413–7.
53. Sinhamahaptra P, Saha SP, Chowdhury A, et al. Visceral afferent hypersensitivity in irritable bowel syndrome – evaluation by cerebral evoked potential after rectal stimulation. Am J Gastroenterol. 2001;96:2150–7.
54. Person B, Wexner SD. Advances in the surgical treatment of faecal incontinence. Surg Innovation. 2005;12(1):7–21.
55. Barber MD, Bremer RE, Thor KB, Dolber PC, Kuehl TJ, Coates KW. Innervation of the female levator ani muscles. Am J Obstet Gynecol. 2002;187(1):64–71.
56. Grigorescu BA, Lazarou G, Olson T, Downie SA, Powers K, Greston WM, Mikhail MS. Innervation of the levator ani muscles: description of the nerve branches to the pubococcygeus, iliococcygeus, and puborectalis muscles. Int Urogynecol J. 2008;19:107–16.
57. Chan CLH, Ponsford S, Scott SM, Swash M, Lunniss PJ. Contribution of the pudendal nerve to sensation of the distal rectum. Br J Surg. 2005;92:859–65.
58. Matzel KE, Schmidt RA, Tanagho EA. Neuroanatomy of the striated muscular anal continence mechanism. Dis Colon Rectum. 1990;33(8):666–73.
59. Fowler CJ, Swinn MJ, Goodwin RJ, Oliver S, Craggs M. Studies of the latency of pelvic floor contraction during peripheral nerve evaluation show that the muscle response is reflexly mediated. J Urol. 2000;163:881–3.
60. Chancellor MB, Chartier-Kastler EJ. Principles of Sacral Nerve Stimulation (SNS) for the treatment of bladder and urethral sphincter dysfunctions. Neuromodulation J Int Neuromodulation Soc. 2000;3:16–26.
61. Blok BF, Groen J, Bosch JL, Veltman DJ, Lammertsma AA. Different brain effects during chronic and acute sacral neuromodulation in urge incontinent patients with implanted neurostimulators. BJU Int. 2006;98:1238–43.
62. Abdel-Halim MR, Crosbie J, Engledow A, Windsor A, Cohen CR, Emmanuel AV. Temporary sacral nerve stimulation alters rectal sensory function: a physiological study. Dis Colon Rectum. 2011; 54:1134–40.
63. Gourcerol G, Vitton V, Leroi AM, Michot F, Abysique A, Bouvier M. How sacral nerve stimulation works in patients with faecal incontinence. Colorectal Dis Off J Assoc Coloproctol Great Britain Ireland. 2011;13:e203–11.
64. Dinning PG, Fuentealba SE, Kennedy ML, Lubowski DZ, Cook IJ. Sacral nerve stimulation induces pancolonic propagating pressure waves and increases defecation frequency in patients with slow-transit constipation. Colorectal Dis Off J Assoc Coloproctol Great Britain Ireland. 2007;9:123–32.
65. Dinning PG, Hunt LM, Arkwright JW, Patton V, Szczesniak MM, Wiklendt L, Davidson JB, Lubowski

DZ, Cook IJ. Pancolonic motor response to subsensory and suprasensory sacral nerve stimulation in patients with slow-transit constipation. Br J Surg. 2012;99:1002–10.

66. Leroi AM, Damon H, Faucheron JL, Lehur PA, Siproudhis L, Slim K, Barbieux JP, Barth X, Borie F, Bresler L, Desfourneaux V, Goudet P, Huten N, Lebreton G, Mathieu P, Meurette G, Mathonnet M, Mion F, Orsoni P, Parc Y, Portier G, Rullier E, Sielezneff I, Zerbib F, Michot F, Club NEMO. Sacral nerve stimulation in faecal incontinence: position statement based on a collective experience. Colorectal Dis. 2009;11(6):572–83.
67. Falletto E, Ganio E, Naldini G, Ratto C, Altomare DF. Sacral neuromodulation for bowel dysfunction: a consensus statement from the Italian group. Tech Coloproctol. 2014;18(1):53–64.
68. Benson JT. Sacral nerve stimulation results may be improved by electrodiagnostic techniques. Int Urogynecol Pelvic Floor Dysfunct. 2000;11:352–7.
69. Spinelli M, Giardiello G, Arduini A, van den Hombergh U. New percutaneous technique of sacral nerve stimulation has high initial success rate: preliminary results. Eur Urol. 2003;43:70–4.
70. Spinelli M, Giardiello G, Gerber M, Arduini A, van den Hombergh U, Malaguti S. New sacral neuromodulation lead for percutaneous implantation using local anesthesia: description and first experience. J Urol. 2003;170:1905–7.
71. Chatoor D, Emmanuel A. Constipation and evacuation disorders. Best Pract Res Clin Gastroenterol. 2009;23:517–30.
72. Borawski KM, Foster RT, Webster GD, Amundsen CL. Predicting implantation with a neuromodulator using two different test stimulation techniques: a prospective randomized study in urge incontinent women. Neurourol Urodyn. 2007;26(1):14–8.
73. Cohen BL, Tunuguntla HS, Gousse A. Predictors of success for first stage neuromodulation: motor versus sensory response. J Urol. 2006;175:2178–80; discussion 2180–81.
74. Govaert B, Melenhorst J, van Gemert WG, Baeten CG. Can sensory and/or motor reactions during percutaneous nerve evaluation predict outcome of sacral nerve modulation? Dis Colon Rectum. 2009;52:1423–6.
75. Altomare DF, Rinaldi M, Lobascio P, Marino F, Giuliani RT, Cuccia F. Factors affecting the outcome of temporary sacral nerve stimulation for faecal incontinence. The value of the new tined lead electrode. Colorectal Dis. 2011;13(2):198–202.
76. Jacobs SLF, Noblett KL. Randomized prospective cross-over study of Interstim lead wire placement with curved vs. straight stylet [abstract]. Female Pelvic Med Reconstr Surg. 2012;18:S52–3.
77. Marcelissen TA, Leong RK, Serroyen J, van Kerrebroeck PE, De Wachter SG. The use of bilateral sacral nerve stimulation in patients with loss of unilateral treatment efficacy. J Urol. 2011;185(3):976–80.
78. Scheepens WA, de Bie RA, Weil EH, van Kerrebroeck PE. Unilateral versus bilateral sacral neuromodulation in patients with chronic voiding dysfunction. J Urol. 2002;168(5):2046–50.
79. Mellgren A, Wexner SD, Coller JA, Devroede G, Lerew DR, Madoff RD, Hull T. Long-term efficacy and safety of sacral nerve stimulation for fecal incontinence. Dis Colon Rectum. 2011;54:1065–75.
80. Maeda Y, Matzel K, Lundby L, Buntzen S, Laurberg S. Postoperative issues of sacral nerve stimulation for fecal incontinence and constipation: a systematic literature review and treatment guideline. Dis Colon Rectum. 2011;54:1443–60.
81. Duelund-Jacobsen J, Lehur PA, Lundby L, Wyart V, Laurberg S, Buntzen S. Sacral nerve stimulation for faecal incontinence – efficacy confirmed from a two-centre prospectively maintained database. Int J Colorectal Dis. 2016;31:421–8.
82. Tan E, Ngo NT, Darzi A, Shenouda M, Tekkis PP. Meta-analysis: sacral nerve stimulation versus conservative therapy in the treatment of faecal incontinence. Int J Colorectal Dis. 2011;26:275–94.
83. Hollingshead JR, Dudding TC, Vaizey CJ. Sacral nerve stimulation for faecal incontinence: results from a single centre over a 10-year period. Colorectal Dis. 2011;13:1030–4.
84. George AT, Kalmar K, Panarese A, Dudding TC, Nicholls RJ, Vaizey CJ. Long-term outcomes of sacral nerve stimulation for fecal incontinence. Dis Colon Rectum. 2012;55:302–6.
85. Lim JT, Hastie IA, Hiscock RJ, Shedda SM. Sacral nerve stimulation for fecal incontinence: long-term outcomes. Dis Colon Rectum. 2011;54:969–74.
86. Wexner SD, Coller JA, Devroede G, Hull T, McCallum R, Chan M, Ayscue JM, Shobeiri AS, Margolin D, England M, et al. Sacral nerve stimulation for fecal incontinence: results of a 120-patient prospective multicenter study. Ann Surg. 2010;251:441–9.
87. Damon H, Barth X, Roman S, Mion F. Sacral nerve stimulation for fecal incontinence improves symptoms, quality of life and patients' satisfaction: results of a monocentric series of 119 patients. Int J Colorectal Dis. 2013;28:227–33.
88. Devroede G, Giese C, Wexner SD, Mellgren A, Coller JA, Madoff RD, Hull T, Stromberg K, Iyer S. Quality of life is markedly improved in patients with fecal incontinence after sacral nerve stimulation. Female Pelvic Med Reconstr Surg. 2012;18:103–12.
89. Duelund-Jakobsen J, van Wunnik B, Buntzen S, Lundby L, Baeten C, Laurberg S. Functional results and patient satisfaction with sacral nerve stimulation for idiopathic faecal incontinence. Colorectal Dis. 2012;14:753–9.
90. Jadav AM, Wadhawan H, Jones GL, Wheldon LW, Radley SC, Brown SR. Does sacral nerve stimulation improve global pelvic function in women? Colorectal Dis. 2013;15:848–57.
91. Leroi AM, Parc Y, Lehur PA, Mion F, Barth X, Rullier E, Bresler L, Portier G, Michot F. Efficacy of sacral nerve stimulation for fecal incontinence: results of a multicenter double-blind crossover study. Ann Surg. 2005;242:662–9.

92. Boyle DJ, Knowles CH, Lunniss PJ, Scott SM, Williams NS, Gill KA. Efficacy of sacral nerve stimulation for fecal incontinence in patients with anal sphincter defects. Dis Colon Rectum. 2009;52:1234–9.
93. Brouwer R, Duthie G. Sacral nerve neuromodulation is effective treatment for fecal incontinence in the presence of a sphincter defect, pudendal neuropathy, or previous sphincter repair. Dis Colon Rectum. 2010;53:273–8.
94. Koughnett JA, Wexner SD. Current management of fecal incontinence: choosing amongst treatment options to optimize outcomes. World J Gastroenterol. 2013;19(48):9216–30.
95. Drossman DA, Li Z, Andruzzi E. U.S. householder survey of functional gastrointestinal disorders. Prevalence, sociodemography, and health impact. Dig Dis Sci. 1993;38(9):1569–80.
96. Xu X, Menees SB, Zochowski MK, Fenner DE. Economic cost of fecal incontinence. Dis Colon Rectum. 2012;55(5):586–98.
97. Deutekom M, Dobben AC, Dijkgraaf MG, Terra MP, Stoker J, Bossuyt PM. Costs of outpatients with fecal incontinence. Scand J Gastroenterol. 2005;40(5):552–8.
98. Leroi AM, Lenne X, Dervaux B, Chartier-Kastler E, Mauroy B, Normand LL, Grise P, Faucheron JL, Parc Y, Lehur PA, et al. Outcome and cost analysis of sacral nerve modulation for treating urinary and/or fecal incontinence. Ann Surg. 2011;253:720–32.
99. Hetzer FH, Bieler A, Hahnloser D, et al. Outcome and cost analysis of sacral nerve stimulation for faecal incontinence. Br J Surg. 2006;93:1411–7.

10 Injectable and Implantable Agents: Current Evidence and Perspective

Carlo Ratto, Angelo Parello, Lorenza Donisi, and Francesco Litta

10.1 Introduction

Multifactorial etiology of fecal incontinence (FI) has a significant impact on the choice of management [1–3]. Sphincter lesions are considered the main cause of FI, particularly in female patients, but frequently the dysfunction occurs also in subjects with intact sphincters. In other cases, neuropathy (either peripheral or central) plays the pivotal role, causing sensory-motor alterations [2–7]. Also the severity of FI can be variable, ranging from soiling, seepage, and incontinence to gas (commonly defined as "minor incontinence") to incontinence to liquid and solid stools (defined as "major incontinence"). Despite the numerous modalities of treatment available, the therapeutic efficacy is still suboptimal for all of them. In fact, "conservative" therapies such as biofeedback have high failure rates, while the success of "minimally invasive" procedures such as bulking agents, radiofrequency, and tibial and sacral nerve stimulation or "aggressive" procedures such as anal sphincteroplasty, graciloplasty, artificial bowel sphincter, and magnetic sphincter ranges from partial success to complete failure [8].

Specifically, injection of bulk-enhancing agents into the anal canal to treat FI has continued to gain popularity. Ideally, any bulking agent for injection should be biocompatible, nonallergenic, non-immunogenic, and easy to inject and should not migrate within the tissues. Traditionally, the bulking agents have been "injected." However, more recently different materials have been introduced in clinical practice and delivered by "implantation."

10.2 Injectable Bulking Agents

Injectable agents have been firstly used for urinary incontinence (UI), with the benefit of an outpatient procedure and low morbidity rate but with variable success. Thereafter, different injectable agents have been attempted for FI.

The use of bulking agents in patients with FI is still controversial, mostly because of conflicting results and lack of agreement regarding adequate indications. Several agents have been used in patients with a wide variety of clinical conditions (weak non-lesioned anal sphincters, limited/extended sphincter lesions). Moreover, different techniques of injection have been performed. It is also debatable whether digitally guided injection is sufficiently accurate or whether endoanal ultrasound (EAUS)-guided injection should be used to significantly improve the procedure.

C. Ratto (✉) • A. Parello • L. Donisi • F. Litta
Proctology Unit, University Hospital
"A. Gemelli", Catholic University,
Largo A. Gemelli, 8, 00168 Rome, Italy
e-mail: carloratto@tiscali.it

M. Mongardini, M. Giofrè (eds.), *Management of Fecal Incontinence*,
DOI 10.1007/978-3-319-32226-1_10

10.2.1 Techniques of Injection

Several agents have been used via injection: Fat, PTQ®, Durasphere®, Coaptite®, NASHA™-Dx, Permacol®, and Bulkamid™. Different techniques of delivery have been described, providing an injection into the anal canal submucosa, intersphincteric or within the sphincter defect scar tissue; the route of injection was transanal/transmucosal, transsphincteric or intersphincteric, at different levels of the anal canal, in two, three, four, or more locations. Pre-postoperative antibiotics, as well as preoperative enemas and postoperative laxatives, have been not routinely used. EAUS seemed able to increase the reliability of the injection of bulking agents [9]. Anesthesia was variably used: no any anesthetic was administered in some studies, while local anesthesia (with or without sedation) in others; general anesthesia was used in the oldest experiences. Patient's position was either the prone, left lateral, or lithotomy.

10.2.2 Safety of Treatment

A number of adverse events have been documented following the bulking agents injection, including infection or abscess formation, ulceration of the anal mucosa, hemorrhagic events, hypersensitivity, pain, and persistent pruritus ani. Although pain is not an unusual event following surgery, it may reflect an underlying problem such as mucosal ulceration, infection, or hematoma formation at the site of injection. Some bulking agents caused granuloma (Polytef®, PTQ™) or potential carcinogenesis (Polytef®). In a recent review on 37 published papers reporting the safety data including 1001 treated patients, Hussain et al. [10] found that adverse events occurred in 139 patients (13.5 %). The most frequent complication was pain (6.5 %) and leakage of injected material (5.6 %).

10.2.3 Clinical Results

Injectable agents for FI were first used in 1993: Shafik [11] injected polytetrafluoroethylene into the anal submucosa in 11 patients and then followed up for 18–24 months. Complete continence was obtained in 64 % and partial improvement in 36 % of them. Subsequently, Shafik [12] used injection of autologous fat in 14 patients and reported 100 % success rate at 2–3 months; in particular, repeat injections allowed continence in those patients presenting incontinence to gas or stool. In this study, no complications were documented; however, other reports of autologous fat use have resulted in death from pulmonary fat embolism, and a randomized clinical trial using fat for UI demonstrated no efficacy over placebo; thus, it is currently not used for FI [13]. In the last 20 years, a number of papers have reported data concerning the clinical effects of numerous injectable agents. Although the results are greatly variable, a few considerations can be done due to those different experiences. Dilution or suspension of bulking agents makes the placement possible by injection (not always easy) and under local anesthesia. However, the major problem presented by the injectable bulking agents is the reduced efficacy due to a variable combination of degradation and/or diffusion through the tissue adjacent to the injection site or, sometimes, far or very far from that site, due to micronized dimension [10, 14, 15]. In terms of durability of results, majority of the previously used bulking agents has not documented a persistence of efficacy in the long term (more than 2 years), and, for most of them, long-term results have never been published. Agents with a diameter of 80 μm or higher should be at lower risk for migration from the injection site, but, on the other hand, agents with a larger particle size require a larger bore needle to inject and, then, at a higher risk for leakage. In a recent study Guerra and colleagues [15] evaluated 19 patients variously "injected" for idiopathic FI. These authors found that, on average, only 14 % of the originally injected volume was still detectable at EAUS performed at a median follow-up of 7 years, and the clinical improvements achieved in the short term had declined significantly.

Table 10.1 reports the summarized results of the published data.

In 2010, a systematic review [43] of the efficacy and safety of injectables for passive FI included 14 heterogeneous series (420 patients); the conclusions drawn were not definitive, although the procedure appeared safe and the improvements significant. A further systematic review [10] analyzed 31 published studies and eight meeting abstracts (1070 patients in total). Pooled analysis showed improved continence in 69.7 % of patients in the postoperative period but in only 45.2 % at the 12-month follow-up. Moreover, in a 2013 Cochrane review, Maeda et al. [14] found only four eligible randomized trials [9, 29, 30, 42], including a total of 176 patients treated with injectable bulking agents (hydrogel cross-linked with polyacrylamide, Bulkamid™ [42]; porcine dermal collagen, Permacol™ [42]; polydimethylsiloxane elastomer implants [29]; silicone biomaterial, PTQ™ [30]; and carbon-coated beads, Durasphere® [30]). Unfortunately, the authors found significant concerns of bias in all trials but one. They were unable to demonstrate a significant effectiveness of perianal injection of bulking agents due to the limited number of identified trials together with methodological weaknesses. Moreover, in a limited follow-up (maximum up to 12 months), only a short-term benefit from injections was reported, regardless of the material used as outcome measures improved over time. A silicone biomaterial (PTQ™) provided some advantages and was safer in treating FI when compared with carbon-coated beads (Durasphere®) in the short term. However, PTQ™ did not show obvious clinical benefit if compared to normal saline injection. Injections made under ultrasound guidance, compared with digital guidance, were clinically more effective. The authors' conclusions were as follows: "No long-term evidence on outcomes was available and further conclusions were not warranted from the available data. None of the studies reported patient evaluation of outcomes and thus it is difficult to gauge whether the improvement in incontinence scores matched practical symptom improvements that mattered to the patients." Reviewing the literature, Hussein et al. [10] did find that in a multivariate analysis, the use of the intersphincteric, instead of transanal or transsphincteric routes of injection, was associated with a higher complication rate. Furthermore, PTQ and Coaptite were significant predictors of short-term outcome, and the use of local anesthesia was associated with a lower likelihood of success.

More recently, another injectable material, the dextranomer in stabilized hyaluronic acid gel, has gained interest. In a multicentre trial [39], 206 patients were randomized in a 2:1 ratio between submucosal injection of dextranomer in stabilized hyaluronic acid gel or sham injection. In the treatment arm, 82.5 % of patients required a double injection to stabilize the results. Adverse events were more frequent in the treatment group. At 6 months, 52 % of patients obtained at least a 50 % reduction in FI episodes; however, surprisingly, the sham injection group showed a 31 % success rate ($p = 0.009$). Results from 112 of 132 patients in the treatment arm were updated in 2014; the same success rate (52 %) was observed at the 36-month follow-up, with significant improvement of both FI severity and QoL scores [40]. La Torre and de la Portilla [41] used the same material in 115 patients with FI and an intact EAS. At 24 months, 32 patients were withdrawn from the study, mostly owing to withdrawal of consent (17 patients), reducing the number of those with 24-month follow-up to 83. Of these, 63 % were considered responders because they experienced at least a 50 % reduction in FI episodes; significant improvement was documented for both the FI severity score and QoL. Although the long-term results from these two series, following the injection of dextranomer in stabilized hyaluronic acid gel, seem interesting, the injectable is comprised of diluted microparticles, and thus the stability of the material at the site of injection needs to be confirmed. Moreover, in these studies, the success rate was also calculated using the criterion "at least 50 % reduction in FI episodes," which is of debatable value.

10.3 Implantable Agents

Recently, a novel approach has been introduced to treat patients with FI, by the placement of implantable agents, in the form of thin cylinders,

Table 10.1 Injectable bulking agents used for treatment of FI: literature review

Agents (commercial name)	Suspension carrier	Agent diameter	Pros	Contras	Clinical results in FI	Adverse events (irrespective of use in FI)
Polytetrafluoroethylene + glycerin + polysorbate (Polytef, Teflon®)		4–100 μm (90 %: 4–40 μm)	First agent injected	Migration to the lymph nodes, lungs, kidneys, spleen, brain [16] Poor durability Chronic granuloma Potentially carcinogenic in animal [17, 18]	*Shafik* [11]: improvement in 11/11 patients	
Autologous fat			Nonallergenic Non-immunogenic	Actually not used for FI due to poor results	*Shafik* [12]: good short-term results in 14 patients	Pulmonary embolism [19, 20] Fatal stroke [21]
Glutaraldehyde collagen (Contigen®)			Easy injection Low antigenicity (~5 %) No granuloma formation Suspected disease transmission	Degradation Decreasing long-term efficacy	*Kumar et al.* [22]: short-term improvement in 11/18 patients. *Stojkovic et al.* [16]: at median 12 months follow-up, improvement in FI score in 63 % of 73 pts. No manometric variations	Suspected disease transmission
Silicone micro-balloons			Expandable micro-balloons No complications	Sterilization issues	*Feretis et al.* [17]: at 8.6 months, mean follow-up, Browning-Parks FI score from 16.6 to 5. No manometric variations	

Polydimethylsiloxane (PTQ™ Macroplastique® Bioplastique®)	Polyvinylpyrrolidone	100–450 µm or smaller		Potential migration of small particles Potential granuloma High viscosity Difficult injection Long-term pain and minor ulceration [9] Abscess [23] Pruritus ani [24]	*Malouf et al.* [18]: at 2 months follow-up, improvement in 6 t 10 pts.; at 6 months only 2 pts. with marked improvement. No manometric variations. *Kenefick et al.* ([19]; retracted): at 18 months follow-up, marked improvement in both FI and QoL in 5 out of 6 pts. No manometric variations. *Tjandra et al.* [9]: at median 6 months follow-up, improvement in FI score, QoL, and maximum resting pressure in 82 pts. *Chan and Tjandra* [20]: improvement of FI score and QoL at 3 and 12 months follow-up in 7 pts. with FI following hemorrhoidectomy. Improvement in maximum resting pressure. *van der Hagen et al.* [21]: resolution in 5 and improvement in 11 out of 24 pts. with fecal soiling. No significant variations in QoL. No manometric variations. *Gett et al.* [25]: at median 9 months follow-up, improvement in 25 pts, no changes in 7, and worsening in 5 pts. out of 37 pts. with passive FI. *Gaj et al.* [23]: at 12 months follow-up, improvement of FI and QoL in 16 pts. *de la Portilla* [24]: Improvement of FI score at 1, 3, 6, and 12 months, but not at 24 months follow-up, in 12 pts. No manometric variations. *Bartlett and Ho* [26]: at 33 months follow-up, 70 % of pts. had complete continence (CCFIS = 0) and in 30 % CCFIS decreased from 12 to 35. Improvement of QoL. Improvement of resting and squeeze pressures and anal canal length.	Pain and ulceration at the injection site

(continued)

Table 10.1 (continued)

Agents (commercial name)	Suspension carrier	Agent diameter	Pros	Contras	Clinical results in FI	Adverse events (irrespective of use in FI)
					Oliveira et al. [27]: In 35 pts CCFIS improved from 11 to 3.5. No improvements od QoL. No manometric improvements. *Maeda et al.* [28]: at 61 months follow-up, some improvement in 3 out 6 pts. *Siproudhis et al.* [29]: at 3 months follow-up, success in 5 of 22 patients (23 %) with CCFIS of 11.7 4.7; no differences in RCT compared with saline solution *Tjandra et al.* [30]: at 12 months follow-up, >50 % improvement of FI in 18 of 20 patients (90 %), significantly higher rate than Durasphere®; improvement of depression/self-perception and embarrassment; 64 % increase of max resting pressure	

Pyrolytic carbon-coated zirconium oxide (Durasphere®)	Water + β-glucan	212–500 μm	Biocompatible Non-degradable Durability	Difficult injection Migration to lymph nodes in urological patients [31]	*Davis et al.* [32]: In 18 pts., no significant benefits up to 6 months; at 12 months, significant improvement of FI scale and QoL. No manometric variations. *Altomare et al.* [33]: at median 20.8 months follow-up, improvement of FI in 10 out of 33 pts. (30.3 %). No improvement of QoL. Improvement of resting and squeeze pressures. *Aigner et al.* [34]: at 2 years follow-up, CCFIS decreased from 12.7 to 4.9 in 11 pts. Improvements of coping and embarrassment (FIQL). Improvement of resting and cough pressures at 1 year follow-up. *Beggs et al.* [31]: at 12 months follow-up, CCFIS improved from 18.7 to 10.9, and FIQL score from 46 to 55.8. Squeeze pressure increased significantly. *Tjandra et al.* [30]: at 12 months follow-up, >50 % improvement of FI in 7 of 20 patients (35 %), significantly lower rate than PTQ™; no improvement of QoL; 32 % increase of max resting pressure	Prolonged pain in 1 pt; perianal fluid collection in 1 pt.
Calcium hydroxylapatite (Coaptite ®)	Gel of sodium carboxymethyl-cellulose + glycerin + water	75–125 μm	Non-antigenic Non-inflammatory Maintenance of volume Easy injection Radiopacity		*Ganio et al.* [35]: at 12 months FU, marked improvement of FI score and QoL in 8 out of 10 pts. (80 %). Improvement of lifestyle and coping and behavior/embarrassment. Improvement of maximum resting pressure	Asymptomatic leakage of Coaptite in 1 pt.
Ethylene vinyl alcohol (EVOH)			Easy injection		*Stephens et al.* [36]: at 12 months follow-up, the FI severity index (FISI) score dropped from 32.8 to 22 CCFIS from 11 to 6.9. Improvement of 2 FIQL subscales. Some increase of anal canal length and resting pressure	

(continued)

Table 10.1 (continued)

Agents (commercial name)	Suspension carrier	Agent diameter	Pros	Contras	Clinical results in FI	Adverse events (irrespective of use in FI)
Dextranomer (Zuidex™ Deflux™ NASHA Dx – Solesta ®)	Hyaluronic acid copolymer	120 μm	Nonallergenic Non-immunogenic Nonmigratory	Degradation	*Dehli et al.* [37]: light decrease of St. Marks' FI score in 4 pts. *Danielson et al.* [38]: at 12 months follow-up, reduction of median number of FI episodes in 34 pts. *Graf et al.* [39]: in a 2:1 randomized trial (compared with sham-operation) including 206 pts, more pts treated with NASHA Dx had 50 % or greater reduction of FI episodes (52 % vs. 31 %, $p=0.009$). Similar improvements between NASHA Dx and sham in CCFIS. Higher improvement in NASHA Dx group only for coping and behavior subscales of FIQL. High retreatment rates in both groups (82 % vs. 87 % of pts). *Mellgren et al.* [40]: at 36 months follow-up, in 112 out of 132 pts treated with NASHA Dx in Graf et al.'s study (…) the same success rate (52 %) was observed, with significant improvement of both FI severity and QoL scores. *La Torre and De la Portilla* [41]: at 24 months follow-up, 32 out of 115 pts withdrawn their consent. 63 % of 83 pts had at least 50 % reduction in FI episodes. Significant improvement of both FI severity score and QoL	NASHA Dx had significantly more adverse events (proctalgia, rectal bleeding, pruritus, diarrhea, constipation, fever, rectal abscess, prostatic abscess)
Porcine dermal collagen (Permacol™)			Biocompatible Nonallergenic Durability Easy injection		*Maeda et al.* [42]: at 6 months follow-up, no any significant improvement of either FI scale or QoL in 5 pts. No manometric variations	
Polyacrylamide (Bulkamid™)	Water		Easy injection Non-reasorbable Nonmigrating Elasticity Nonallergenic		*Maeda et al.* [42]: at 6 months follow-up, no any significant improvement of either FI scale or QoL in 5 pts. No manometric variations	

FI fecal incontinence, *QoL* quality of life, *n.a.* not available

within the sphincteric complex. The THD Gatekeeper™ was the first device used, but very recently the THD SphinKeeper™ has been available for implantation.

10.3.1 Gatekeeper

Gatekeeper™ implants are made of a unique material (HYEXPAN™) that is solid at the time of delivery but slowly absorbs water and expands once implanted. Within 48 h, the prosthesis has reached its final size and shape. At this stage the consistency of the material has changed from hard to soft with shape memory, giving the implant a pliable texture that makes it compliant to external pressures without losing its original shape. For these reasons, it was decided to place the implants in the intersphincteric space, in the belief that this would achieve a more effective distribution of a presumed "bulking effect" than would be achieved with submucosal positioning, thus exploiting the physical characteristic of the implant most effectively. However, the "bulking effect" should be not the only and/or main effect contributing to the therapeutic efficacy. The intersphincteric location should also minimize the potential risk of erosion, ulceration, fistulation of the anal canal, and possible displacement of the prosthesis. This is particularly important in view of the solid state of the prostheses at the time of implantation.

10.3.1.1 Techniques of Implant

Preferably, the procedure should be performed under local anesthesia using a posterior perineal block with the patient placed in the lithotomy position. In the first preliminary experience [44], four 2-mm skin incisions were made at 3, 6, 9, and 12 o'clock positions in the perianal area 2 cm from the anal verge. With an Eisenhammer retractor inserted in the anal canal, a dedicated introducer formed by an introducer guide and an external sheath were tunneled from the skin incision to the intersphincteric margin and advanced into the intersphincteric space until the tip of the introducer reached the level of the puborectalis muscle. The introducer guide was removed, leaving the sheath in the intersphincteric space. The prosthesis was inserted into the lumen of the introducer sheath and advanced. When the prosthesis reached the middle-upper anal canal, the introducer sheath was removed, leaving the prosthesis in place. The same procedure was repeated for all four positions. All prosthesis placement steps were carried out under direct vision and under EAUS guidance. At the end of procedure, the correct positioning of the prostheses was confirmed by EAUS. All patients received oral antibiotic prophylaxis for 3 days. Following this pilot study [44], the delivery system of Gatekeeper™ implant was significantly improved (Fig. 10.1) and the implant configuration changed [45]. Six minimal perianal skin incisions were made at 1, 3, 5, 7, 9, and 11 o'clock for the implantation of 6 Gatekeeper™ prostheses. A specially designed delivery system (THD Gatekeeper™ Delivery System; THD SpA) (Fig. 10.1) was used providing the automatized implantation procedure, under visual, digital, and ultrasonographic control.

10.3.1.2 Feasibility and Safety of Implant

Some cautions were adopted (and still suggested) for an optimal implant of Gatekeeper™ prostheses, valid also for the following SphinKeeper™ procedure. Skin incisions were made about 2 cm away from the anal verge to minimize the risk of wound contamination during bowel movements. The nonlinear tunneling through the soft subcutaneous tissues to reach the intersphincteric plane from the

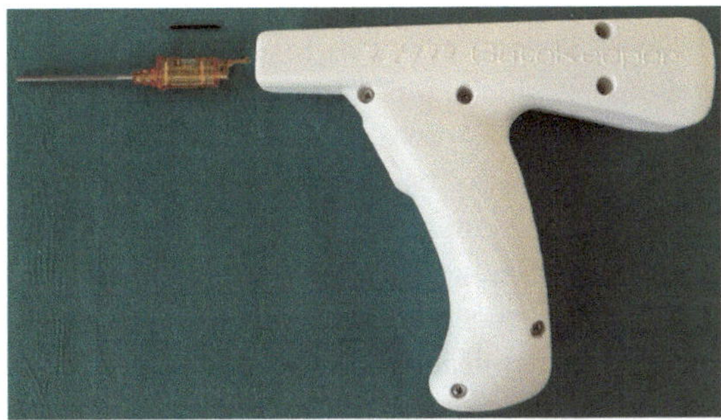

Fig. 10.1 Device for THD Gatekeeper™ implantation, including both the delivery system and dispensers in which a single prosthesis is placed

skin incision should also avoid possible prosthesis extrusion along the track. Prosthesis placement was performed under EAUS guidance, to control the procedure step by step and ensure correct positioning of the prostheses. The operator could easily reach the intersphincteric space and decide on the exact position for each implant. Moreover, the introducer could be followed by direct vision and digital palpation and visualized by EAUS. Therefore, lesions in the rectoanal mucosal/submucosal layer could be avoided. The contribution of EAUS during Gatekeeper™ placement was fundamental in guiding the prosthesis placement.

In the first report [44], the mean duration of operation to implant 4 prostheses in 14 pts was 35 ± 7 min; the procedure was easy and safe, and no intraoperative complications were observed. Moreover, neither postoperative morbidity nor prostheses dislodgement was noted. Patients experienced no anal discomfort either at rest or during defecation. The application of Gatekeeper in larger population (54 pts) in a multicentre study [45] demonstrated similar positive intra- and postoperative results. The mean duration of operation was 31.0 ± 13.4 min. In three patients (6 %), a single prosthesis was extruded spontaneously immediately after placement and was replaced. There were no postoperative complications or long-term sequelae. Throughout the entire follow-up, dislodgement of a single prosthesis was documented in three patients (6 %), but replacement was not required. At the 1- and 3-month and 1-year follow-up, EAUS confirmed that neither acute nor chronic peri-prosthesis inflammation was present.

10.3.1.3 Clinical Results

In the preliminary report [44], 14 patients (6 men, 8 women) were submitted to implant of 4 prostheses. Overall median follow-up was 33.5 ± 12.4 (range 5–48) months. All but one patient reported a significant improvement and regarded the treatment as successful. The mean total number of episodes of major FI (incontinence to liquids or solids) decreased significantly immediately after surgery, and the improvement was maintained over time, with a change from 7.1 per week before operation to 1.4, 1.0, and 0.4 per week at 1-month, 3-month, and last follow-up, respectively ($p = 0.002$). Post-evacuation soiling and ability to postpone defecation also improved significantly. Mean Cleveland Clinic FI score (CCFIS) and Vaizey score were significantly reduced at the 1- and 3-month and last follow-up ($p < 0.001$ and $p = 0.010$, respectively); only 2 of 13 patients had a CCFIS higher than 7 at the final evaluation. After implantation of Gatekeeper™, there was a significant increase in mean scores of the physical function, role-physical, general health, social function, role-emotional, and mental health domains of the SF-36. All FIQL questionnaire items showed a significant improvement in values at final follow-up compared with baseline. Mean anal manometric values did not change compared with baseline during follow-up. A slight increase was noted in mean functional anal canal length and rectal sensation, but there were no statistically significant changes. In this series the ultrasonographic surveillance for a mean of almost 3 years confirmed that none of the implants had become displaced. The ultrasound results also showed that the size of all prostheses remained virtually unchanged over time, thus confirming the durability of the Gatekeeper™. This cohort included not only patients with an intact IAS but also those with an IAS tear or both IAS and EAS defects; patients with isolated EAS defects, however, were excluded. The prostheses were placed in the same position in all patients, irrespective of the location of the sphincter lesion.

Fifty-four patients (17 men and 37 women) were enrolled in the following multicenter study [45], between June 2011 and November 2013. Preoperative EAUS demonstrated no sphincter injury in 48 patients (89 %) and an isolated IAS defect (range 30–60°) in 6 (11 %). All patients were evaluated at 1, 3, and 12 months after implantation. A statistically significant decrease of the number of FI episodes (gas, liquid and solid stools, and soiling) was observed at different follow-up stages compared with preimplantation features (Fig. 10.2). At baseline, 31 patients (57 %) could defer defecation for less than 5 min, whereas 1 year after Gatekeeper™ implantation 43 patients (80 %) had the ability to defer defecation for at least 5 min. At the final 1-year follow-up, 30 patients (56 %) had improvement of at least 75 % in all FI parameters; among them, seven patients (13 %) obtained full anal continence; using "at least 50 % improvement" criterion as the cut-off

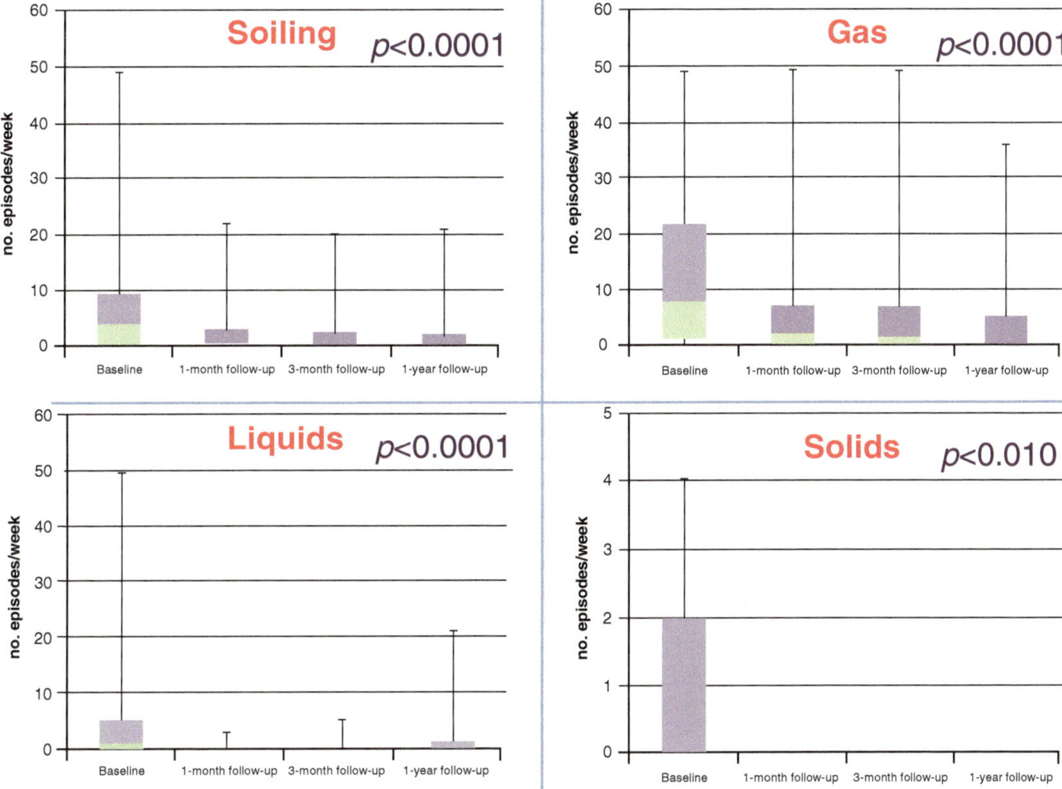

Fig. 10.2 Episodes of soiling and incontinence to gas, liquid stools, and solid stools at baseline and during follow-up after Gatekeeper™ implantation. Median values, interquartile ranges and ranges are denoted by *horizontal bars*, *boxes*, and *error bars*, respectively. An outlier (49 episodes/week at baseline) has been omitted from "solids" diagram. "Soiling," "gas," and "liquids": $p<0.001$; "solids": $p=0.010$ [45]

for success, 38 (70%) of the 54 patients would have been classified as responders. All of the scores measuring FI severity were reduced significantly throughout follow-up compared with baseline values (Fig. 10.3). Patients' QoL, as assessed throughout each follow-up stage, was significantly improved for all FIQL questionnaire items (lifestyle, coping and behavior, depression and self-perception, and embarrassment). Evaluation of the patients' generic health status (by SF-36® questionnaire) did not show any significant differences at follow-up compared with baseline.

10.3.2 SphinKeeper

SphinKeeper™ is the result of multiple innovations in the treatment of FI, concerning both the device and the implantation procedure, providing the implantation of 8–12 prostheses all around the entire circumference of the anal canal. Therefore, the title definition of "new artificial anal sphincter" was deserved. Ratto et al. have recently reported preliminary results (concerning only feasibility and safety of the implant procedure) of using the new device (always providing 10 implants) in 10 FI patients [46]. In terms of biomechanics, SphinKeeper™ prostheses have been made of the same material of Gatekeeper™. Also the site of placement (in the intersphincteric space at the upper-middle thirds of the anal canal) has been replicated, where, physiologically, the rectoanal inhibitory reflex is elicited, starting the cascade of defecation events. Again the placement has been performed under the guidance of EAUS using similar technology of delivery than Gatekeeper™ implant (Figs. 10.4 and 10.5). The ultimate model of prostheses have been long

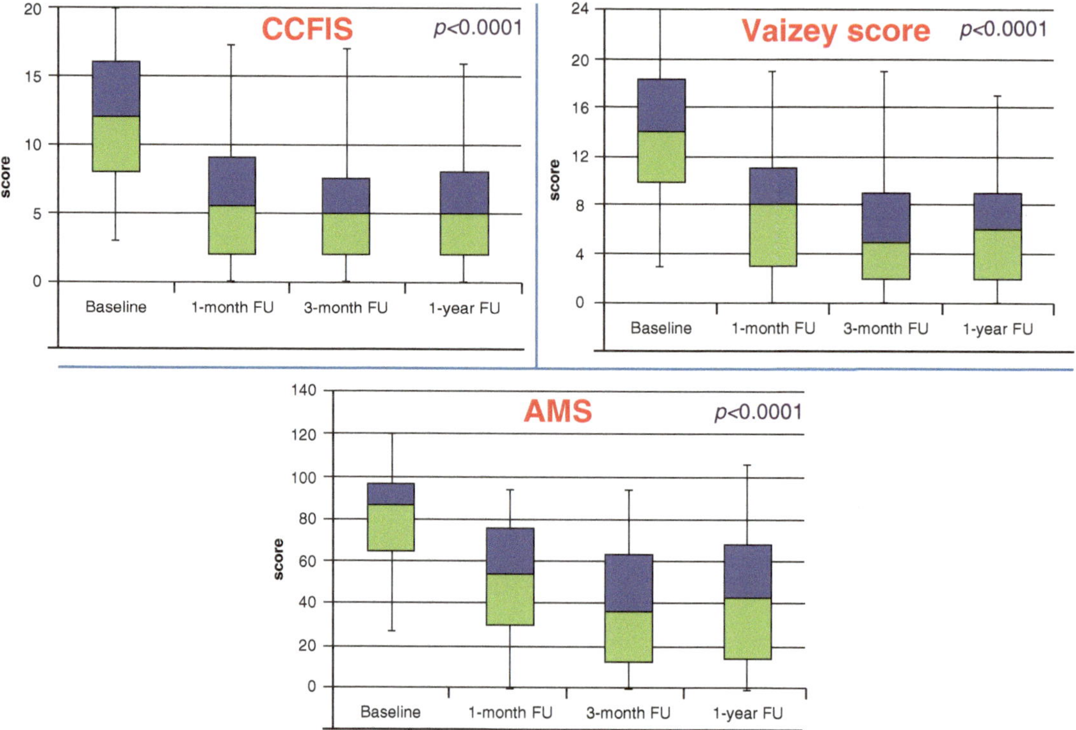

Fig. 10.3 Fecal incontinence severity scores at baseline and during follow-up after Gatekeeper™ implantation: Cleveland Clinic Fecal Incontinence Score (CCFIS), Vaizey score, and American Medical Systems (AMS) score. Median values, interquartile ranges, and ranges are denoted by *horizontal bars*, *boxes*, and *error bars*, respectively. "CCFIS," "Vaizey," and "AMS": $p<0.001$ [45]

enough (23 mm in the final length) to reconstitute the normal anal canal length and wide enough (7 mm in the final diameter) to ensure a significant filling ability. Compared to Gatekeeper™, in SphinKeeper™ the higher number of prostheses implanted reached a very high final volume of implanted material (8650 mm^3, approximately 480 % increase in size of the native sphincter), surrounding the anal canal and playing the role of an "additional" sphincter. Moreover, it was documented the expansion of SphinKeeper™ prostheses also within the scar tissue, giving the opportunity to treat also patients with sphincter defects. These aspects should be further investigated in large number of patients.

As regards postoperative complications, SphinKeeper™ implant was very safe in this study; in fact, no acute sepsis at the site of implantation and around the prostheses was documented within 90-day period. No patient had long-lasting symptoms (including anorectal pain and discomfort) directly or indirectly related to the implanted prostheses. On the other hand, no obstruction developed during the stool passage.

10.3.3 Mechanisms of Action of Implantable Agents

The changes in the sphincter anatomy due to the Gatekeeper™ and SphinKeeper™ implantation (as confirmed by endosonographic imaging) are expected to play a physiologic role. The hypothetical positive interaction between the prostheses and the adjacent IAS and EAS is interesting. Under physiological conditions, central input (neural drive to the muscle) and muscle length (microscopically, sarcomere length) are the key determinants of tension and force generated by the skeletal muscles [46]. It has been well demonstrated that EAS muscle operates at a short sarcomere length in both rabbits and humans; in other

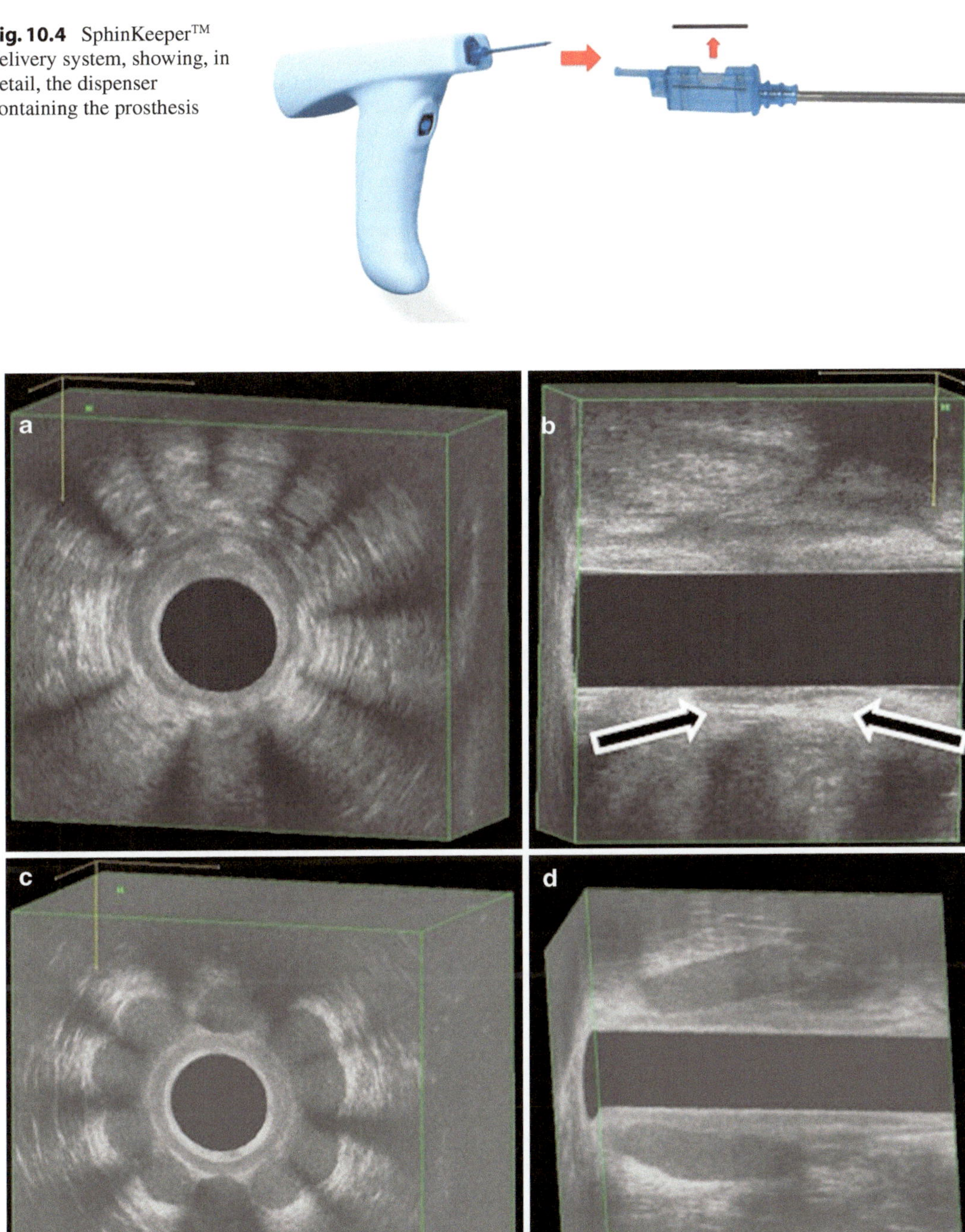

Fig. 10.4 SphinKeeper™ delivery system, showing, in detail, the dispenser containing the prosthesis

Fig. 10.5 3D-endoanal ultrasound showing the implanted SphinKeeper™ prostheses as imaged at the end of operation (**a**, **b**) and 1 week after (**c**, **d**)

words, increasing its in vivo length increases its contraction [47–51]. Hypothetically, the large volume of Gatekeeper™ and, much more, SphinKeeper™ implants, placed between EAS and IAS (pushing the EAS outward and the IAS inward), may increase the muscle fiber length and therefore increase their contractility. Further studies will definitely elucidate this mechanism of action. These properties make of Gatekeeper™ and, much more, SphinKeeper™ an attractive alternative to the "external" artificial anal sphincters (ABS, i.e., artificial bowel sphincter, dynamic graciloplasty, slings, magnetic anal sphincter). In fact, in the case of ABS and dynamic graciloplasty, only the release of the closure system, operated by the patient, can permit the defecation, while, in the case of anal slings and magnetic anal sphincter, the pressure of the rectal content allows the anal canal opening. The implantable agents, as embedded into the anal canal, may improve sphincter contractility by increasing sarcomere length as well as increase the length of the anal canal and provide a powerful "bulking effect."

Following this hypothesis, in patients with loose, patulous, funnel-like, or keyhole-shaped anal canal, SphinKeeper™ could offer the opportunity to reconstitute the cylindrical shape of the anal canal, while in patients with sphincteric lesions, it could reinforce the area of scarring improving the contribution to the continence by the remaining intact sphincters. Finally, not insignificant could be the role played by Gatekeeper™ or, much better, by SphinKeeper™ as adjunctive therapy in patients with incomplete resolution of symptoms after other procedures for FI.

References

1. Paquette IM, Varma MG, Kaiser AM, Steele SR, Rafferty JF. The American Society of Colon and Rectal Surgeons' clinical practice guideline for the treatment of fecal incontinence. Dis Colon Rectum. 2015;58:623–36.
2. Hayden DM, Weiss EG. Fecal incontinence: etiology, evaluation, and treatment. Clin Colon Rectal Surg. 2011;24:64–70.
3. Hull T. Fecal incontinence. Clin Colon Rectal Surg. 2007;20:118–24.
4. Brown HW, Wexner SD, Segall MM, Brezoczky KL, Lukacz ES. Accidental bowel leakage in the mature women's health study: prevalence and predictors. Int J Clin Pract. 2012;66:1101–8.
5. Brown HW, Wexner SD, Lukacz ES. Factors associated with care seeking among women with accidental bowel leak-age. Female Pelvic Med Reconstr Surg. 2013;19:66–71.
6. Bharucha AE, Fletcher JG, Melton LJ, Zinsmeister AR. Obstetric trauma, pelvic floor injury and fecal incontinence: a population-based case-control study. Am J Gastroenterol. 2012;107:902–11.
7. Nelson RL. Epidemiology of fecal incontinence. Gastroenterology. 2004;126:S3–7.
8. Van Koughnett JA, Wexner SD. Current management of fecal incontinence: choosing amongst treatment options to optimize outcomes. World J Gastroenterol. 2013;19:9216–30.
9. Tjandra JJ, Lim JF, Hiscock R, Rajendra P. Injectable silicone biomaterial for fecal incontinence caused by internal anal sphincter dysfunction is effective. Dis Colon Rectum. 2004;47:2138–46.
10. Hussain ZI, Lim M, Stojkovic SG. Systematic review of perianal implants in the treatment of faecal incontinence. Br J Surg. 2011;98:1526–36.
11. Shafik A. Polytetrafluoroethylene injection for the treatment of partial fecal incontinence. Int Surg. 1993;78:159–61.
12. Shafik A. Perianal injection of autologous fat for treatment of sphincteric incontinence. Dis Colon Rectum. 1995;38:583–7.
13. Lee PE, Kung RC, Drutz HP. Periurethral autologous fat injection as treatment for female stress urinary incontinence: a randomized double-blind controlled trial. J Urol. 2001;165:153–8.
14. Maeda Y, Laurberg S, Norton C. Perianal injectable bulking agents as treatment for faecal incontinence in adults. Cochrane Database Syst Rev. 2013;(2):CD007959.
15. Guerra F, La Torre M, Giuliani G, Coletta D, Amore Bonapasta S, Velluti F, et al. Long-term evaluation of bulking agents for the treatment of fecal incontinence: clinical outcomes and ultrasound evidence. Tech Coloproctol. 2015;19:23–7.
16. Stojkovic SG, Lim M, Burke D, Finan PJ, Sagar PM. Intraanal collagen injection for the treatment of faecal incontinence. Br J Surg. 2006;93:1514–8.
17. Feretis C, Benakis P, Dailianas A, Dimopoulos C, Mavrantonis C, Stamou KM, Manouras A, Apostolidis N, Androulakis G. Implantation of microballoons in the management of fecal incontinence. Dis Colon Rectum. 2001;44:1605–9.
18. Malouf AJ, Vaizey CJ, Norton CS, et al. Internal anal sphincter augmentation for fecal incontinence using injectable silicone biomaterial. Dis Colon Rectum. 2001;44:595–600.
19. Kenefick NJ, Vaizey CJ, Malouf AJ, et al. Injectable silicone biomaterial for faecal incontinence due to internal anal sphincter dysfunction. Gut. 2002;51:225–8. Retraction in: Kenefick NJ, Vaizey CJ, Malouf AJ et al. Gut. 2006;55:1824.
20. Chan MK, Tjandra JJ. Injectable silicone biomaterial (PTQ) to treat fecal incontinence after hemorrhoidectomy. Dis Colon Rectum. 2006;49:433–9.
21. van der Hagen SJ, van Gemert WG, Baeten CG. PTQ implants in the treatment of faecal soiling. Br J Surg. 2007;94:222–3.
22. Kumar D, Benson MJ, Bland JE. Glutaraldehyde cross-linked collagen in the treatment of faecal incontinence. Br J Surg. 1998;85:978–9.
23. Gaj F, Trecca A, Crispino P. Efficacy of PTQ agent in the treatment of faecal incontinence. Chir Ital. 2007;59:355–9.

24. de la Portilla F, Fernandez A, Leon E, Rada R, et al. Evaluation of the use of PTQ(™) implants for the treatment of incontinent patients due to internal anal sphincter dysfunction. Colorectal Dis. 2008;10: 89–94.
25. Gett RM, Gyorki D, Keck J, et al. Managing faecal incontinence: the role of PTQ injections. ANZ J Surg. 2007;77 suppl 1:A16.
26. Bartlett L, Ho YH. Ptq anal implants for the treatment of faecal incontinence. Br J Surg. 2009;96:1468–75.
27. Oliveira LC, Neves Jorge JM, Yussuf S, Habr-Gama A, Kiss D, Cecconello I. Anal incontinence improvement after silicone injection may be related to restoration of sphincter asymmetry. Surg Innov. 2009;16:155–61.
28. Maeda Y, Vaizey CJ, Kamm MA. Long-term results of perianal silicone injection for faecal incontinence. Colorectal Dis. 2007;9:357–61.
29. Siproudhis L, Morcet J, Lainè F. Elastomer implants in faecal incontinence: a blind, randomized placebo-controlled study. Aliment Pharmacol Ther. 2007;25:1125–32.
30. Tjandra JJ, Chan MK, Yeh HC. Injectable silicone biomaterial (PTQ) is more effective than carbon-coated beads (Durasphere) in treating passive faecal incontinence – a randomized trial. Colorectal Dis. 2009;11:382–9.
31. Beggs AD, Irukulla S, Sultan AH, Ness W, Abulafi AM. A pilot study of ultrasound guided durasphere injection in the treatment of faecal incontinence. Colorectal Dis. 2010;12:935–40.
32. Davis K, Kumar D, Poloniecki J. Preliminary evaluation of an injectable anal sphincter bulking agent (Durasphere) in the management of faecal incontinence. Aliment Pharmacol Ther. 2003;18:237–43.
33. Altomare DF, La Torre F, Rinaldi M, Binda GA, Pescatori M. Carbon-coated microbeads anal injection in outpatient treatment of minor fecal incontinence. Dis Colon Rectum. 2008;51:432–5.
34. Aigner F, Conrad F, Margreiter R, Oberwalder M, Group CW. Anal submucosal carbon bead injection for treatment of idiopathic fecal incontinence: a preliminary report. Dis Colon Rectum. 2009;52:293–8.
35. Ganio E, Marino F, Giani I, et al. Injectable synthetic calcium hydroxylapatite ceramic microspheres (Coaptite) for passive fecal incontinence. Dis Colon Rectum. 2008;12:99–102.
36. Stephens JH, Rieger NA, Farmer KC, Bell SW, Hooper JE, Hewett PJ. Implantation of ethylene vinyl alcohol copolymer for faecal incontinence management. ANZ J Surg. 2010;80:324–30.
37. Dehli T, Lindsetmo RO, Mevik K, Vonen B. Anal incontinence – assessment of a new treatment. Tidsskr Nor Laegeforen. 2007;127:2934–6.
38. Danielson J, Karlbom U, Sonesson AC, Wester T, Graf W. Submucosal injection of stabilized nonanimal hyaluronic acid with dextranomer: a new treatment option for fecal incontinence. Dis Colon Rectum. 2009;52:1101–6.
39. Graf W, Mellgren A, Matzel KE, Hull T, Johansson C, Bernstein M, NASHA Dx Study Group. Efficacy of dextranomer in stabilised hyaluronic acid for treatment of faecal incontinence: a randomised, sham-controlled trial. Lancet. 2011;377:997–1003.
40. Mellgren A, Matzel KE, Pollack J, Hull T, Bernstein M, Graf W, Nasha Dx Study Group. Long-term efficacy of NASHA Dx injection therapy for treatment of fecal incontinence. Neurogastroenterol Motil. 2014;26:1087–94.
41. La Torre F, de la Portilla F. Long-term efficacy of dextranomer in stabilized hyaluronic acid (NASHA/Dx) for treatment of faecal incontinence. Colorectal Dis. 2013;15:569–74.
42. Maeda Y, Vaizey CJ, Kamm MA. Pilot study of two new injectable bulking agents for the treatment of faecal incontinence. Colorectal Dis. 2008;10:268–72.
43. Luo C, Samaranayake CB, Plank LD, Bissett IP. Systematic review on the efficacy and safety of injectable bulking agents for passive faecal incontinence. Colorectal Dis. 2010;12:296–303.
44. Ratto C, Parello A, Donisi L, Litta F, De Simone V, Spazzafumo L, Giordano P. Novel bulking agent for faecal incontinence. Br J Surg. 2011;98(11): 1644–52.
45. Ratto C, Buntzen S, Aigner F, Altomare DF, Heydari A, Donisi L, Lundby L, Parello A. Multicentre observational study of Gatekeeper for faecal incontinence. Br J Surg. 2016;103(3):290–9.
46. Gordon AM, Huxley AF, Julian FJ. The variation in isometric tension with sarcomere length in vertebrate muscle fibres. J Physiol. 1966;184:170–92.
47. Rajasekaran MR, Jiang Y, Bhargava V, et al. Length-tension relationship of the external anal sphincter muscle: implications for the anal canal function. Am J Physiol Gastrointest Liver Physiol. 2008;295: G367–73.
48. Rajasekaran MR, Jiang Y, Bhargava V, Ramamoorthy S, Lieber RL, Mittal RK. Sustained improvement in the anal sphincter function following surgical plication of rabbit external anal sphincter muscle. Dis Colon Rectum. 2011;54:1373–80.
49. Mittal RK, Sheean G, Padda BS, Lieber R, Rajasekaran MR. The external anal sphincter operates at short sarcomere length in humans. Neurogastroenterol Motil. 2011;23:643 (e258).
50. Rajasekaran MR, Jiang Y, Bhargava V, Lieber RL, Mittal RK. Novel applications of external anal sphincter muscle sarcomere length to enhance the anal canal function. Neurogastroenterol Motil. 2011;23:70–5 (e7).
51. Kim YS, Weinstein M, Raizada V, et al. Anatomical disruption and length-tension dysfunction of anal sphincter complex muscles in women with fecal incontinence. Dis Colon Rectum. 2013;56:1282–9.

11 Artificial Bowel Sphincter

Filippo La Torre, Giuseppe Giuliani, Diego Coletta, Francesco Guerra, and Marco La Torre

Abbreviations

ABS Artificial bowel sphincter
FI Fecal incontinence

11.1 Introduction

Given the complexity and the multiplicity of factors involved on fecal incontinence etiology, in the last 20 years, several procedures, less or more invasive, have been developed to improve the strategy of FI treatment.

Although the treatment of medically refractory severe FI remains challenging, to date, FI surgery is still young, associated with elevated morbidity and with variable long-term outcomes [1]. Among the different surgical approaches, the artificial bowel sphincter (ABS) is still considered an optional treatment together with dynamic graciloplasty and sacral nerve stimulation (SNS) for refractory conservative treatment and severe FI.

Christiansen and Lorentzen, for the first time, reported in 1987 a perianal implantation of an artificial urinary sphincter (AMS 800, America Medical System) for a patient with fecal incontinence [2].

In 1996 a paper of Lehur and colleagues described the results obtained with an artificial bowel sphincter designed specifically for FI (Acticon Neosphincter – American Medical System) [3].

To date, despite the good results reported in literature, in terms of improved continence and quality of life, the rate of surgical explantation and procedures for infections of ABS still remains high [4]. These were the reasons that reduced a wide acceptance of ABS in coloproctology practice.

In accordance with Wexner et al., the cumulative risk of device explant increases with time but less dramatically in the longer follow-up [5]. Moreover, Wong et al. have shown, in long-term follow-up, as after explantation for infection the reimplantation can be performed without difficulty [6].

The aim of this chapter is to describe the indications, the technical approach for implantation, and finally the results reported by the literature on ABS.

11.2 Indications and Technique

ABS implantation represents the last resort after failure of conservative and less-invasive surgical procedures in fecal incontinence [7].

F. La Torre (✉) • G. Giuliani • D. Coletta • F. Guerra • M. La Torre
DEA – Department of Surgical Sciences, SAPIENZA Rome University, Policlinico Umberto I, Viale del Policlinico 155, 00161 Rome, Italy
e-mail: filippo.latorre@uniroma1.it

M. Mongardini, M. Giofrè (eds.), *Management of Fecal Incontinence*,
DOI 10.1007/978-3-319-32226-1_11

Colostomy can be considered the real final option if also the ABS fails. It is best indicated for patients with substantial sphincter injury or with sphincter surgically excised for patients with congenital malformation or with significant neurological dysfunction [8]. In order to achieve long-term satisfying results and to use the device completely and competently, potential candidates must not have recent or active perineal infection and should not have manual limitations [9, 10].

Artificial sphincter was used before for treating urinary incontinence and later modified for fecal incontinence. The ABS, Acticon Neosphincter (American Medical Systems, Minnetonka, MN, USA), aims to control incontinence by mimicking the natural action of the sphincter muscle. The device composed of three components: an inflatable cuff that serves as the new sphincter and occludes the anal canal, a control pump, and a pressure-regulating balloon that also functions as a fluid reservoir connected by two special tubes system [11]. The patient is placed in the lithotomy position under general anesthesia. The cuff is positioned creating a tunnel around the rectum; the balloon is implanted anterior to the bladder in the space of Retzius and the pump is inserted into the major labia in women or inside the scrotum in men [3, 10, 12, 13]. The purpose of the device is to take over from the muscle to control the opening and closing of the anus. When a patient wishes to defecate, the bulb on the control pump is manually squeezed and released several times. This transfers the fluid from the cuff to the balloon through the tube, thereby deflating the cuff and allowing the stool to pass. Pressure from the balloon slowly forces the fluid back into the cuff over several minutes and consequently closes the anus regaining continence [14]. Antibiotic prophylaxis is recommended also after surgery for a few days. It is advised to activate the implanted device at least 2 months after the operation to ensure complete wound healing and consolidate the prevesical space made to house the pressure balloon [12, 15, 16].

11.3 Results

The safety and efficacy of ABS have been evaluated in terms of effectiveness for the treatment of fecal incontinence and in terms of outcomes related to the implantation of the device. The effectiveness in treating fecal incontinence has been evaluated studying the efficacy in controlling the fecal incontinence episodes, the quality of life (QOL), the anal pressure data (anal manometry), and the percentage of functioning device at the end of follow-up. The outcomes related to the implantation of the device are studied as surgical revision and explant of the device, infection, erosion or local ulceration, and evacuatory difficulty [4, 15].

11.3.1 Device-Related Outcomes

There were no mortality cases related to the ABS implantation [4].

Complications were treated with observation excluding only one major complication of a total colectomy due to pseudomembranous colitis after implantation [17]. Most other complications were treated with antibiotics, device revision, replacement, or explantation.

Surgical revision was defined as the total number of device revisions, including explantation and reimplantation. The most common reason for surgical revision was device malfunction, such as cuff rupture, balloon and pump leak, or cuff unbuttoning [17]. The surgical revision rate was 69 % when a maximum follow-up of 5 years was considered; however, when the follow-up is increased up to 5 years, the revision rate increased to 94 % of cases (range 74–99 %) [15, 18].

A definite explant was registered in 39 % of cases (range 29–49 %) with a follow-up minimum of 5 years defined as the number of patients who had undergone permanent removal of the device [4]. The most common reason of device explant was device infection and erosion [3, 5, 6, 13, 15–29].

Evacuatory difficulty at last follow-up among patients with an implanted device is a common device complication encountered by several authors and usually related to a short cuff, device malfunction, or short opening time of the sphincter. Most evacuatory difficulty was relieved by laxatives, enemas, or treatment deactivation and in a small series of cases by anesthesia, surgical revision, or admission for fecal disimpaction. The evacuatory difficulty rate was 34 % (27–42 %) and the rate of surgical revision for evacuatory difficulty was as low as 8 % [4, 15].

11.3.2 Functional Outcomes

Fecal incontinence was studied pre- and postoperatively by using different validated FI scoring methods. When Williams score was used, a substantial (>50 %) improvement in FI rate was registered; when the American Medical Systems score was adopted, the improvement rate after implantation was 63 % (45–77 %); and finally when Cleveland Clinic Fecal Incontinence (CC-FI) score was used, the improvement rate after implantation was 65 % (56–73 %). Even those patients who had a functional device at last follow-up experienced decreased continence that deteriorated with increasing time [4].

All study populations revealed significant improvements in QOL after implantation and specifically at long-term follow-up, two studies revealed considerable improvement of QOL after implantation [15, 29].

Functional outcomes intended as anal manometry data comparing resting anal pressure before and after implantation were evaluated by the majority of the published studies.

A substantial increase in resting anal pressure occurred after implantation. Five study populations compared anal squeeze pressure before and after implantation with the ABS cuff closed [23, 26, 28, 30, 31]. In three study populations [23, 28, 30], there was a considerable increase in anal squeeze pressure after implantation; otherwise, in two study populations [26, 31], there was no difference in anal squeeze pressure between preoperative and postoperative values.

11.4 Discussion

The management of severe FI that is refractory to behavioral and medical treatment remains a clinical challenge [4, 10, 32]. However, the last decade has seen dramatic advances in the field of minimally invasive procedures for FI [7, 10]. The injection of perianal bulking agents (BA) together with sacral nerve stimulation (SNS) is the most striking example of such progress. As a result, possible indications for more invasive procedures such as graciloplasty and ABS implantation are currently strictly limited to large sphincter disruptions or congenital defects in those few patients with no other viable alternatives [4, 10, 15].

Since its first implantation for the treatment of FI in 1987 [2], the use of ABSs has been reported by several groups [2, 6, 17, 19, 21–26], yielding encouraging results. Although the methods employed to assess functional outcomes have been mostly not univocal, a number of reports showed notable results in terms of continence function and quality of life. As far as continence is concerned, both manometric data and clinical scores showed to be significantly improved and well preserved over time on the short term in most cases of well-tolerated ABSs.

However, despite the initial enthusiasm, long-term outcomes are now generally considered disappointing [4, 5, 7, 27].

The first concern regarding the implantation of ABSs was noted to be the significant rate of device-related complications, mostly due to a combination of infection or erosion of the device [4, 5]. Indeed, in a recent systematic review including more than 500 patients [4], Hong and coworkers found that 5 years after the original implantation, surgical revision was required in nearly all patients and, globally, about 40 % of patients had their ABS definitively explanted. In addition, even in those patients with a functioning device, continence function seems to decrease over time [4, 5].

Finally, it is to be considered that a significant percentage of patients who receive ABS implantation may experience other adverse events such as evacuatory difficulties and chronic pain possibly requiring prolonged medications [4–6, 27].

To date, the available inherent literature fails to provide strong evidence, mostly due to the lack of well-conducted, controlled studies [4–6]. Of note, there is no analysis comparing the employ of the ABS with the dynamic graciloplasty, which should be considered the *conventional* surgical alternative [4]. Moreover, no evidence is currently available on the clinical outcomes of patients who had their device explanted so that the real effectiveness on an intention-to-treat basis cannot be assessed [5, 6]. As a consequence, it has precluded the possibility to draw definitive conclusions on the safety and effectiveness of ABS for FI and thus on its role in clinical practice. Nonetheless, taken together, all data from the inherent literature seem to suggest that ABS implantation is burdened by high late morbidity rates and significant progressive decline in therapeutic effect.

Currently, the use of the ABS to treat FI is still to be considered controversial. Its application is burdened by several safety issues and by the fact that clinical results seem to decline with time and long-term outcomes are essentially unknown.

References

1. Finlay JM, Maxwell-Armstrong C. Posterior tibial nerve stimulation and faecal incontinence: a review. Int J Colorectal Dis. 2011;26:265–73.
2. Christiansen J, Lorentzen M. Implantation of artificial sphincter for anal incontinence. Lancet. 1987;2:244e245.
3. Lehur PA, Michit F, Denis P, Grise P, Leborgne J, Teniere P, et al. Results of artificial sphincter in severe anal incontinence. Report of 14 consecutive implantations. Dis Colon Rectum. 1996;39:1352–5.
4. Hong KD, Dasilva G, Kalaskar SN, et al. Long-term outcomes of artificial bowel sphincter for fecal incontinence: a systematic review and meta-analysis. J Am Coll Surg. 2013;217(4):718–25.
5. Wexner SD, Jin HY, Weiss EG, et al. Factors associated with failure of the artificial bowel sphincter: a study of over 50 cases from Cleveland Clinic Florida. Dis Colon Rectum. 2009;52:1550e1557.
6. Wong MT, Meurette G, Wyart V, et al. The artificial bowel sphincter: a single institution experience over a decade. Ann Surg. 2011;254:951–6.
7. Lee YY. What's new in the toolbox for constipation and fecal incontinence? Front Med (Lausanne). 2014;1:5.
8. Galandiuk S, Roth LA, Greene QJ. Anal incontinence sphincter ani repair: indications, techniques, outcome. Langenbecks Arch Surg. 2009;394(3):425–33.
9. Tan JJ, Chan M, Tjandra JJ. Evolving therapy for fecal incontinence. Dis Colon Rectum. 2007;50(11):1950–67.
10. Edden Y, Wexner SD. Therapeutic devices for fecal incontinence: dynamic graciloplasty, artificial bowel sphincter and sacral nerve stimulation. Expert Rev Med Devices. 2009;6:307–12.
11. Person B, Wexner SD. Advances in the surgical treatment of fecal incontinence. Surg Innov. 2005;12(2):182.
12. Altomare DF, Dodi G, La Torre F, Romano G, Melega E, Rinaldi M. Multicentre retrospective analysis of the outcome of artificial anal sphincter implantation for severe faecal incontinence. Br J Surg. 2001;88(11):1481–6.
13. La Torre F, Masoni L, Montori J, et al. The surgical treatment of fecal incontinence with artificial anal sphincter implant. Preliminary clinical report. Hepatogastroenterology. 2004;51:1358–61.
14. Wang M, Zhou Y, Zhao S, Luo Y. Challenges faced in the clinical application of artificial anal sphincter. J Zhejiang Univ Sci B. 2015;16(9):733–42.
15. Mundy L, Merlin TL, Maddern GJ, Hiller JE. Systematic review of safety and effectiveness of an artificial bowel sphincter for faecal incontinence. Br JSurg. 2004;91(6):665–72.
16. Romano G, La Torre F, Cutini G, et al. Total anorectal reconstruction with the artificial bowel sphincter: report of eight cases. A quality-of-life assessment. Dis Colon Rectum. 2003;46:730–4.
17. Finlay IG, Richardson W, Hajivassiliou CA. Outcome after implantation of a novel prosthetic anal sphincter in humans. Br J Surg. 2004;91:1485–92.
18. Chittawatanarat K, Koh DC, Seah AA, et al. Artificial bowel sphincter implantation for faecal incontinence in Asian patients. Asian J Surg. 2010;33:134–42.
19. Ortiz H, Armendariz P, DeMiguel M, et al. Prospective study of artificial anal sphincter and dynamic graciloplasty for severe anal incontinence. Int J Colorectal Dis. 2003;18:349–54.
20. Christiansen J, Rasmussen OO, Lindorff-Larsen K. Long-term results of artificial anal sphincter implantation for severe anal incontinence. Ann Surg. 1999;230:45–8.
21. Lehur PA, Roig JV, Duinslaeger M. Artificial anal sphincter: prospective clinical and manometric evaluation. Dis Colon Rectum. 2000;43:1100–6.
22. Savoye G, Leroi AM, Denis P, et al. Manometric assessment of an artificial bowel sphincter in 12 patients. Gastroenterology. 2000;118:A1028–9.
23. Devesa JM, Rey A, Hervas PL, et al. Artificial anal sphincter: complications and functional results of a large personal series. Dis Colon Rectum. 2002;45:1154–63.
24. Ortiz H, Armendariz P, DeMiguel M, et al. Complications and functional outcome following

artificial anal sphincter implantation. Br J Surg. 2002;89:877–81.
25. Michot F, Costaglioli B, Leroi AM, et al. Artificial anal sphincter in severe fecal incontinence: outcome of prospective experience with 37 patients in one institution. Ann Surg. 2003;237:52–6.
26. Parker SC, Spencer MP, Madoff RD, et al. Artificial bowel sphincter: long-term experience at a single institution. Dis Colon Rectum. 2003;46:722–9.
27. Altomare DF, Binda GA, Dodi G, et al. Disappointing long-term results of the artificial anal sphincter for faecal incontinence. Br J Surg. 2004;91:1352–3.
28. Melenhorst J, Koch SM, van Gemert WG, et al. The artificial bowel sphincter for faecal incontinence: a single centre study. Int J Colorectal Dis. 2008;23:107–11.
29. Ruiz Carmona MD, Alos Company R, Roig Vila JV, et al. Long-term results of artificial bowel sphincter for the treatment of severe faecal incontinence. Are they what we hoped for? Colorectal Dis. 2009;11:831–7.
30. Michot F, Lefebure B, Bridoux V, et al. Artificial anal sphincter for severe fecal incontinence implanted by a transvaginal approach: experience with 32 patients treated at one institution. Dis Colon Rectum. 2010;53:1155–60.
31. Casal E, San Ildefonso A, Carracedo R, et al. Artificial bowel sphincter in severe anal incontinence. Colorectal Dis. 2004;6:180–4.
32. Ratto C, Buntzen S, Aigner F, Altomare DF, Heydari A, Donisi L, Lundby L, Parello A. Multicentre observational study of the Gatekeeper™ for faecal incontinence. Br J Surg. 2016;103(3):290–99. doi:10.1002/bjs.10050.

12 Surgical Treatments

Massimo Mongardini and Manuel Giofrè

12.1 Introduction

In the treatment of fecal incontinence, surgical invasive procedures are ordinarily reserved for patients with whom conservative or minimally invasive treatments were unsuccessful [1]. A careful selection of patients and an accurate and consistent identification of disorders, which lie at the root of the condition, are essential to the treatment's success. In cases of fecal incontinence which are associated with or caused by disease which alter the anatomy and sphincter system function, such as hemorrhoids or rectal prolapse, perianal fistula, rectovaginal fistula, and cloacal lesions, these diseases must be treated first, as their resolution often leads to an improvement in or the resolution of incontinence.

Reconstructive surgery is indicated more specifically in cases of fecal incontinence incurred by anal sphincter lesions, abnormalities, or deformities, as well as sphincter deficiency with no evident lesions and abnormalities of the pelvic floor.

M. Mongardini, MD, PhD (✉) • M. Giofrè, MD
Department of Surgical Sciences, "Sapienza" University of Rome, Viale Regina Elena 241, Rome, Italy
e-mail: massimo.mongardini@uniroma1.it; manuelgiofre@libero.it

The following are several reconstructive techniques:

- Sphincteroplasty
- Suture of the levator ani
- Reconstruction of the sphincter complex using muscle repair

12.2 Sphincteroplasty

Sphincter suture repair techniques which result in a direct repair are only indicated when lesions are located in the external anal sphincter.

The leading cause of sphincter lesions is obstetric trauma. Despite the lack of any particular continence consequences caused by parturition, 1–4 % of deliveries result in lesions of the sphincter complex or of the pelvic floor (lesions of the third and fourth degrees – see, Cap. 2) [2–5]. The main risk factors include fetus weight, surgical median incision of the perineum performed in order to ease childbirth (episiotomy), the use of forceps, and breech presentation [6–8]. Obstetric sphincter lesions can be detected immediately postpartum and are caused by third-degree laceration. In approximately 40 % of cases [9], continence disorders are detected as early as 6 months postdelivery [6]. The compensation of the pelvic muscles frequently disguises sphincter

M. Mongardini, M. Giofrè (eds.), *Management of Fecal Incontinence*,
DOI 10.1007/978-3-319-32226-1_12

function deficit; however, with time, abnormalities deviously evolve along with muscle weakening, most frequently during menopause, and are discovered years later [10, 11]. Other causes for sphincter damage are consequences related to proctological surgery and accidental trauma (road accidents, impalements, sexual abuse).

The most frequently performed surgical procedure for the treatment of obstetric lesions is direct anterior sphincter suture repair [1, 12]. Optimal timing for the repair is within 3–4 months following the trauma [2]. However, the surgical procedure is often performed years later (even if the results are less effective) when the clinical evidence of incontinence symptoms leads to ultrasound diagnosis of a previously hidden lesion.

Anal sphincter repair can be performed using the "end-to-end" technique, thereby facing the two laps after resecting scar tissue, as well as through the "overlapping" technique, which is performed by overlaying the residual functional extremities. The first technique is generally used to repair recent lesions in which a scar that has outdistanced the extremities of the muscles is not yet formed, thus allowing for the facing of the extremities without excessive tension. In long-standing lesions, the sphincter defect is often substantial, and a direct approximation of the extremities is to be avoided at all cost, as it would be invariably destined to failure.

The overlapping technique is generally quite safe for sphincter suture repair; this technique consists of the mobilization of the two muscular extremities which are subsequently overlapped. Similarly, it is appropriate to associate preanal sutures of the levator ani, used most often in the delayed repair of extended defects, as it allows for the reduction of tension on the sutures dispersing it on a greater length.

The patient is placed in a lithotomy position. The incision is made at the inferior margin level of the vagina, horizontally, in the ischium direction or circumferentially on the perianal skin along the anal anterior side (Fig. 12.1). In cases of preanal sutures of the levator ani, the rectovaginal cleavage that leads to the peritoneal floor leaves the external anal sphincter of the anus posteriorly and the vaginal flap anteriorly. The levator ani muscles are now visible laterally. Therefore, preanal sutures of the levator ani are obtained with two–three polypropylene sutures 2/0 located far behind on the muscles so as to avoid tightening the vagina and potential dyspareunia.

The anterior quadrant of the anal external sphincter, often sclerotic and with poor tropism, is then dissected (Fig. 12.2), detached from the internal sphincter, and placed on a ribbon (Fig. 12.3). The scar is followed laterally until the identification of the residual muscles/extremities is performed, on which two traction sutures can be made. When using the "end-to-end" technique, in order to restore the anatomical continuity and functional external anal sphincter as well as to restore its tension, a few approximation-interrupted sutures are needed (two or three polypropylene sutures 2/0 or 0/0, depending on the

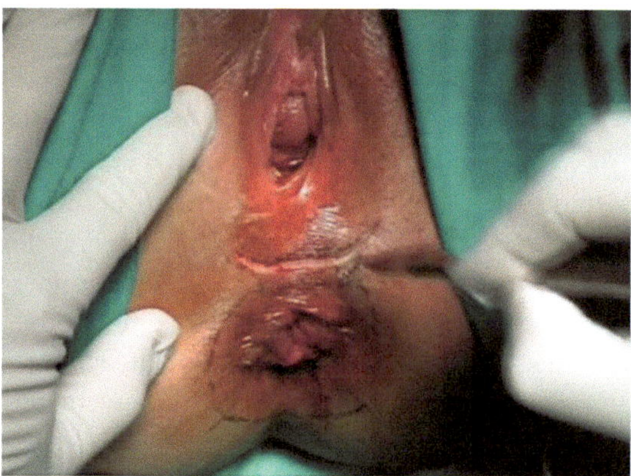

Fig. 12.1 Anterior perineal incision

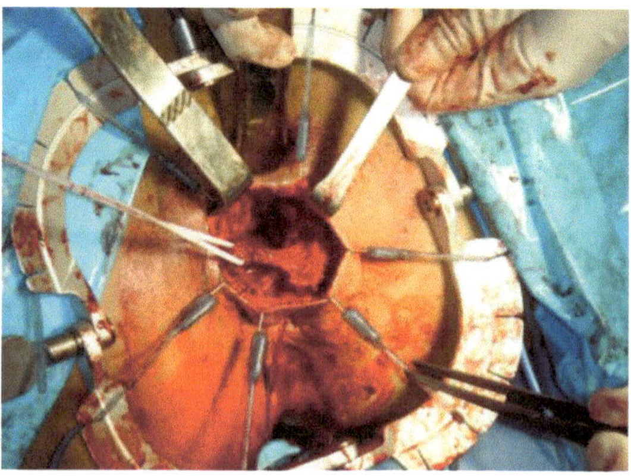

Fig. 12.2 External anal sphincter dissection

muscle fiber volume which needs to be attached) (Fig. 12.4).

When using the "overlapping" technique, the sphincter extremities are dissected by approximately 3 cm, while carefully maintaining the vascular nerves. At this point, it is possible to remove the sclerotic scar tissue, which still maintains the muscles/extremities aligned or, as is often preferred, to fold the scar in order to prevent an interfering tissue regeneration caused by the incision. By crossing the two traction sutures, the sphincter extremities are exposed as to ensure that they are sufficiently mobilized and to obtain an overlapping of at least 2 cm without tension. At this point, an overlapping structure is achieved, as is expected when using this technique (Fig. 12.5).

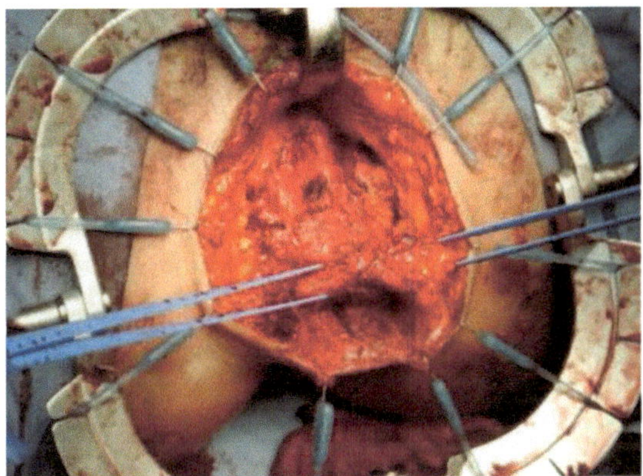

Fig. 12.3 The external sphincter is preparing and placing on two ribbons

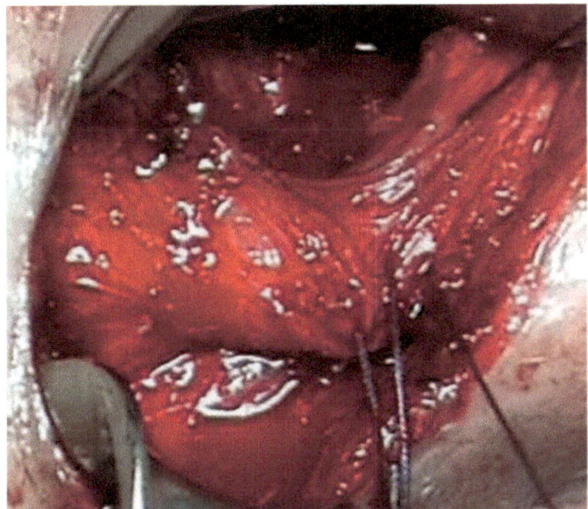

Fig. 12.4 The external anal sphincter is repaired affixing some sutures in the end-to-end technique

Before definitive closure, it is appropriate to calibrate the anal circumference by inserting the pinky finger and/or by using a 15 mm dilator. The surgical procedure is completed with subcutaneous and skin sutures. Based on the complexity of the procedure, positioning a drain can be useful. The drain will be removed within 24–48 h.

The consequences of iatrogenic or accidental trauma can affect any quadrant of anal circumference. The lesions may be identified clinically, upon observing the anal margin, scar, or the absence of radiated folds, as well as through the use of ultrasound. In such cases, the reconstructive surgical technique is identical to that of an anterior repair; however, the local conditions may vary; sclerosis is often more severe than in cases of obstetric lesions and makes identifying the muscle margins more challenging.

The short-term results of this technique have been quite favorable, with good to excellent functional results in 80 % of the cases [12, 13]. In literature, the outcomes of treated cases are controversial and differ within a range of 30–85 % [12, 14, 15]. The results are accompanied by an improvement of the manometry of the sphincter conditions [16]. In addition, postsurgical ultrasound images are compatible with the results obtained; in the event of failure, the persistence of the defect is a sign of an incomplete or an

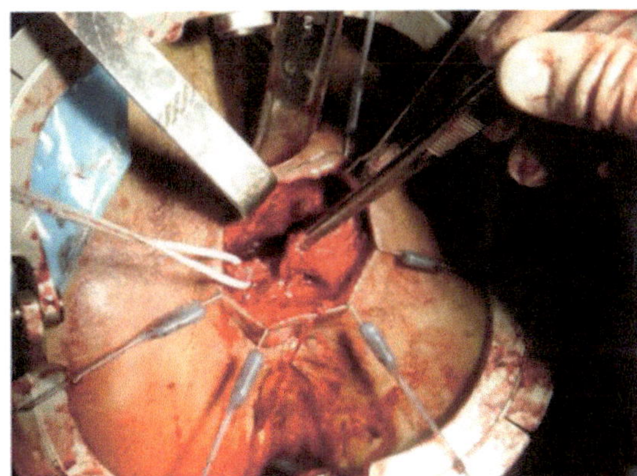

Fig. 12.5 Overlapping of 2 cm of the external anal sphincter extremities

insufficient repair [2, 17]. In cases of sphincter repair carried out at an early stage of postobstetric incontinence, the results are generally better and long lasting. Within a 5–10 year range in patients who were treated only with sphincteroplasty decades after a trauma, a gradual decline of defecatory function may be reported, with incomplete gas and solid stool incontinence. However, the level of patient satisfaction reported is 40–85 % [13, 18–22].

Lamblin (2014) reports a study of 23 female patients (at an average age of 52 at the time of treatment) who underwent a sphincteroplasty using the "overlapping" technique [12]. Six years following the repair, only 48 % of cases reported a preserved complete continence, yet 85 % of the patients consider themselves satisfied with the procedure.

Several factors can predict postoperative results. Anatomically, the localized and isolated nature of the lesions which are clinically diagnosed must be confirmed by ultrasound. According to our experience, the interrupted area should not be greater than 90–120° of the anal circumference in order to allow for an efficient repair. A sufficient and functional remaining muscle mass must be present. Furthermore, the conventionally pejorative significance attributed to aging, former duration of incontinence, and previous sphincter repair was not confirmed by recent studies [23].

In a Cochrane review from 2013, Fernando compares the "end-to-end" technique with that of the "overlapping" technique in the treatment of sphincter obstetric lesions [2]. In spite of the inhomogeneity of the data and patient recruitment from various studies, a major improvement is noted regarding fecal urgency in 6–12 months, in patients that had an overlap repair. A corresponding improvement in gas incontinence in both groups was seen (although a better result was reported at 6 months using the "end-to-end" technique). An equal Wexner incontinence score after 6 months was significantly lower after 12 months in patients who had undergone an overlapping repair, thereby suggesting a greater stability of the functional effects achieved with this technique, which seems to be less affected by deterioration. Based on the invalidating data, the authors conclude that both techniques may be used at the surgeon's discretion.

The most suitable time to perform a sphincter repair is still under debate. There are no studies which compare an immediate post-trauma repair with one carried out days or months later.

When treating lesions of a third and fourth degrees, repair is usually performed immediately postpartum. However, the data which analyze this choice does not seem to support it. Nielsen [24] reports that within 12 months after an immediate reconstruction, there is 58 % persistence of the defect evidenced on ultrasound, with 30 % of patients reporting incontinence symptoms. Walsh [25] reports 37 % of lesion persistence seen on ultrasound after 3 months and 13.5 % of incontinence. Sultan [26] finds that between 42 and 651 days after reconstruction, 85 % of cases have defects seen on ultrasound, 41 % of patients with incontinence symptoms, and 26 % experience urgency. Such data seems to imply that the primary repair tends to deteriorate within a short time and to suffer a high percentage of lesion persistence and incontinence symptoms. The edematous and traumatized tissue in immediate postpartum is most likely not suitable for a prompt reconstruction. It is preferred to allow for a complete healing of the wound, with a resolution of a potential bacterial superimposed infection that might lead to the formation of an abscesses and dehiscence. Reconstruction may be performed using an overlap repair within a few weeks and may have a greater possibility of success.

12.3 Suture of the Levator Ani

Suture repairs of the pelvic muscles, performed alone or with a sphincteroplasty, are carried out in order to treat muscle deficit or defects. The objective of this type of repair is the restoration of tension to the functionally deficient sphincter muscles through the use of plication (reefing technique). The goal is to achieve a better efficiency of continence mechanisms, thanks to anatomical modifications preformed during the procedure.

In the history of surgery, the first recommended and validated procedure was the postanal repair, presented by Parks in 1971 and subsequently modified [20]. This procedure was at first suggested to patients with neurogenic or idiopathic fecal incontinence, with no sphincter defects. Its purpose was the lengthening of the anal canal and the repair of the anorectal angle. The rationale behind this technique was that the obtuse anorectal angle should cause these types of incontinence; however, there was no proven correlation with the modification of the anorectal angle. Nevertheless, several authors have reported favorable outcomes of incontinence, however very inhomogeneous, showing success of 27–87 % [27–29]. According to Bartolo, the effect on continence is determined by levator fibrosis caused by the procedure itself and which increases resistance during the passage of stool [30, 31].

The patient is placed in a gynecological position, with the lower limbs spread wide and resting on thigh holders. After a horizontal or a "V" incision is made in the postanal area (Fig. 12.6), halfway between the anus and the coccyx and halfway between the ischial tuberosities, we proceed with the dissection of the lower edges of the internal and the external anal sphincters (Fig. 12.7). Often, these limits are not easily identified. However, the surgeon's experience and the accurate preparations of the anatomical structures rapidly lead to the identification of the various muscle components. After the incision, an intersphincteric cleavage is made in the existent embryological avascular plane between the internal muscles (originally endodermic) and the externals (originally ectodermal). This access allows lesions to be avoided in the neurovascular branches leading to the sphincters.

The midplane is prepared simply, and subsequent release is then easily executed by 180°, sectioning the rectum's longitudinal muscle fibers. Subsequently, a retractor is used in order to move the rectum anteriorly until reaching the pelvic aponeurosis of Waldeyer (Fig. 12.8). The latter is an appendix of the parietal pelvic fascia that covers and inserts on the raphe or the

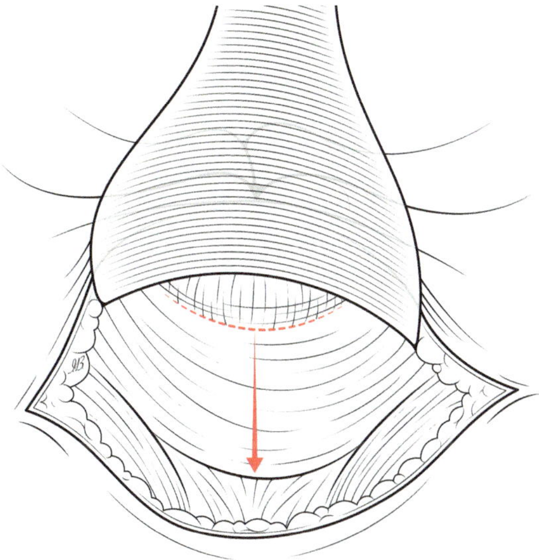

Fig. 12.7 Dissection of the lower edges of the internal and the external anal sphincter

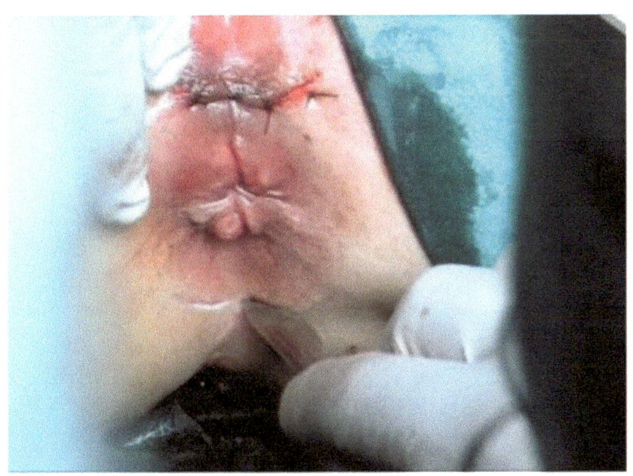

Fig. 12.6 Postanal incision

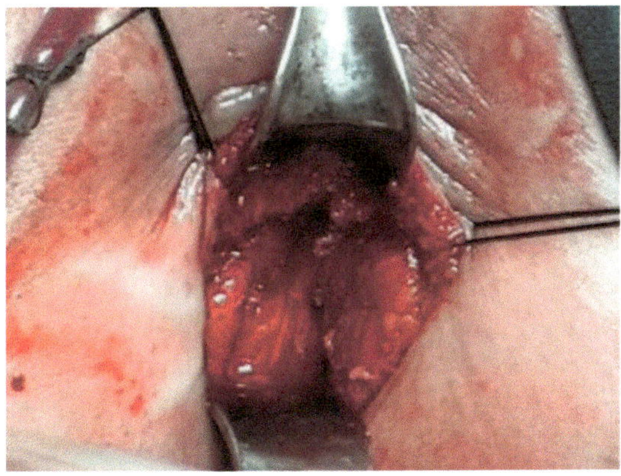

Fig. 12.8 A retractor moves the rectum anteriorly

anococcygeal ligament that runs from the distal extremity of the coccyx to the anal canal. This aponeurosis will be sectioned providing an access to the retrorectal space (Fig. 12.9).

With the finger or forceps-holding gauze, we are able to release the internal margins and the upper fascia of the levator hiatus (Fig. 12.8). We proceed to the retroanal suture performing a plication of the pelvic floor muscles in three successive planes using polypropylene 0/0. The inner plane formed by the iliococcygeal and the pubococcygeal bundles is sutured from front to back, typically using interrupted sutures (Fig. 12.10). The puborectal intermediate plane is similarly tightened and plicated with interrupted sutures (Fig. 12.11). The superficial plane of the external sphincter is plicated in the same manner (Fig. 12.12). In the past, the internal anal sphincter muscles were also anteriorly plicated. However, several studies have shown that such a procedure is worthless. At the end of the procedure, the cutaneous incision is closed, and a drain is positioned.

The anterior levatorplasty procedure is often performed to treat pelvic trauma frequently resulting from obstetric injury. We proceed by performing a curvilinear incision in correspondence with the perineum, anteriorly to the anal orifice (Fig. 12.1).

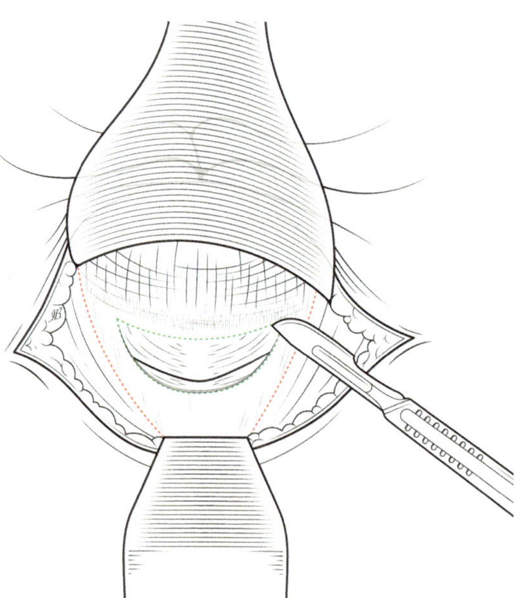

Fig. 12.9 Waldeyer's aponeurosis is sectioned providing an access to the retrorectal space

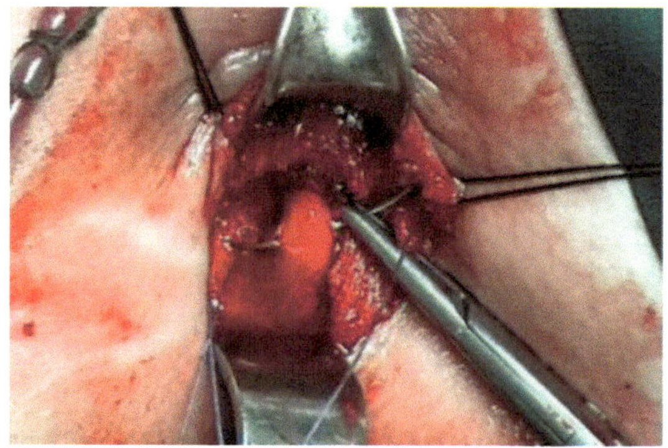

Fig. 12.10 Retroanal suture performing a plication of the pelvic floor muscles

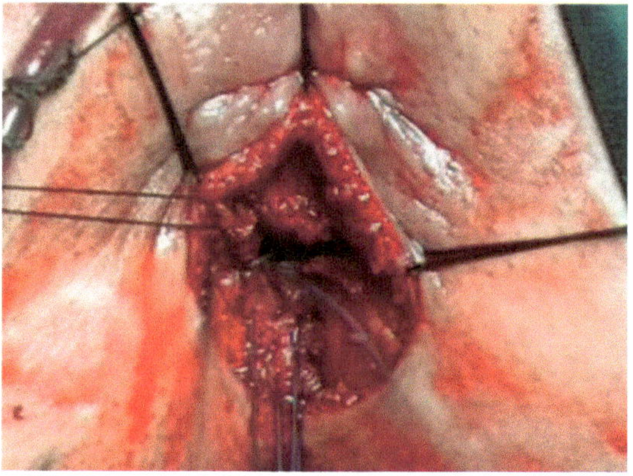

Fig. 12.11 Puborectal muscle plication

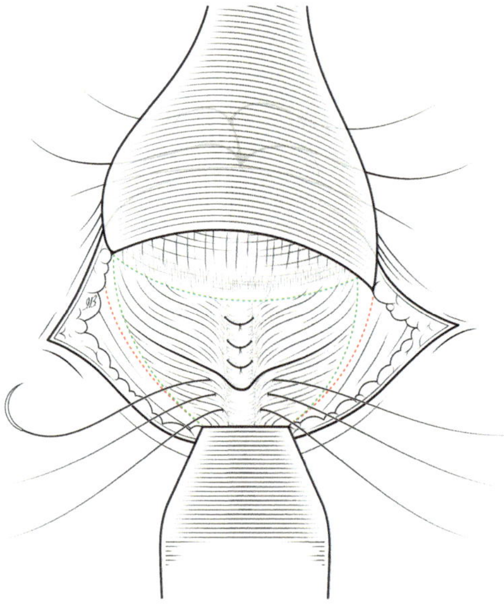

Fig. 12.12 Postanal repair

This site corresponds to the inferior margin of the vagina. Subsequently, we continue incising horizontally toward the ischium, then follow the recto-vaginal cleavage until the peritoneum is reached, leaving behind the external anal sphincter.

The intervention is preceded by a plication of the external sphincter (Fig. 12.13 – Fig. 12.14).

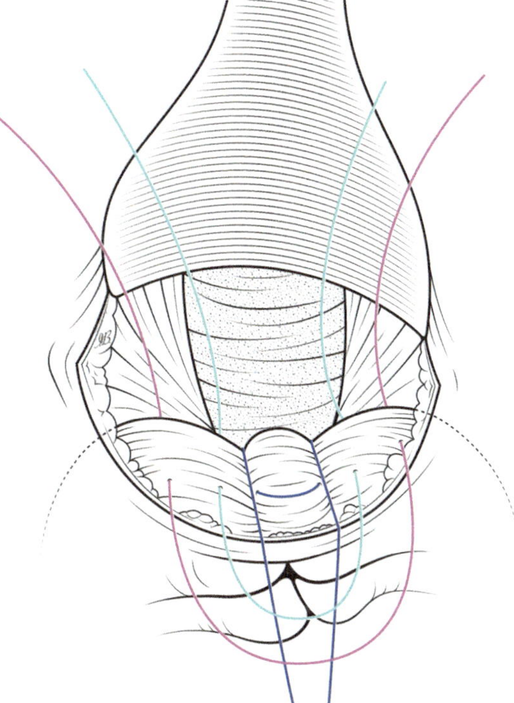

Fig. 12.13 Anterior plication of external anal sphincter

Proceeding thusly, we identify the levator muscles located on both sides of the rectum, upon which a series of interrupted sutures will be affixed and later placed in traction (Fig. 12.15).

The aforementioned sutures are needed to approximate and medialize the puborectalis muscles as well as to increase pressure applied on the anal canal (Fig. 12.16). Thus, we are able to restore tension to the pelvic muscles and reestablish fecal continence while at the same time lengthen the anal canal.

An alternate solution is the total pelvic floor repair which is performed through the merging of the two previous techniques. Typically, an anterior incision is made beginning on the inferior margin of the vagina, and subsequently the posterior stage is performed.

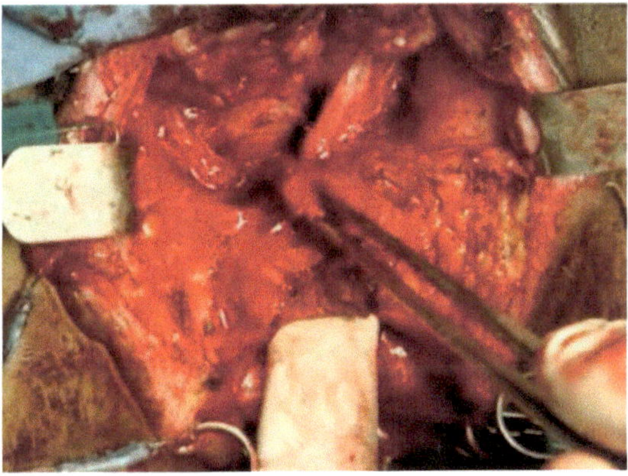

Fig. 12.14 Plication of external anal sphincter in cloacal lesion

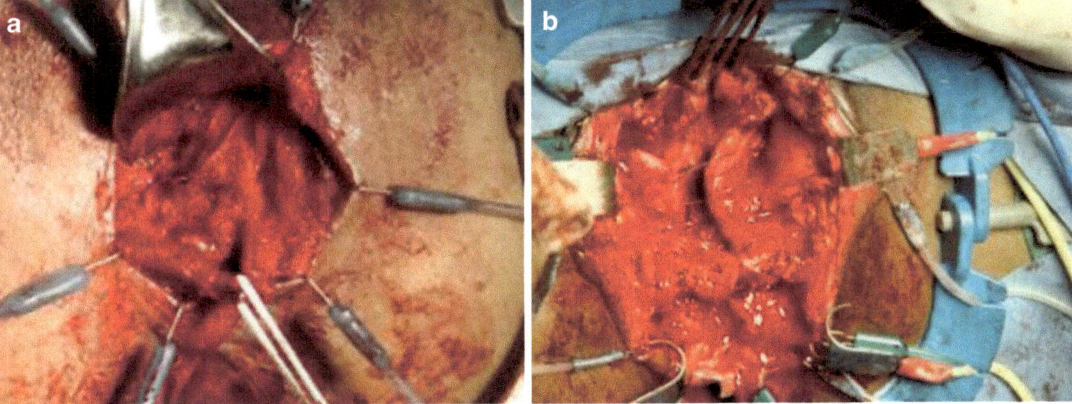

Fig. 12.15 Anterior levatorplasty with intact perineum anatomy and in cloacal lesion

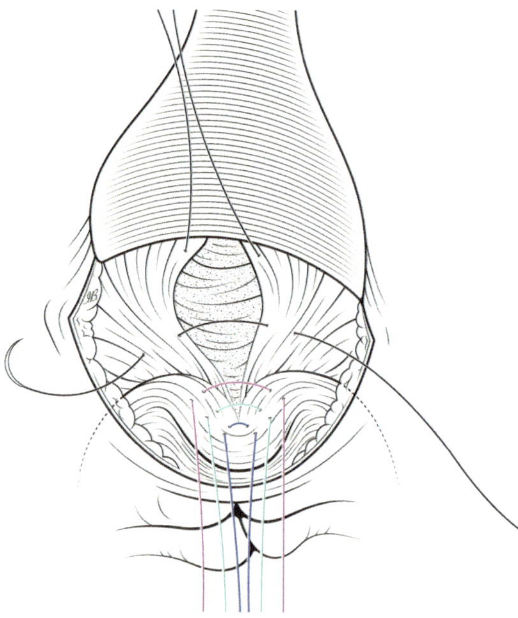

Fig. 12.16 Puborectal muscle medialization after external anal sphincter plication

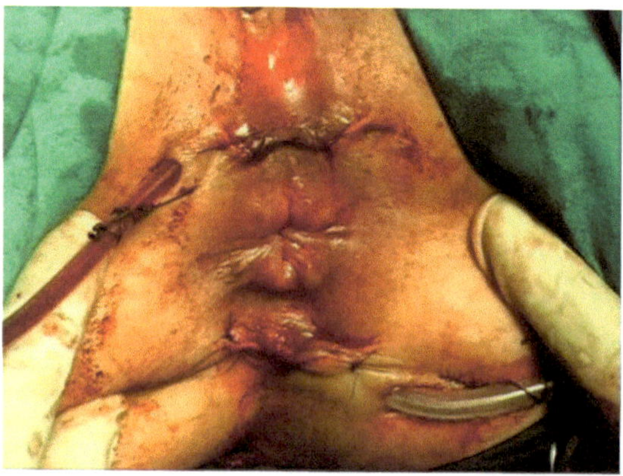

Fig. 12.17 Placement of drainages at the end of the procedure

At the end of the procedure, it is useful to place anteriorly and posteriorly a drainage (Fig. 12.17).

The muscle suture repair was invented initially to treat patients suffering from incontinence with an intact but nonfunctioning anal sphincter. The cause of this incontinence was initially unknown (idiopathic incontinence) and in the 1980s was attributed to the progressive denervation of the pelvic floor and the sphincter apparatus (neurogenic incontinence). The improvement of anal continence was dependent upon in varying degrees, and according to various authors, the lengthening of the high-pressure area, the anorectal angle accentuation, the improvement of the sphincter pressure during rest and/or voluntary contractions, and the improvement of the anal canal and the distal rectum sensibilities would allow for a better perception of the need to defecate.

12.4 Complex Sphincter Reconstruction with Muscle Repair

These types of surgical procedures are performed when an attempt to reconstruct the sphincter using the aforementioned technique has not led to any effective results. The logic behind this strategy is to recreate the anal sphincter by replacing degenerative tissue with ectopic muscle located at the perineal level or by using a prosthetic device [15].

Muscle transposition and prosthetic replacement are two different techniques, yet both utilize the same functionality: to create an area with high pressure around the terminal part of the gastrointestinal tract by tightening around the distal rectum. Muscle transposition corresponds to perianal autologous repair, which can be performed using one or both of the gracilis muscles. Another option is the muscle of the lower limb, which extends from the ischium to the knee joint, also called "rectus femoris muscle" alternatively; the gluteus maximus muscle may be used. In the past, also the palmaris longus muscle and the flexor carpi radialis muscle were used. These techniques have since been abandoned. Today, electrical stimulation is used to complete transposition [32–34].

Dynamic graciloplasty is often indicated as the type of procedure with the most favorable outcomes, above all thanks to its anatomical characteristics that predispose its transposition [34]. This surgical procedure is performed in two stages. "Graciloplasty" represents the first stage, and it begins with muscle mobilization after the patient has been placed in a gynecological position with the lower limbs properly divaricated and resting in thigh holders. The "donor" lower limb is included in the operative field. The muscle is identified through an incision made at the anatomical reference points that corresponds to the insertion of the gracilis muscle on the "goosefoot" at the level of the medial side of the anterior tibial tuberosity (Fig. 12.18).

Two to four incisions on the internal side level of the thigh allow for the mobilization of the muscle, while being careful to not damage the upper vascular pedicle, which is fundamental to the muscle's blood supply and to the positive outcomes of the procedure. A lower incision at the tibial level allows for the interruption of the distal tendon in the vicinity of its insertion on the tibial tuberosity [15]. During the dissection, it is important to mind the neural and vascular networks of the thigh. Upon concluding mobilization, the gracilis muscle will be dissected along almost the entire muscle extension and remain attached only at the proximal pedicle in correspondence with the ischial side (Figs. 12.19, 12.20, 12.21, and 12.22). Subsequently, a perianal access will be created, starting from the two lateral incisions or from the anterior and posterior incisions made at about 3 cm from the anal margin (Fig. 12.23). The tunnel must be large enough in order to allow the gracilis muscle to pass through it without being compressed (Fig. 12.24). The transposition of the muscle is performed by holding the distal

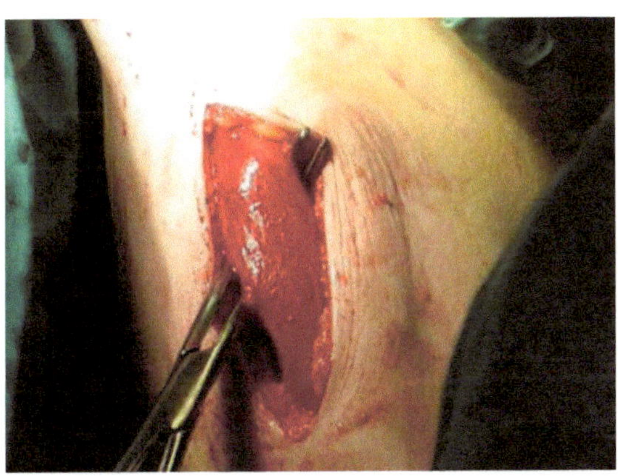

Fig. 12.18 Right Gracilis muscle identification

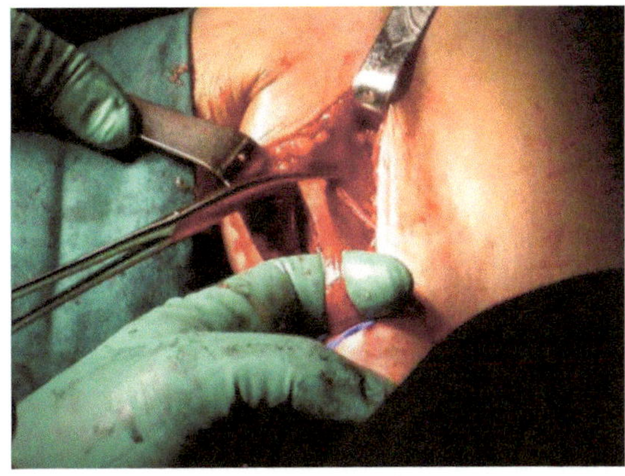

Fig. 12.19 Interruption of the Gracilis muscle tendon

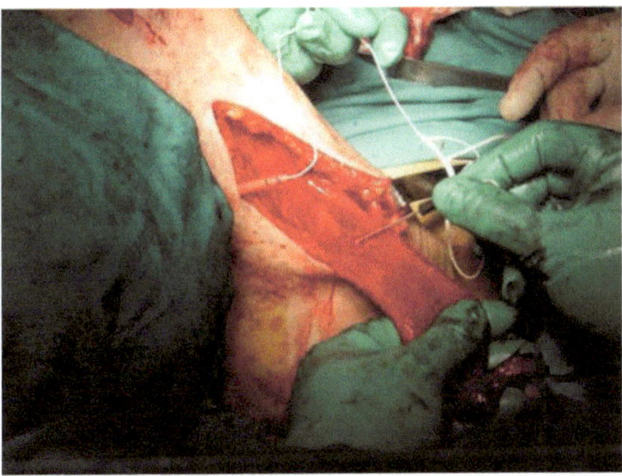

Fig. 12.20 Evaluation of the functional integrity of the muscle (middle part)

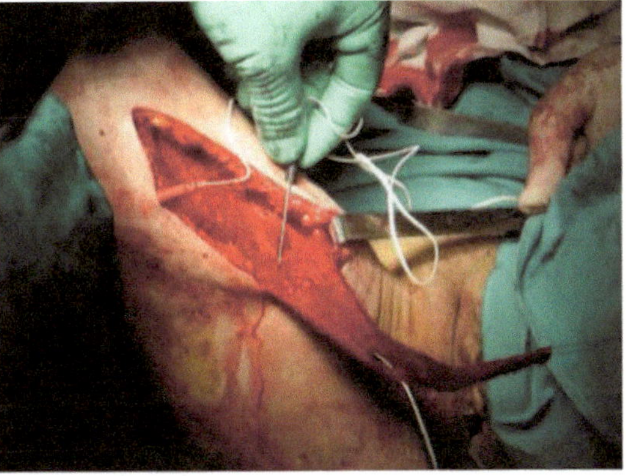

Fig. 12.21 Evaluation of the functional integrity of the muscle (ischial side)

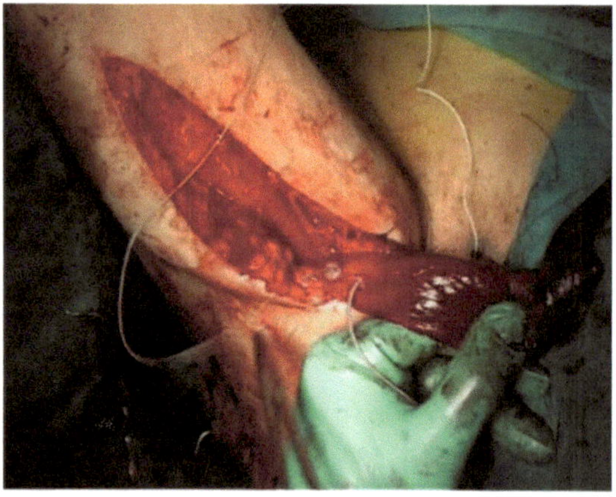

Fig. 12.22 Stimulation test of the muscle

extremity of the tendon and passing it through the previously created tunnel toward the anus (Figs. 12.25, 12.26, 12.27, and 12.28). The muscle will now be wrapped around the anal canal in a 360° counterclockwise manner if the right gracilis is used or clockwise if the left gracilis is used (Fig. 12.29). An anal cerclage is made and must be wrapped around the entire anal circumference, while trying carefully not to englobe the tendon; should this not occur, a high-tension area ulcerating the mucosa may be inadvertently created. The gracilis muscle will now be fixed on the contralateral ischial tuberosity. The muscle must be put in tension in such a way as it tightens the

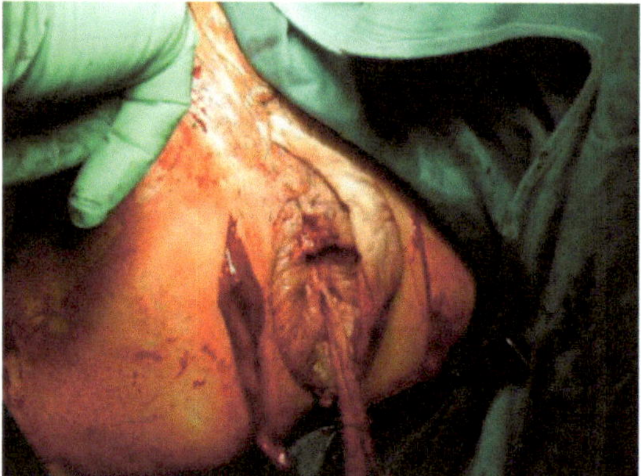

Fig. 12.23 Perianal incisions to allow the transposition of the muscle

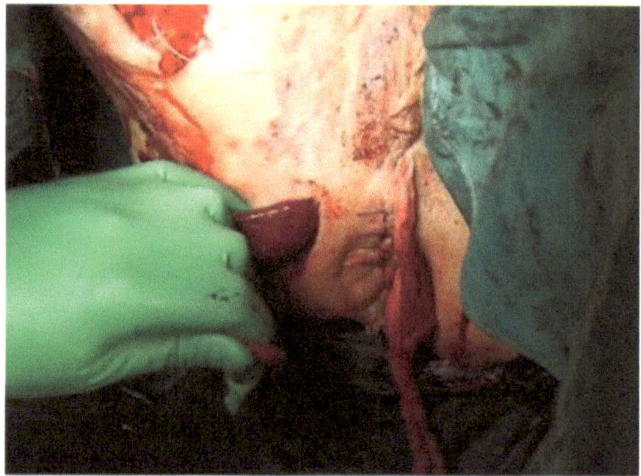

Fig. 12.25 Transposition of the muscle performed by holding the distal extremity

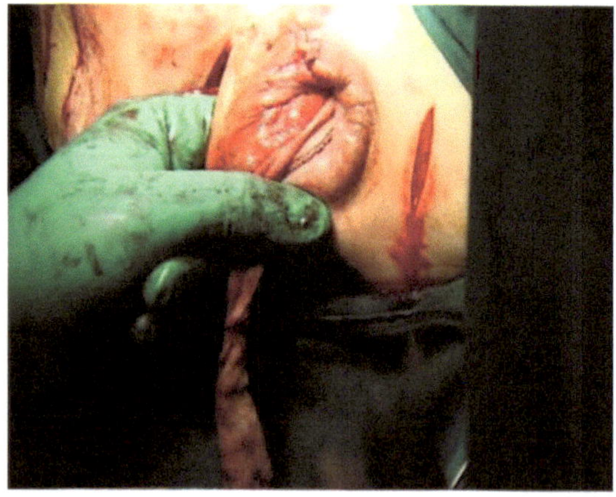

Fig. 12.24 Creation of tunneling

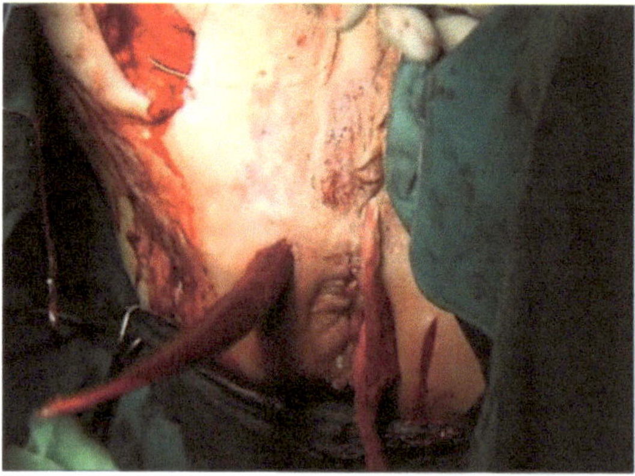

Fig. 12.26 Muscle transposed

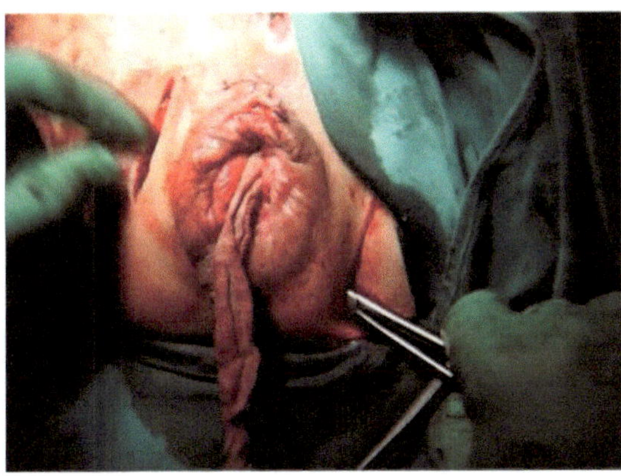

Fig. 12.27 The muscle is wrapped around the anal canal

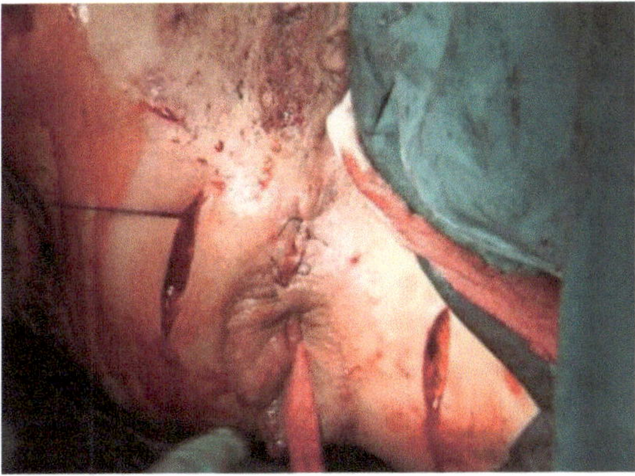

Fig. 12.28 The right Gracilis muscle is wrapped in a counterclockwise manner around the entire anal circumference

canal. In order to allow this to happen, the "donor" thigh will be put into maximum adduction in favor of maintaining this indispensable condition. The incisions will then be sutured.

The second surgical stage involves the implantation of a stimulator (Fig. 12.30) and allows for the beginning of the graciloplasty's dynamic function. This second stage is an innovation of the classical graciloplasty procedure, which used to consist of only one stage. Continued electric stimulation radically modifies transposition results. It is accomplished, thanks to an implanted and programmed neurostimulator. Due to the continued stimulation of the striated muscle fibers, which are subject to fatigue and are able to contract rapidly but briefly, these fibers are transformed into a muscle with permanent contraction, resistant to fatigue and fit to maintain an extended and toned contraction. The muscle will therefore replace the insufficient anatomical sphincter in every aspect. Defecation will occur by inhibiting the sub-tetanus contraction of the muscle and blocking the input sent to the neosphincter by the neurostimulator. Typically, implantation of the neurostimulator is performed at the same time as the graciloplasty. In some cases, it is implanted at a subsequent date, approximately 2 or 3 months later.

A study conducted by Ronger compares the outcomes of dynamic graciloplasty performed in

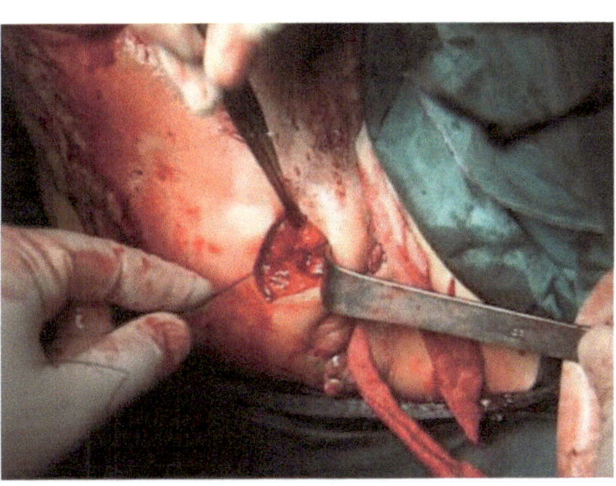

Fig. 12.29 The Gracilis muscle is fixed

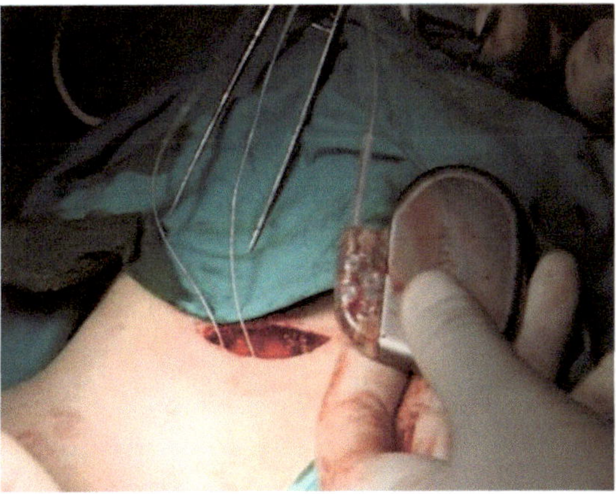

Fig. 12.30 Implantation of the stimulator

a single-stage procedure with its two-stage counterpart. In the study, the neurostimulator implantation was performed approximately 6 weeks following the transposition. Differences were detected regarding the morbidity, quality of life, and fecal incontinence; however, these values were not relevant or significant; from a symptomatic point of view, the two methods almost overlap. However, the preferred choice should still be the single-stage method in order to avoid the consequences of a second surgical procedure. It is important to perform a protective colostomy at the time of the graciloplasty, which can be removed only after the neurostimulator has improved the neosphincter.

The neurostimulator consists of monopolar electrode terminations implanted directly on the gracilis nerve or on the neuromuscular junction. Typically, the latter technique is preferred as implanting the electric stimulator along the gracilis nerve can damage the vascular pedicle, causing ischemia and denervation of the muscle.

During the procedure, tests are carried out in order to initially control the vitality of the prepared muscle structure (Images 12.16, 12.17, and 12.18) and, secondly, the correct positioning of the electrodes and the stimulus threshold, which must be reached in order to contract the muscle. These electrodes are then connected to the neurostimulator which, in turn, will be placed in a subcutaneous or subaponeurotic pocket on the abdomen (Fig. 12.26), usually in the right iliac fossa. After its positioning, "muscle conditioning" is carried out for 6 weeks using electric stimulation at a low frequency (15–25 Hz). The duration of the stimulation is gradually increased until a continuous stimulation is reached at a frequency of 15 Hz following 8 weeks of conditioning. After such training, the muscle will be able to maintain a painless and ongoing sub-tetanus contraction, which keeps the anus closed.

We would like to emphasize that a graciloplasty without neurostimulation has less positive outcomes, especially for frequent muscle hypotonicity/atrophy and the failure of the muscle structure to adapt to a persistent closure effort. Thus currently, this variant is more frequently preferred in comparison to its older counterpart. In cases in which we choose not to use neurostimulation, the procedure may be performed by strengthening the repair using a bilateral transposition. We must however emphasize that dynamic graciloplasty is suitable only for particular cases and carried out by few surgical teams only, consisting of highly expert groups. Dynamic graciloplasty is often used after all other techniques prove unsuccessful or as a result of trauma sequels.

12.5 Magnetic Anal Sphincter

The magnetic anal sphincter (MAS; Fenix™ Torax Medical, Inc., MN, USA) is a recent device proposed for the management of severe fecal incontinence (FI). The rational operation of the MAS has caused from a similar device used in the treatment of gastroesophageal reflux disease, the LINX™ Reflux Management System. The MAS consists of string of titanium beads with magnetic cores linked together with a titanium wire to form an annular structure [35].

The MAS is placed around the external anal sphincter in a circular fashion. At rest, the magnets pull together, which serves to occlude the anal orifice, and the force during Valsalva provides an adequate aperture for defecation. Therefore, the MAS is not a replacement but an enhancement technique of the natural sphincter pressure.

The device is manufactured in different lengths based on the number of beads to accommodate the variation in anal canal circumferences in different individuals.

Lehur in 2010 reported an initial study on 14 females implanted with the magnetic anal sphincter. Adverse events were reported in 50 %. At 6-month follow-up, five patients had a greater than 90 % reduction in the number of FI episodes and significant improvement in Cleveland Clinic Incontinence Score (CCFIS) [36].

Barussaud et al. reported on a study of 23 patients with a median follow-up of 17.6 months. The device was explanted in two patients due to complications. Median preoperative CCFIS decreased from 15.2 to 6.9 at 6 months; about 70 % of the patients were satisfied with this therapy [37].

The long-term efficacy of MAS implantation is still unknown. The procedure appears technically simple, especially if compared with the replacement of the anal sphincter techniques. It will be necessary to evaluate the incidence of adverse events in the future. The few studies available suggest good efficacy of the technique as significant improvement of the patients' QoL.

Note: The figures 12.7, 12.9, 12.12, 12.13, and 12.16 have been realized by Ilaria Bondi.

References

1. Rao SSC. Current and emerging treatment options for fecal incontinence. J Clin Gastroenterol. 2014; 48(9):752–64.
2. Fernando RJ, Sultan AH, Kettle C, Thakar R. Methods of repair for obstetric anal sphincter injury. Cochrane Database Syst Rev. 2013 Dec 8;(12).
3. Sultan AH. Obstetric perineal injury and anal incontinence. Clin Risk. 1999;5:193–6.
4. Koelbl H, Igawa T, Salvatore S, Laterza RM, Lowry A, Sievert KD, et al. Pathophysiology of urinary incontinence, faecal incontinence and pelvic organ prolapse. In: Abrams P, Cardozo L, Khoury S, Wein A, editors. Incontinence. 5th ed. [place unknown]: ICUD-EAU; 2013. p. 261–359.
5. Premkumar G. Perineal trauma: reducing associated postnatal maternal morbidity. RCM Midwives. 2005;8(1):30–2.
6. Fornell EU, Matthiesen L, Sjodahl R, Berg G. Obstetric anal sphincter injury ten years after: subjective and objective long term effects. BJOG. 2005;112:312–6.
7. Rieger N, Wattchow D. The effect of vaginal delivery on anal function. Aust N Z J Surg. 1999;69:172–7.
8. Valsky DV, Lipschuetz M, Bord A, Eldar I, Messing B, Hochner-Celnikier D, Lavy Y, Cohen SM, Yagel S. Fetal head circumference and length of secondary stage ah labor are risk for levator ani muscle injury, diagnosed by 3-dimensional transperineal ultrasound in primiparous women. Am J Obstet Gynecol. 2009;201:91–7.
9. Midwifery J, McCandlish R. Perineal trauma: prevention and treatment. Womens Health. 2001;46(6): 396–401.
10. Snooks SJ, Swash M, Mathers SE, et al. Effect of vaginal delivery on the pelvic floor: a five-year follow-up. Br J Surg. 1990;2:1358–60.
11. Gyhagen M, Bullarbo M, Nielsen TF, Milsom I. Faecal incontinence 20 years after one birth: a comparison between vaginal delivery and caesarean section. Int Urogynecol J. 2014;25(10):1411–8.
12. Lamblin G, Bouvier P, Damon H, Chabert P, Moret S, Chene G, Mellier G. Long-term outcome after overlapping anterior anal sphincter repair for fecal incontinence. Int J Colorectal Dis. 2014;29:1377–83.
13. Johnson E, Carlsen E, Steen TB, Backer Hjorthaug JO, Eriksen MT, Johannessen HO. Short- and long-term results of secondary anterior sphincteroplasty in 33 patients with obstetric injury. Acta Obstet Gynecol Scand. 2010;89(11):1466–72.
14. Power D, Fitzpatrick M, O'Herlihy C. Obstetric anal sphincter injury: how to avoid, how to repair: a literature review. J Fam Pract. 2006;55:193–200.
15. Brown SR, Wadhawan H, Nelson RL. Surgery for faecal incontinence in adults. Cochrane Database Syst Rev. 2013 Jul 2;(7).
16. Gleason JL. Anal sphincter repair for fecal incontinence: effect on symptom severity, quality of life, and anal sphincter squeeze pressure. Int Urogynecol J. 2011;22:1587–92.
17. Faltin D, Boulvain M, Irion O, Bretones S, Stan C, Weil A. Diagnosis of anal sphincter tears by postpartum endosonography to predict fecal incontinence. Obstet Gynecol. 2000;95:643–7.
18. Glasgow SC, Lowry AC. Long-term outcomes of anal sphincter repair for fecal incontinence. Dis Colon Rectum. 2012;55:482–90.
19. Halverson AL, Hull TL. Long-term outcome of overlapping anal sphincter repair. Dis Colon Rectum. 2002;45:345–8.
20. Parks AG, McPartlin JF. Late repair of injuries of the anal sphincter. Proc R Soc Med. 1971;64(12): 1187–9.
21. Riss S, Stift A, Teleky B, Rieder E, Mittlböck M, Maier A, et al. Long-term anorectal and sexual function after overlapping anterior anal sphincter repair: a case-match study. Dis Colon Rectum. 2009;52:1095–100.
22. Barisic GI, Krivokapic ZV, Markovic VA, Popovic MA. Outcome of overlapping anal sphincter repair after 3 months and after a mean of 80 months. Int J Color Dis. 2006;21:52–6.
23. Young CJ, Mathur MN, Eyers AA, Solomon MJ. Successful overlapping anal sphincter repair: relationship to patient age, neuropathy, and colostomy formation. Dis Colon Rectum. 1998;41:344–9.
24. Nielsen MB, Dammegaard L, Pedersen JF. Endosonographic assessment of the anal sphincter after surgical reconstruction. Dis Colon Rectum. 1994;37(5):434–8.
25. Walsh KA, Grivell RM. Use of endoanal ultrasound for reducing the risk of complications related to anal sphincter injury after vaginal birth. Cochrane Database Syst Rev. 2015 Oct 29;(10).
26. Sultan AH, Monga AK, Kumar D, Stanton SL. Primary repair of obstetric anal sphincter rupture using the overlap technique. Br J Obstet Gynaecol. 1999;106(4):318–23.
27. Setti Carraro P, Kamm MA, Nicholls RJ. Long-term results of postanal repair for neurogenic faecal incontinence. Br J Surg. 1994;81(1):140–4.
28. Matsuoka H, Mavrantonis C, Wexner SD, et al. Postanal repair for fecal incontinence – is it worthwhile? Dis Colon Rectum. 2000;43(11):1561–7.

29. Mackey P, Mackey L, Kennedy ML, et al. Postanal repair – do the long-term results justify the procedure? Colorectal Dis. 2010;12(4):367–72.
30. Bartolo DC, Paterson HM. Anal incontinence. Best Pract Res Clin Gastroenterol. 2009;23(4):505–15.
31. Bartolo DC. Point of view: anal incontinence in men. Gastroenterol Clin Biol. 2008;32(11):949–52.
32. Wexner SD, Bleier J. Current surgical strategies to treat fecal incontinence. Expert Rev Gastroenterol Hepatol. 2015;9(12):1577–89.
33. Shi GG, Wang H, Wang L, Zhang ZX, Wang H. Two different gracilis loops in graciloplasty of congenital fecal incontinence: comparison of the therapeutic effects. Int J Colorectal Dis. 2015;30(10):1391–7.
34. Walega P, Romaniszyn M, Siarkiewicz B, Zelazny D. Dynamic versus adynamic graciloplasty in treatment of end-stage fecal incontinence: is the implantation of the pacemaker really necessary? 12-month follow-up in a clinical, physiological, and functional study. Gastroenterol Res Pract. 2015;2015:698516.
35. Mantoo S, Meurette G, Podevin J, Lehur PA. The magnetic anal sphincter: a new device in the management of severe anal incontinence. Expert Rev Med Devices. 2012;9:483–90.
36. Lehur PA, McNevin S, Buntzen S, et al. Magnetic anal sphincter augmentation for the treatment of fecal incontinence: a preliminary report from a feasibility study. Dis Colon Rectum. 2010;53(12):1604–10.
37. Barussaud ML, Mantoo S, Wyart V, et al. The magnetic anal sphincter in faecal incontinence: is initial success sustained over time? Colorectal Dis. 2013;15(12):1499–503.

13 Ostomy in Fecal Incontinence

Livia de Anna, Raffaele Merola, and Claudia Donello

13.1 Fecal Diversion

Although fecal diversion may be considered a failure of fecal incontinence (FI) treatment, it is an effective, safe, and appropriate operation for certain patients with severe incontinence, although aesthetically less preferable [1].

Indications of colostomy or ileostomy include spinal cord injury, complete pelvic floor denervation, severe perianal trauma, and radiation-induced FI that can lead to severe neurogenic incontinence. It is also performed on patients immobilized with skin problems or other complications [1, 2] or on those who are physically or mentally incapable without any bowel control resulting in a poor quality of life [3]. The creation of a colostomy or ileostomy provides definitive control of fecal incontinence.

An ileostomy may be considered in patients with colonic transit abnormalities, but colostomy is the standard ostomy utilized in the treatment of FI.

In many patients ostomy can be created using a laparoscopic approach to improve recovery time. Even though an ostomy is not without short- and long-term risks, such as bleeding, anesthesia-related cardiac or respiratory morbidities, and parastomal hernia, it is a safe and effective treatment of severe FI.

It is generally performed only if other treatment modalities have failed. Patients are usually understandably very reluctant to the idea of a permanent ostomy, fearing it will be difficult to manage, due to the great impact on self-image and social interactions. When patients who had undergone ostomy creation were surveyed, general quality of life was actually higher in the ostomy group than in other patients [4].

Patients generally reported high satisfaction with their stomas, with over 80% stating that they would likely or definitely choose to undergo the procedure again [5].

Compared to other surgical treatments of severe incontinence (dynamic graciloplasty and artificial bowel sphincters), a British study found ostomy to be the most effective in terms of quality-adjusted life years [6]. While fecal diversion is not commonly performed in the majority of patients, it is a viable, definitive, and well-tolerated treatment which offers good quality of life. Knowledge of these currently used treatments is essential to honest and thorough counseling of the patient with FI to improve treatment success. Together with the patient, the surgeon can select the best treatment from the five available categories of repair, replacement, augmentation, stimulation, and diversion.

L. de Anna (✉) • R. Merola • C. Donello
Department of Surgery R. Paolucci,
Sapienza – University of Rome, Rome, Italy
e-mail: livia.deanna@uniroma1.it

M. Mongardini, M. Giofrè (eds.), *Management of Fecal Incontinence*,
DOI 10.1007/978-3-319-32226-1_13

13.2 Preoperative Design

When the operation is planned in advance, a specialist stoma nurse should be firstly consulted, in order to define suitable locations for the stoma.

The practice of performing a preoperative design is still a key element in the prevention of complications due to wrong positioning.

Having a stoma poorly positioned can negatively affect the quality of life of the patient: it can often cause anxiety and it can arouse fear of leaving the house and/or of eating. Not to mention the difficult management of the stoma with the possible occurrence of premature detachment of the garrison, with leaking enteric material and subsequent psychological trauma of the patient.

The preoperative design is the key to improve the quality of life in the postoperative phase, promoting their independence and reducing the rate of postoperative complications.

The correct position will have to be far away from the costal margin, umbilicus, previous scars, fat folds, waistline, main surgical incisions, iliac crest, and skin changes (skin diseases, naevi, other).

By applying an adhesive label (you can also use a "sticker" instead of a normal plate of ostomy) representing the ostomy, you will have to verify the exact positioning in three different basic postures: supine, sitting, and standing. It can also be useful to try the squatting position and overlapping the leg. Clothing, religion, and way of life will also be kept on account, though they cannot be binding.

Patients who have undergone the procedure of the preoperative drawing of the stomal site have significantly suffered fewer postoperative complications, and these results are independent from the type of stoma (permanent or temporary).

13.3 Ileostomy

Ileostomy may be terminal or derivative.

The technique of wrapping ileostomy is much faster because it is sufficient to drill a small circular skin access (or racket) to pull out the last ileal loop.

In case of a loop ileostomy, the stoma has two openings: the former is connected to the functioning part of the bowel and the latter to the "inactive" part, leading to the rectum which produces only small amounts of mucus.

The stoma will appear large at first, as the effects of surgery cause swelling. It usually shrinks during the first weeks after surgery, reaching its final size after about 8 weeks. The stoma will be red and moist. It has no nerve endings, therefore touching is painless. It may bleed when touched but this is entirely normal and it is not a reason for concerning.

In some cases, a support device (called a rod or bridge) may be used to hold the loop in place while it heals. The supporting rod is removed approximately 7–10 days after surgery, when healing has occurred. It will prevent the loop of bowel from retracting into the abdomen.

13.3.1 Disadvantages

The acidity and the fluid consistency of the feces that can easily get under the plate facilitate the onset of dermatitis around the stoma, and there is no type of control on the emission of the enteric fluid.

Lacking the resorption of fluids and salts from part of the colon, the most evident consequence is dehydration and loss of electrolytes.

13.3.2 Technique

The skin hole must be necessarily circular, about the size of 2.5–3 cm diameter.

The loop must be fixed to the peritoneum and to the muscular fascia with absorbable suture wire to prevent herniation.

The stoma must be open directly to the operating table, so as to allow a correct packaging.

The end of the bowel wall is sutured to the skin by means of a 3/0 absorbable suture which first passes through the skin, followed by a seromuscular bite, taken 1.5 cm proximal to the end of the bowel. The suture is then passed through the full thickness of the end of the bowel wall, according to Brooke technique. Four of these sutures are placed at quarterly intervals and then secured. Additional sutures are placed as required, passing solely between the skin and the end of the bowel.

In case of loop ileostomy, the supporting rod is removed approximately 7–10 days after surgery. When healing has occurred, it will prevent the loop of bowel from retracting into the abdomen.

13.4 Colostomy

The terminal colostomy is the best choice among the various types of ostomy in the treatment of fecal incontinence.

13.4.1 Technique

The ideal seat from the functional point of view is that paramedian, at the level of the external margin of the rectus abdominis muscle, with the loop that passes through the fibers of the latter, with perfectly perpendicular course. The loop should always be carefully attached to the peritoneum, fascia, and skin to prevent prolapse or retraction.

The thickness of the subcutaneous layer should be taken into consideration especially in the case of obese patients.

Ideal colostomy is flat. It is important to perform a sufficient mobilization of the loop externalized, so as to prevent its retraction.

13.4.2 Advantages

It is possible to control the release of stool through diet and irrigation; the feces are not "aggressive" for the surrounding skin, and therefore complications are fewer.

13.5 Laparoscopic Colostomy

The patient is placed in the supine position and in the Trendelenburg position with the operating bed rotated slightly to the right. This requires three trocars of the following size: 10, 10–12, and 5 mm. The technique indeed provides for the use of the trocar 10 mm for the camera, in umbilical level, a second 5 mm trocar between the appendix xiphoid and the umbilicus and the use of a grasping forceps. Finally, a third trocar from 10 to 12 mm in suprapubic for the use of bipolar and the introduction of the Endo GIA. After adequate exploration of the abdominal cavity, the intervention starts with the partial opening of the left paracolic gutter, so as to obtain an adequate mobilization of the descending colon and sigmoid.

When a terminal colostomy is performed, the meso and the tract of the intestine chosen are sectioned with Endo GIA. The proximal stump is externalized and the distal one is left in the pelvis.

When it is decided for a colostomy "on gun barrels," a small fenestration is carried out, with the bipolar forceps on the mesocolon, in correspondence of which the bowel will be led out, without interrupting the colic continuity.

One proceeds then to the sectioning of the parietal peritoneum in the proximity of the site chosen for the colostomy. The stump of the colon is maintained with grasping forceps. Then the skin and fascia are opened with the help of transillumination. The stoma is then packaged as a rule.

13.6 Morbidity and Mortality Rates

Complications after ostomy surgery can occur. The doctor should be made aware of any of the following problems after surgery:

- Increased pain, swelling, redness, drainage, or bleeding in the surgical area
- Headache, muscle aches, dizziness, or fever
- Increased abdominal pain or swelling, constipation, nausea or vomiting, or black, tarry stools

Stomal complications can also occur. They include:

Death (necrosis) of stomal tissue. Caused by inadequate blood supply, this complication is usually visible 12–24 h after the operation and may require additional surgery.

Retraction (stoma is flushed with the abdomen surface or has moved below it). Caused by insufficient stomal length, this complication may be managed by the use of special pouching supplies. Elective revision of the stoma is also an option.

Prolapse (stoma increases length above the surface of the abdomen). Most often, this results from an overly large opening in the abdominal wall or inadequate fixation of the bowel to the abdominal wall. Surgical correction is required when blood supply is compromised.

Stenosis (narrowing at the opening of the stoma). This is often associated with infection around the stoma or scarring. Mild stenosis can be removed under local anesthesia; severe stenosis may require surgery for reshaping the stoma.

Parastomal hernia (bowel causing bulge in the abdominal wall next to the stoma). This occurs due to placement of the stoma where the abdominal wall is weak or an overly large opening in the abdominal wall was made. The use of an ostomy support belt and special pouching supplies may be adequate. If severe, the defect in the abdominal wall should be repaired and the stoma moved to another location.

Mortality rates for colostomy patients vary according to the patient's general health upon admittance to the hospital. Even among higher-risk patients, mortality is about 16 %. This rate is greatly reduced (between 0.8 and 3.8 %) when the colostomy is performed by a board-certified colon and rectal surgeon.

13.7 Colostomy and Irrigation

People with colostomies who have ostomies of the sigmoid colon or descending colon may have the option of irrigation, an enema of the colon in order to promote mechanical continence, or a free interval from the issue of feces of 36–48 h, which allows for the person not to wear a pouch but rather just a gauze cap over the stoma.

Getting this condition will improve the comfort and well-being of the person with an ostomy and it will drastically reduce the risk of skin complications.

Peristomal contact with feces reduces health care costs for the management of the stoma.

13.7.1 Technique of Irrigation

A catheter is placed inside the stoma, flushed with 1.5–2 l of warm water, to allow the feces to come out of the body into an irrigation sleeve.

Most patients irrigate once a day or every other day, though this depends on their personal choice, on their food intake, and on their health.

The practice of irrigation has to be repeated at regular intervals, usually on alternate days, in order to be effective.

Following this kind of rehabilitation, the patient can use only a little cap (Fig. 13.1).

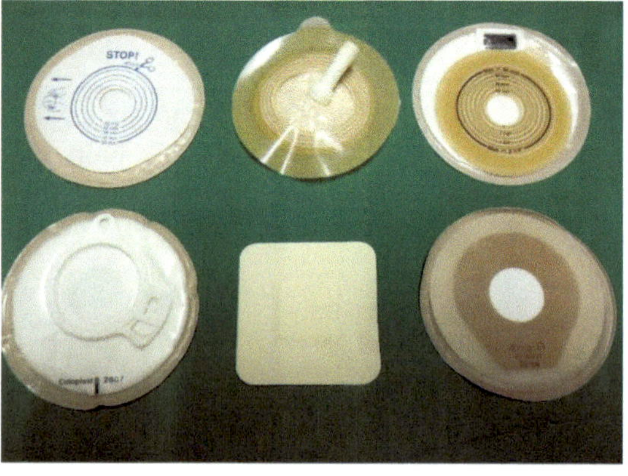

Fig. 13.1 Post-irrigation mini cap

13.8 The Malone Procedure

The antegrade continence enema procedure [7] is used to control fecal soiling in both adults and children, but it is most commonly used and reported in the pediatric population. Firstly described by Malone et al. in 1990 [8], it consists of fashioning a cecostomy button or appedicostomy, which allows antegrade washing out of the colon.

It may be suitable for children and patients with neurological conditions, such as spina bifida, resulting in neurogenic bowel and urinary symptoms [9].

While the antegrade continence enema may be helpful in pure fecal incontinence, most often patients who undergo this procedure have the combination of constipation or colonic dysmotility with associated overflow FI.

Patients also undergo urological procedures to control neurogenic bladder symptoms, with good results for these combined indications [10]. In adults, good functional outcomes are better in this setting, when compared to those patients who undergo the procedure for constipation alone [11]. An antegrade continence enema does not alter anorectal physiology or anatomy, and moreover, it provides a mechanism to empty the colon in a controlled way, allowing patients to perform their daily activities with little worry about fecal soiling or incontinence episodes.

Since Malone's original description, various techniques have been described for the creation of an antegrade continence enema. The appendix, ileum, cecum, and left colon may successfully be used as the access point for irrigation [12, 13]. The appendix is most commonly used, where it is inverted and fixed to the skin at the umbilicus or at the right lower quadrant. This can be opened or laparoscopically performed with good results [14]. The access point is left intubated with a catheter for about 3 weeks after the operation, before beginning intermittent intubations. Then, patients or their caregivers intubate the bowel daily or every few days and perform colonic irrigation with tap water or an electrolyte solution. The volume of irrigation is gradually increased and the timing and frequency of irrigation may be easily performed by patients themselves.

In the pediatric patients, the operation is performed around the age of 10 years. Persistent leakage, stoma stenosis, and surgical site infections are common complications, which require a 13 % of stoma revision [15–16].

Since the antegrade continence enema is not often performed in adults, these patients require long-term follow-up and attention to possible complications. Fibrosis of the stoma site may lead to a loss of response, even though overall success rate of 61 % has been reported at an average follow-up of 3.5 years [17].

References

1. Vaizey CJ, Kamm MA, Nicholls RJ. Recent advances in the surgical treatment of faecal incontinence. Br J Surg. 1998;85:596–603.
2. Senapati A, Phillips RK. The trephine colostomy: a permanent left iliac fossa end colostomy without recourse to laparotomy. Ann R Coll Surg Engl. 1991;73:305–6.
3. Poirier M, Abcarian H. Fecal incontinence. In: Cameron JL, editor. Current surgical therapy. Philadelphia: Mosby Elsevier; 2008. p. 285–91.
4. Colquhoun P, Kaiser R, Efron J, Weiss EG, Nogueras JJ, Vernava AM, Wexner SD. Is the quality of life better in patients with colostomy than patients with fecal incontinence? World J Surg. 2006;30:1925–8.
5. Norton C, Burch J, Kamm MA. Patients' views of a colostomy for fecal incontinence. Dis Colon Rectum. 2005;48:1062–9.
6. Tan EK, Vaizey C, Cornish J, Darzi A, Tekkis PP. Surgical strategies for faecal incontinence – a decision analysis between dynamic graciloplasty, artificial bowel sphincter and end stoma. Colorectal Dis. 2008;10:577–86.
7. Malone PS, Ransley PG, Kiely EM. Preliminary report: the antegrade continence enema. Lancet. 1990;336:1217–8.
8. Duel BP, Gonzalez R. The button cecostomy for management of fecal incontinence. Pediatr Surg Int. 1999;15:559–61.
9. Van Koughnett JAM, Wexner SD. Current management of fecal incontinence: choosing amongst treatment options to optimize outcomes. World J Gastroenterol. 2013;19(48):9216–30.
10. Teichman JM, Harris JM, Currie DM, Barber DB. Malone antegrade continence enema for adults with neurogenic bowel disease. J Urol. 1998;160:1278–81.

11. Gerharz EW, Vik V, Webb G, Leaver R, Shah PJ, Woodhouse CR. The value of the MACE (Malone antegrade colonic enema) procedure in adult patients. J Am Coll Surg. 1997;185:544–7.
12. Tackett LD, Minevich E, Benedict JF, Wacksman J, Sheldon CA. Appendiceal versus ileal segment for antegrade continence enema. J Urol. 2002;167:683–6.
13. Ellison JS, Haraway AN, Park JM. The distal left Malone antegrade continence enema – is it better? J Urol. 2013;190:1529–33.
14. Herndon CD, Rink RC, Cain MP, Lerner M, Kaefer M, Yerkes E, Casale AJ. In situ Malone antegrade continence enema in 127 patients: a 6-year experience. J Urol. 2004;172:1689–91.
15. Yerkes EB, Cain MP, King S, Brei T, Kaefer M, Casale AJ, Rink RC. The Malone antegrade continence enema procedure: quality of life and family perspective. J Urol. 2003;169:320–3.
16. Hoekstra LT, Kuijper CF, Bakx R, Heij HA, Aronson DC, Benninga MA. The Malone antegrade continence enema procedure: the Amsterdam experience. J Pediatr Surg. 2011;46:1603–8.
17. Curry JI, Osborne A, Malone PS. How to achieve a successful Malone antegrade continence enema. J Pediatr Surg. 1998;33:138–41.

14 Stem Cells

Mario Ledda, Antonella Lisi, and Alberto Giori

14.1 Stem Cell Biology

14.1.1 Stem Cell Classification

The German biologist Ernst Haeckel first introduced the term "stem cell" in the scientific literature in 1868 with the term "Stammzelle" (stem cell) to describe the unicellular ancestor progenitor of all organisms. In the nineteenth century, Theodor Boveri and Valentin Häcker instead used the same term to describe "cells committed to give rise to the germline" [1],and 4 years later, Edmund B. Wilson made the term "stem cell" universal by reviewing Hacker's and Boveri's work in his book entitled *The Cell in Development and Inheritance* [2].

Around 100 years later, Gail Martins of the University of California, Martin Evans and Matthew Kaufman of the University of Cambridge, independently isolated stem cells from mouse embryos and coined the term "embryonic stem cells" (ESCs). In 2007, Mario Capecchi, Martin Evans, and Oliver Smithies shared the Nobel Prize in Physiology and Medicine for the great achievement in the field of ESCs obtained in the mid-1980s. In 1995, Jamie Thompson of the University of Wisconsin cultured monkey ESCs for the first time and later, in 1999, human embryonic stem cells.

All tissues are composed by highly specialized cells derived from an initial pool of stem cells generated during early embryonic development, which provides a reserve for injured tissue repair and replaces the cells lost daily in the lifespan. Stem cells are unspecialized cells that have two key properties that distinguish them from other types of cells; they have the capacity of self-renewal and the ability of generating differentiated cells [3, 4]. These cells are capable of generating daughter cells for long periods identical to their mother cells (self-renewal). They are also able of differentiating, under specific physiological conditions, into many types of mature cell, which make up totally all our organs and tissues.

This area of interest includes different types of stem cells, which can be isolated during different phases of the development of an organ-

M. Ledda • A. Lisi (✉)
Institute of Translational Pharmacology, National Research Council (CNR), Rome, Italy
e-mail: antonella.lisi@ift.cnr.it

A. Giori
Department of General Surgery, San Paolo University Hospital, Milan, Italy

M. Mongardini, M. Giofrè (eds.), *Management of Fecal Incontinence*,
DOI 10.1007/978-3-319-32226-1_14

ism. In the initial stage of the embryo development, stem cells (ESCs) can be found in the blastocyst (50–100 cells), whereas in the adult stage, tissue stem cells can be found almost in all body tissue. These adult stem cells (ASCs) can also be found in the fetus and in babies. Finally, induced pluripotent stem cells (iPS cells) derived from specialized cells (e.g., skin cells) can be "in vitro" engineered, or "reprogrammed," to become pluripotent cells like embryonic stem cells (Fig. 14.1).

Specifically, embryonic stem cells are derived from preimplanted embryos after the formation of the blastocyst [5]; this is made up of an outer layer of cells, an internal fluid-filled space, and an inner cell mass where the ESCs reside. They are defined "pluripotent" because of their ability to differentiate toward all the different types of body cells and tissues, except for extraembryonic organs such as the placenta, yolk sac, and umbilical cord. On the contrary, embryonic stem cells that immediately arise in the first few divisions of the fertilized egg, and defined "totipotent," are able to totally generate a viable embryo including extraembryonic organs.

Instead, adult stem cells are committed cells able of differentiating into all mature cell lineages typical of the tissues or organs in which they reside and for this reason described as "multipotent." For example, stem cells within the adult brain are able to differentiate in neurons and into other two types of cells, astrocytes and oligodendrocytes. Adult stem cells have been found in several organs, mostly those that continuously replenish themselves, such as the blood, skin, muscle, and liver, in large quantity but also in other, less regenerative organs such as the heart and brain.

Finally, induced pluripotent stem cells were "in vitro" produced in 2006 [6] by using viruses for the insertion inside somatic cells of four genes (Oct4, Sox2, c-myc, and Klf4) known to be important for the embryonic stem cell development. These pluripotent stem cells share many characteristics of embryonic stem cells, including the ability to differentiate toward all the cell types in the body. How these four "reprogramming" genes are able to induce pluripotency is not yet well known, and this question is the object of current studies [7]. In addition, recent research is concentrated on finding an alternative way to reprogram somatic

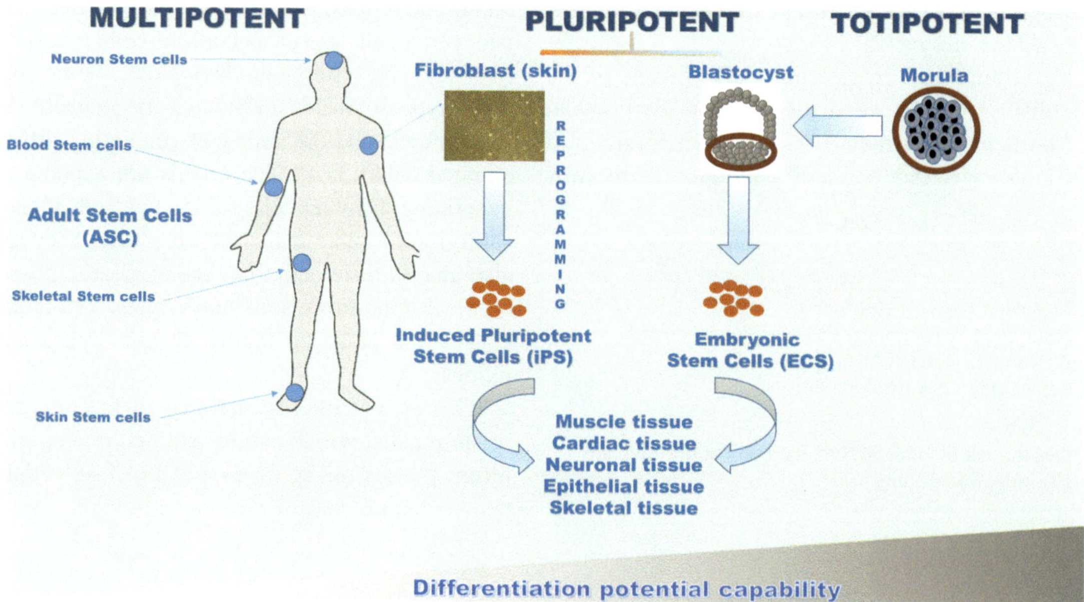

Fig. 14.1 Classification of stem cell sources and definition of differentiation potential capability

cells using safer approaches in clinical sceneries [8, 9].

14.1.2 Stem Cells' Potential Use: Advantages and Disadvantages

Several challenges must be addressed before stem cells can be used in regenerative medicine applications. The first important issue to be addressed is the identification, isolation, and growth of stem cells which are not easy procedures in the case of rare adult stem cells. The following reports and discusses the positive and negative aspects of the three main promising stem cells types, currently the object of worldwide research and investment.

Pluripotent embryonic stem cells that are easily isolated and have the advantage of an unlimited in vitro growth also have the capability of a great differentiating potential through strictly controlled processes. On the contrary, their clinical use has important limitations, due to their genetic instability, potential tumorigenic risk, and ethical considerations related to their origin [10]. For this last reason, in Europe there are rigorous laws that forbid destructive embryo research, while federal laws in the USA instead allow embryo use only in the case of it being discarded after in vitro fertilization [11].

Induced pluripotent stem cells, deriving from reprogrammed somatic cells with standard protocols, are able to differentiate into the three germ layer cell types [12], but still have a very low reprogramming efficiency. These cells could be a good option in autologous transplant applications, overcoming the tissue rejection; however, like the ES cells, they have an important genetic instability and a high tumorigenic [13] risk. Therefore, the standard and safe use in cell therapies of both stem cell types is still a target to reach which needs extensive research and effort.

Finally, multipotent adult stem cells can be used in autologous transplantation in which the patient's own cells are expanded and differentiated in vitro. They are then implanted in the same person, avoiding the host's immune rejection and protecting the patients from viral, bacterial, or other types of donor's contamination. The disadvantage of ASCs is a very short life in culturing and expansion and a weaker differentiating potential in comparison with embryonic stem cells.

Although significant progress has been made in the stem cell research field and many preclinical studies have highlighted the great therapeutic potential of these cells, among the stem cells types, only the adult stem cells are currently used in some clinical applications. In particular, the bone marrow stem cells have been employed for more than 50 years, giving excellent results especially in the hematopoietic and immune system pathologies, which are addressed in the next section.

14.1.3 Current Clinical Applications Using Multipotent Adult Stem Cells

Presently, in some cases, this clinical protocol is replaced by autologous transplantation of stem cells; as a matter of fact, in the area of therapeutic implantation, it is very important to have a strong compatibility between the donor and the host tissue, in order to minimize the risk of rejection and at the same time deliver and engraft the stem cells to the target damaged tissue to improve the stem cell integration.

In successful clinical applications, the stem cells used were the blood (hematopoietic) stem cells from the bone marrow for the treatment of leukemia, lymphoma, and several inherited blood disorders. Umbilical cord blood, like bone marrow, is also collected as a source of blood stem cells and then used as an alternative to bone marrow transplantation, especially for the treatment of diseases in children. Other stem cell treatments which proved safe and effective involved bone, skin, and corneal diseases or injuries.

14.1.3.1 Bone Marrow Stem Cells in Transplants

Bone marrow stem cell therapy has been in routine use since the 1970s [14] and is able to treat a patient's diseased blood. Although it presents a direct complication, due to the donor's immune cells that sometimes can react to the patient's tissues (graft-versus-host disease or GVHD) [15, 16], and an indirect complication, due to a risk of infection in chemotherapy pretreated patients [17], many thousands of people benefit from this kind of treatment every year.

14.1.3.2 Umbilical Cord Blood Stem Cells in Transplants

The umbilical cord blood stem cells (UCSCs) have the advantage of being less rejected by the immune system, compared to conventional bone marrow transplants. UCSCs, adequately cryopreserved in cell banks, are presently used for treating cancer blood disorders in children, such as leukemia, and genetic blood diseases like Fanconi anemia [18, 19].

14.1.3.3 Skin Stem Cells in Transplants

Skin stem cells have been used since the 1980s for the in vitro growth of new skin sheets for treating patients with severe burns [20]. However, the new skin has no hair follicles, sweat glands, or sebaceous (oil) glands, so this approach is used only for saving the lives of patients with third-degree burn over very large areas of their bodies [20].

14.1.3.4 Eye Stem Cells in Transplants

Clinical studies have shown that adult stem cells isolated from the limbus area of the eye can be used to repair damaged cornea. As matter of fact, the limbal stem cells can be taken from the patients, in vitro cultured and transferred back to their injured eye [20]. The treatment, safe and effective in early stage trials [20], is limited if both eyes have been seriously damaged for the impossibility to obtain the patients' limbal stem cells. The safe and routine use of adult stem cells in clinical therapies needs a considerable research work and for this scope the public funds are required.

14.1.4 Multipotent Mesenchymal Stem Cells

Among the adult stem cells, multipotent mesenchymal stem cells (MSCs) are a promising cell source for tissue engineering and cell-based therapies due to their ability of self-renewal and of differentiating into specific cell lineages. Human Mesenchymal Stem Cells (hMSCs) have aroused great interest in the scientific community since their use in clinical applications does not imply neither ethical problems nor teratoma-risk formation. The number of clinical trials in which hMSCs have been tested has been increasing since 2004 [21], opening up their potential employment in the future treatment of numerous diseases, mainly tissue injuries and immune disorders. These non-hematopoietic adult stem cells, first isolated and studied by Friedenstein in 1971 [22], are able to differentiate into various mesoderm lineages, such as osteocytes, chondrocytes, and adipocytes, as well as ectodermic and endodermic cell lineages [23–27]. MSCs originate from the mesoderm but have a wide distribution in organs and can be isolated from many tissues such as the bone marrow, adipose tissue, muscle, liver, lung, and extraembryonic tissues [28–32].

These stem cells, involved in normal human tissue renewal, wound healing, and in physiological responses to injuries [33], have shown repairing effects for the treatment of damaged tissues and degenerative diseases [34–39]. In patients with cirrhosis disease due to hepatitis B, the autologous transplant of mesenchymal stem cells from the bone marrow (BM-MSCs) has showed encouraging results being able to improve the liver function [40, 41]. BM-MSCs have also provided positive responses in the treatment of muscular-skeletal diseases, periodontal tissue defects, diabetic critical limb ischemia, and burnt skin repair [42–44]. In addition, some preclinical studies have reported tissue regeneration through an anti-inflammatory effect of BM-MSCs in myocardial infarction treatment [45], cornea damage, and other tissue injuries, such as the brain, spinal cord [46], and lung [47–49].

For a long time, the main and traditional source of hMSCs for clinical application uses has been the bone marrow, but their employment is still limited not only because the procedures to isolate hMSCs are highly invasive and the cell quantity obtained is low but also because the proliferating and differentiating potential decreases as the donor's age increases [50]. For this reason, the identification of an alternative source of hMSCs has been an important and necessary issue that still needs to be explored, and for this aim, a promising choice could be adipose tissue and neonatal tissues, including placenta.

14.1.5 hMSCs from Neonatal Tissue

Placental tissue is involved in important functions such as nutrition, respiration, and excretion and the maintenance of fetomaternal tolerance. It is made up of the chorionic plate, which is in close contact with the uterine decidua, and the fetal membranes (amnion and chorion), which spread from the borders of the chorionic plate and enclose the fetus in the amniotic cavity. The amniotic membrane (AM) encloses two types of stem cells, epithelial and mesenchymal, which have different embryological origins. The human amniotic epithelial cells (hAECs), derived from the embryonic ectoderm, form a continuous monolayer in contact with the amniotic fluid. The human amniotic mesenchymal stromal cells (hAMSCs), deriving from the embryonic mesoderm, are instead spread in the stromal layer underlying the amniotic epithelium. Stem cells deriving from AM have a great differentiating potential since these two layers originate at day 8–9 after fertilization, in a very early stage of the embryonic development. This has been extensively verified by several studies that report the capability of hAECs and hAMSCs to differentiate toward different cell lineages belonging to all three germ layers [51, 52]. The recovery of these stem cell types does not require any invasive procedures for the donor and does not rise any ethical issue; furthermore, the fact that the placenta is generally discarded after birth and is available in large supplies makes these stem cells an excellent candidate for their eventual use in cell therapy approaches [51]. The scientific interest for the use of these stem cells in regenerative medicine is also generated by their low immunogenicity characteristics; this is confirmed by the clinical applications that use the AM as biologic bandages in surgical procedures [53] for the treatment of corneal or conjunctival destructive loss [54].

The low immunogenic and the immunomodulatory properties of hAECs and hAMSCs can be explained by their low or limited levels of the HLA-ABC expression and the absence of the HLA-DR expression together with the co-stimulatory molecules [55–57]. All these immunological characteristics make them particularly suitable for the use in allogenic transplantations for the recovery of the damaged tissue through anti-inflammatory, anti-fibrotic, and pro-regenerative effects, minimizing the risk of rejection. This procedure is less invasive compared to autologous transplants and have all the advantages of allogenic transplantations in which the stem cells can be previously isolated and cryopreserved, making them readily available for possible clinical uses. This fact shortens the time of transplantation, offering the advantage of intervening timely on the damaged tissue before the fibrotic process irreversibly compromises the tissue regeneration.

14.1.5.1 Potential Use of hAMSC in Muscle Repair

The capability of muscle tissues to regenerate in response to injury stimuli represents an essential homeostatic process, in which the cell turnover plays an important role and in the case of small injuries due to contusions, the muscle is able to self-repair its damage through four correlated time-dependent phases: degeneration, inflammation, regeneration, and remodeling repair [58]. The injury of myofibers results in the rapid necrosis in which the influx of extracellular calcium induces the proteolysis of the myofibers [59]. The necrotic fibers activate an inflammatory response characterized by the recall of specific cell populations into the muscle [60]. The inflammatory response is then followed by a regenerative phase, characterized by satellite stem cell activation and by the presence of regenerating fibers [61]. In the final phase, the maturation of the regenerated myofibers, and the contraction and reorganization of the scar tissue occur, recovering the functional performance of the injured muscle [62]. On the contrary, in the case of severe muscle injuries, the muscle function results permanently damaged for the formation of dense scar tissue (fibrosis) [63, 64] that can diminish the ability of full recovery leading to muscle contracture and chronic pain [65]. Up to date, optimal treatment strategies for severe muscle injuries have not yet been identified, and for this scope, a new strategy needs to be developed. In this context, AM-derived mesenchymal stem cell could be a promising option for their anti-inflammatory, anti-fibrotic, and pro-regenerative intrinsic characteristics.

In our laboratory, the hAMSCs isolated from AM are being studied to investigate their possible use in severe muscle injury also with the goal of sphincter incontinence regeneration. These cells are isolated from the term amnion and dissected from the part connected to the umbilical cord to minimize the presence of maternal cells. Homogenous hAMSC populations are obtained by a two-step procedure: the amniotic membrane is treated with trypsin to remove hAECs and the remaining mesenchymal stem cells are then released by digestion with collagenase [66]. The quantity obtained from the term amnion is about one million hAMSCs [67], a great amount that is possible to cryopreserve. After isolation, the hAMSCs are characterized according to the minimal and univocal criteria indicated by the Mesenchymal and Tissue Stem Cell Committee of the International Society for Cellular Therapy [68]. The first cell requirement needed is the plastic-adherent ability when maintained in standard culture conditions; they must also express *CD105, CD73, CD29, and CD90* and lack the expression of *CD45* and *CD31* surface molecules, and finally, they must show a differentiating potential toward osteoblast, adipocyte, and chondroblast lineages after specific in vitro chemical treatments. Based on this, we demonstrated by phase-contrast analysis on isolated hAMSCs the ability to adhere to plastic Petri dishes (Fig. 14.2a), and by trypan blue assay, they resulted able to exponentially grow from day 1 to day 4 (Fig. 14.2b). Actin fluorescence staining also revealed (Fig. 14.3) their typical fibroblast-like morphology (Fig. 14.3). The presence of MSC markers (*CD90, CD44, CD73, CD54, CD105,* and *CD29*) and a very low expression of hematopoietic markers such as *CD31, CD34,* and *CD45* were also highlighted by their immunophenotypical characterization (Table 14.1). Moreover, a widespread expression of the mesenchymal ubiquitous *Vimentin* marker was revealed, by fluorescence microscopy analysis (Fig. 14.4) together with the capability to achieve osteogenic, adipogenic, and chondrogenic commitments when growing in appropriate and specific differentiating mediums as highlighted by specific assays (data not shown).

The mRNAs' expression of early and late muscle differentiation markers has been also investigated in hAMSCs after the treatment of chemical and physical differentiating stimuli. The ongoing results confirmed their muscle commitment, suggesting their potential use in cell therapy leading us to suppose that these cells' engraftment could be enhanced compared to other uncommitted transplanted stem cells. This hypothesis is presently under investigation in various muscles injury animal models in order to understand the most efficient differentiating level to be used to improve muscle repair.

14.1.6 hMSCs from Adipose Tissue

The adipose tissue was for a long time considered only for its energy storage function [69, 70], but in 1994 after the discovery of leptin, the first adipokine, it became clear that this tissue is also an endocrine organ playing an important role for several inflammatory diseases in physiopathology [71]. Adipose tissue is widely distributed in the adult human body and is found in the bone marrow; intra-articular, subcutaneous, and visceral depots; and ectopic sites such as intrahepatic and intramuscular tissues. The worldwide diffusion of obesity has contributed to increase the scientific interest toward this tissue. Even though the mature adipocytes are their main component, it is also composed by other cell types that contribute to its cellular heterogeneity. These different cell components are usually isolated from surgical specimens or lipoaspirates by collagenase enzyme digestions [72, 73] followed by centrifugation to separate the floating mature adipocytes from the remain-

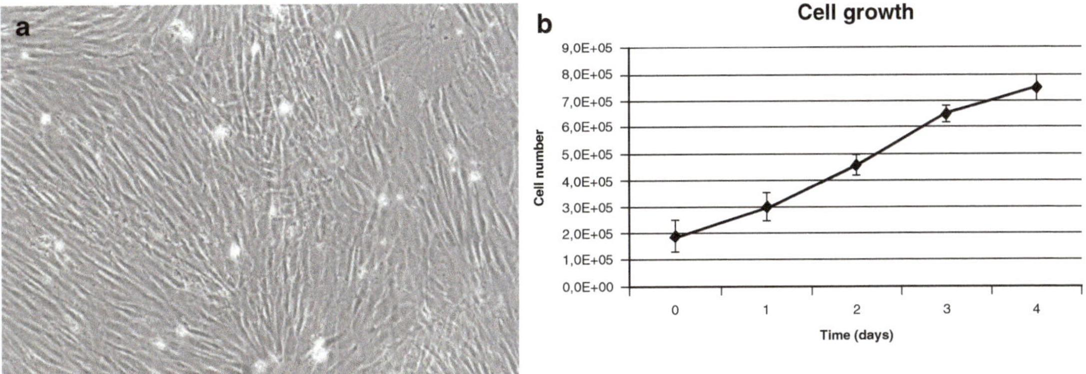

Fig. 14.2 (a) Plastic Petri dishes adherence ability of hAMSCs by phase-contrast microscope analysis (20× objective). (b) hAMSCs exponential growth trend from day 1 to 4, by trypan blue cell assay

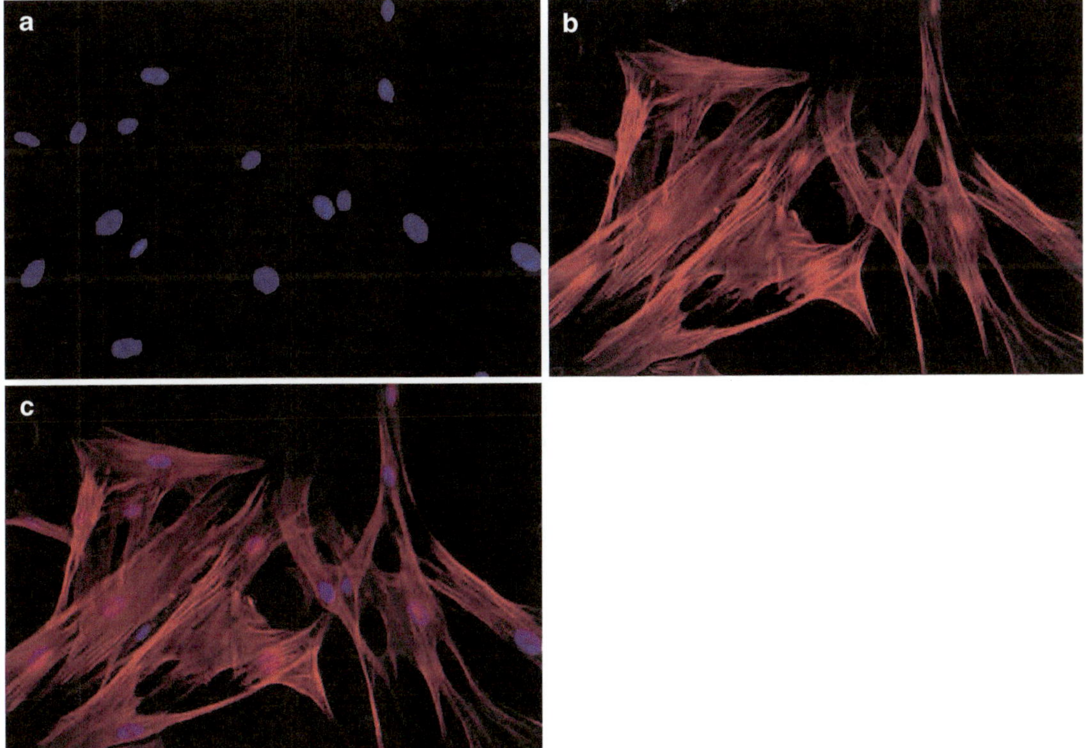

Fig. 14.3 hAMSCs typical fibroblast-like morphology by actin fluorescence analysis (a) Hoechst nuclei staining, (b) phalloidin actin staining, and (c) merged image (20× objective)

ing cells, forming a stromal vascular fraction (SVF) pellet [73]. It contains endothelial cells, macrophages, fibroblasts, B- and T-lymphocytes, myeloid cells, pericytes, smooth muscle cells, pre-adipocytes, and adipose-derived stem cells (ADSCs). After about 1 week of expansion in specific medium, it is possible to obtain from one milliliter of human lipoaspirate between 0.2 and 0.4×10^6 of ADSCs which are able to differentiate toward the adipocyte, chondrocyte, and osteoblast lineages [74, 75]. Since many patients routinely undergo liposuction annually, it is easy to isolate hundreds of million ADSCs from a single donor, making them particularly interesting for regenerative medicine applications. Recently, the International Federation for Adipose Therapeutics and Science (IFATS) have provided minimal criteria for the characterization of ASC based on functional and quantitative features [76], and many companies have developed closed system devices designed for ADSC isolation [77]. These automated devices have improved the methods to obtain reproducibility of results and their safety in clinical application uses.

The clinical translation of ADSCs still remains object of intensive research [78], but some very promising findings have been already reported. Finnish and collaborators at the Universities of Helsinki and Tampere, for example, used autologous human ADSCs to repair hard palate defect

Table 14.1 hAMSC mesenchymal and hematopoietic markers immunophenotypical characterization by FACS Cytometer analysis

Mesenchymal markers		Hematopoietic markers	
CD90	96 %	CD31	0 %
CD44	97 %	CD34	3 %
CD54	99 %	CD45	0 %
CD29	95 %		
CD105	96 %		
CD73	98 %		

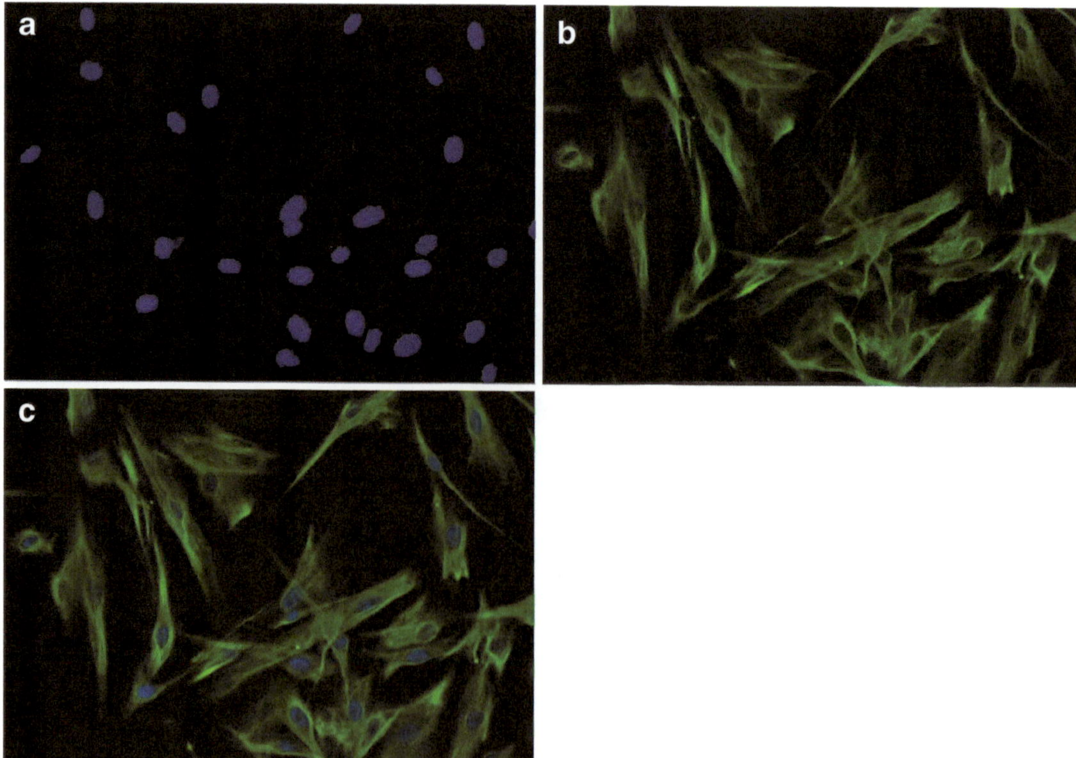

Fig. 14.4 hAMSCs mesenchymal Vimentin expression by fluorescence microscopy analysis: (**a**) Hoechst nuclei staining, (**b**) Vimentin fluorescence analysis, and (**c**) merged image (20× objective)

[79], reporting the encouraging results of a full recovery of the oral function and independent groups have shown similar results [80, 81].

14.2 Clinical Applications

14.2.1 Stem Cells and Sphincters Dysfunctions of the Pelvis

At present there are more than 350 clinical trials involving human MSCs for very different entities (www.clinicaltrials.gov). Most of these studies involve the use of mesenchymal stem cells from the bone marrow and adipose tissue, and no significant adverse effects were observed in all studies. Relatively few studies were performed to treat a degenerated sphincter muscle in humans with MSCs or MSC-like cells.

Based on the promising preclinical "in vitro" and "in vivo studies" [82–84], MSCs have been also investigated for their potential therapeutic applications in sphincter dysfunctions of the pelvic floor, both in the proctologic and in the urogynecological field [21, 85–88]. As a matter of fact, the use of MSCs for fecal and urinary incontinence treatments may be a major step forward in clinical efficacy with minimal risks, especially compared to surgical repair treatments [89–96].

The incontinence, both fecal and urinary, may result from the loss of the sphincter function due to muscle damage and peripheral nerve lesions, with various combinations of both. The rebuilding of the muscle fibers and nerve endings by a regenerative therapy employing mesenchymal stem cells is then an ideal treatment concept, especially because clinical use of these stem cells appears free of ethical concerns and risk of tumor formations [97].

Autologous and heterologous MSCs are used for "in vivo" studies on animals, while only autologous MSCs are employed in human trials. The most widely used technique for the production of adequate amounts of MSCs provides for their harvesting from several adult tissues, such as the bone marrow, muscle, and adipose tissue. Subsequently, MSCs are "in vitro" expanded, until desired cell numbers are achieved ready to transplantation to regenerative therapy [98]. However, the use of MSCs in clinical practice is still not widespread, and the clinical application in patients remains an important goal. Certainly, this is not due to the low consideration of physicians for this procedure but rather to the complex production method of expanding some types of stem cells and to their high costs [99].

The gynecological field of urinary incontinence was the first that received the attention of the scientific community, and only later researchers focused their interest on fecal incontinence. The first MSCs application in a rat urinary incontinence model was published in 2000 by Chancellor et al. [100], and only 8 years later Carr published the first study on patients affected by stress urinary incontinence [101].

14.2.2 Urinary Incontinence

14.2.2.1 Animal Models

Different animal models have been used to mimic the injuries that can produce urinary incontinence. The first model, introduced by Lin in 1998 [102], utilized vaginal distension in female rats to simulate the trauma of childbirth with damage to surrounding muscles and nerves. Subsequent other models have been developed to investigate the incontinence mechanism, including nerve injury (transection of pudendal or sciatic nerve), direct urethral injury (urethral transection or cryo-chemo injury), and pelvic ligament injury. However, female Sprague–Dawley rats are the most used in these experiments [103–105].

In preclinical studies reported, two main approaches have been used for MSC transplants: the systemic administration by intravenous injection and local injections by direct puncture [21, 106–108]. The advantage of the first method is characterized by the simplicity of the technique and the ability of MSCs to migrate "in vivo" to specific inflammatory tissue and concentrate at the site of the lesion, thanks to the capacity of MSCs to "homing" into the site of injury in several disease models. Cruz et al. in 2012 [109], and Dissaranan et al. in 2014 [110], showed, by intravenous injection of MSCs in a rat model, the homing of these cells in the urethra and a facilitated recovery of continence. However, additional studies have shown limits to this technique as reported by Rombouts and Ploemacher in 2003 [111] due to the fact that the increasing age and passage number in stem cell culture reduce the homing effect and the efficiency of MSCs engraftment. Furthermore, Fischer et al. in 2009 [112] reported that systemically infused MSCs often suffer from a first-pass effect where the larger cells become trapped in capillary beds of various tissues, decreasing their therapeutic bioavailability and functionality. Therefore, for increasing the number of mesenchymal stem cells and the efficiency of differentiation into the damaged sites, researchers have used local injections of MSCs, as reported by several pilot studies [43].

Functional analysis and histological examinations were performed to evaluate the therapy outcome, before and after treatment. Measurements of leak point pressure and bladder capacity were monitored to detect changes in urinary incontinence. To confirm the survival and differentiation of transplanted cells, histological sections of animal urethra were studied by immunohistochemistry–immunofluorescence analysis.

Although not all evaluation methods were uniform, in almost all studies performed on animal models of urinary incontinence, positive results are reported that showed both the improvement of the functional sphincter activity and the regeneration of new muscle and neuronal cells in the injured area.

Some of the most significant studies on animal model of urinary incontinence are summarized in Table 14.2.

14.2.2.2 Clinical Study

The clinical trial studies were performed using autologous muscle-derived mesenchymal stem cells (MDSCs) or adipose-derived mesenchymal stem cells (ADSCs) which can be obtained in large quantities from patients with an easy and low-invasive biopsy under local anesthesia. In these trials, the direct injection of MSCs was the most widely used procedure, performed by a local intrasphincteric injection by transurethral or periurethral approach using cystoscopy or ultrasonography guidance, both in females and in males. Clinical outcome was commonly based on 3-day leakage diary, 24 h pad test, quality-of-life score, and urodynamic test by urethral pressure measurement at rest and in squeezing.

In 2008, Carr et al. from the University of Toronto [101] reported the first clinical trial and published the results of 1-year follow-up on eight women in which urinary incontinence was treated with local injection of MDSCs. In this study, autologous muscle cells obtained from the thigh of patients, using a percutaneous needle technique, were expanded in culture and concentrated into a single-use dose containing $18–22 \times 10^6$ cells for injection in patients. This pilot study reported an improvement in urinary incontinence, especially between 3 and 8 months after the initial injection. Moreover, this study proved to be safe and with the absence of adverse events related to MDSCs transplant.

Later, Sebe et al. in 2011 [126], Gotoh et al. in 2013 [127], and other authors reported that MSCs are able to reduce urinary incontinence symptoms and improve quality of life of patients. Results of 11 clinical trials in a total of 456 women and 241 men, published in peer-reviewed journals [128], showed that MDSCs are safe for the treatment of urinary incontinence, suggesting their potential use in cell therapies. However, only a restricted number of studies have focused on the number of stem cells to be used, and in this context, a multicenter study of Carr, Chancellor, and colleagues, published from 2008 to 2014 [88, 100, 101, 129–133], reported that treatment outcomes depend on the number of transplanted cells. These authors reported that in all groups, there was a statistically significant reduction in stress leaks within 1–3 months of treatment that was maintained through the 12-month follow-up, suggesting that the efficacy of MSCs is related to cell dose. In particular patients who received higher doses (200×10^6 cells) appeared to have better efficacy outcomes than those who received lower doses (10×10^6) [133].

The most significant clinical studies on urinary incontinence are reported in Table 14.3.

Table 14.2 Summary of stem cell studies in animal models of urinary incontinence

	Author	Stem cell type	Animal	Injury/injection	Outcome	Conclusion
1	Chermansky et al. [113] (2004)	MDSCs	Female rat	Urethral cauterization Periurethral injection 1 week after injury	Increases in LPP at 2, 4, and 6 weeks MDSC integration in urethral striated muscle	Periurethral MDSC injection improves sphincter function in rats with sphincter deficiency
2	Fu et al. [114] (2010)	ADSCs	Female rat	Vaginal distension Periurethral injection 4 weeks after injury	Increases in max bladder capacity and LPP. Muscle thickness increased at 1 and 3 months	This procedure can be used to treat stress incontinence, with the advantages of minimal invasion and fast recovery
3	Kinebuchi et al. [115] (2010)	BMSCs	Female rat	Combined urethrolysis and toxin injection Periurethral injection 1 week after injury	During the following 12 weeks LPP increased but not significant vs control group Skeletal muscle and ganglia were significantly greater than in the control group	Transplanted cells survived and differentiated into striated muscle cells and peripheral nerve cells
4	Lim et al. [116] (2010)	HUCB	Female rat	Periurethral electrocautery Periurethral injection 1 week after injury	Increases in LPP at 2 and 4 weeks Sphincter muscle restored	HUCB is a easy and safely stem cells therapy applicable with noticeable therapeutic efficacy
5	Lin et al. [117] (2010)	ADSCs	Female rat	Vaginal distension Periurethral or intravenous injection 1 week after injury	Improvement in LPP with either transplantation method Higher urethral elastin and smooth muscle content in treated animals	Transplantation of ADSC via urethral or intravenous injection is effective in the treatment of SUI in a preclinical animal model
6	Xu et al. [118] (2010)	MDSCs (–/+ fibrin glue)	Female rat	Bilateral pudendal nerve transection Intraurethral injection 4 week after injury	Increases in LPP at 1 and 4 weeks MDSCs with fibrin glue increased muscle and microvessel density	MDSCs with fibrin glue may restore the histology and function of the urethral sphincter

(continued)

Table 14.2 (continued)

	Author	Stem cell type	Animal	Injury/injection	Outcome	Conclusion
7	Zou et al. [119] (2010)	BMSCs	Female rat	Bilateral proximal sciatic nerve transaction Implantation of tissue-engineered sling seeded with BMSCs, sling, or no sling, 4 week after injury	The tissue-engineered sling group had normal LPP, higher collagen content, and higher failure force at 12 weeks after treatment	MSC have potential for use in the next generation of prosthetic devices
8	Kim et al. [120] (2011)	BMSCs	Female rat	Bilateral pudendal nerve dissection Periurethral injection 2 weeks after injury	LPP were restored to the control values at 4 weeks Injected MSCs positive for muscle-specific markers	MSCs might differentiate into muscle lineage cells and may contribute to the repair of damaged muscle tissue
9	Corcos et al. [121] (2011)	BMSCs	Female rat	Bilateral pudendal nerve transection Periurethral injection 4 week after injury	LPP were restored to the control values at 4 weeks New tissue organization with striated skeletal muscle cells	MSCs significantly improved LPP and partially restored damaged external urethral sphincters
10	Imamura et al. [122] (2011)	BMSCs	Female rabbit	Urethral cryoinjury Intraurethral injection 1 week after injury	LPP significantly higher vs. control group at 1 and 2 weeks Growing of striated and smooth muscle-like cells	BMSCs can reconstruct functional urethral sphincters
11	Wu et al. [123] (2011)	ADSCs	Female rat	Bilateral pudendal nerve transection Periurethral injection 3 weeks after injury	Improvements in MBV, LPP, CP, FUL vs. control group at 2 weeks Significantly improvement of striated urethral muscles	ADSCs significantly strengthened local urethral muscle layers and significantly improved the morphology and function of sphincters
12	Zhao et al. [124] (2011)	ADSCs +/− nerve growth factor (NGF)	Female rat	Bilateral pudendal nerve transection Periurethral injection	ADSCs + NGF resulted in significant improvements in LPP and RUPP as well as the amount of muscle and ganglia, at 2, 6, and 8 weeks	NGF could enhance the therapeutic efficacy of ADSC transplantation

	Author	Stem cell type	Animal	Injury/injection	Outcome	Conclusion
13	Cruz et al. [109] (2012)	BMSCs – GFP labeled	Female rat	Vaginal distension Intravenous injection 1 h after injury	Significantly more MSCs home to the pelvic organs than control group at 4 and 10 days	The study provides basic science evidence that intravenous administration of MSCs could provide an effective route for cell-based therapy to facilitate repair after injury
14	Chun et al. [125] (2014)	hAFSCs early differentiated into muscle, neuron, and endothelial progenitor cells	Female ICR mice	Bilateral pudendal nerve transection Periurethral injection 2 weeks after injury	Increases in LPP and CP at 2 and 4 weeks High levels of myogenic, neuronal and endothelial marker expression	Early-differentiated hAFSCs may have synergic effects on myogenesis, neuromuscular junction formation, and angiogenesis in the regeneration of the damaged urethral sphincter

ADSCs adipose-derived mesenchymal stem cells, *BMSCs* bone marrow-derived mesenchymal stem cells, *CP* closing pressure, *FUL* functional urethral length, *GFP* green fluorescent protein, *hAFSCs* human amniotic fluid stem cells, *HUCB* human umbilical cord blood, *MDSCs* muscle-derived mesenchymal stem cells, *LPP* leak point pressure, *MBV* maximum bladder volume, *NGF* nerve growth factor, *RUPP* retrograde urethral perfusion pressure

14.2.3 Fecal Incontinence

14.2.3.1 Animal Models

Based on animal and clinical experiences of MSCs therapy for the treatment in urinary incontinence, in 2008 Lorenzi et al. and Kang et al. published the results of the first two in vivo studies with induced anal lesion.

In his study, Lorenzi treated an experimental rat model of anal sphincters injury followed by surgical repair with intrasphincteric injection of expanded rat bone marrow mesenchymal stem cells (BMSCs). The results indicate that, 30 days later, the injection of BMSCs led to an increase of muscle tissue in the injured area of the external and internal anal sphincter in which it is possible to observe abundant muscle cells of different sizes and irregularly disposed. Furthermore, functional studies highlighted an improved contractility of muscle fibers [135].

Kang injected 3×10^6 MDSCs into the anal sphincter in rats with cryoinjured anal sphincters, as a fecal incontinence model. One week after treatment, the anal sphincter was trimmed and functional tests and microscopic examination were evaluated. In the MDSCs injection group, contraction amplitude was higher than in the control group but not significantly. By immunohistochemical staining, regenerating muscle fibers were observed in variable orientation, both smooth and skeletal [136].

Two years later, White et al. published their study on 120 rats to estimate the effect of myogenic stem cells on contractile function of the external anal sphincter after transection with or without surgical repair. He noted that, in the sphincter repair group, injection of myogenic stem cells induced the enhancement of the contractile function [137]. Aghaee-Afshar et al. in 2009 [138] and Kajbafzadeh et al. in 2010 [139] focused their study on the use of stem cell transplantation in sphincter injury model without subsequent surgical repair. A stem cell injection was performed respectively 2 and 3 weeks after injury, and results were obtained at different intervals from the treatments, showing significant improvement in the electrical activity and in the mean resting pressure of the anal canal. Furthermore, histopathologic evaluation showed regenerated myotubes and a significant decrease in interstitial fibrosis.

In 2012, Pathi et al. [140] published an interesting randomized study on 204 female rats with external anal sphincter laceration and repair. Animals were treated with direct or intravenous injection of 4×10^6 heterologous BMSCs. The contractile function of sphincters and the parameters of wound healing were analyzed up to 21 days after injury, showing that the direct injection of MSCs into the injured anal sphincter leads to full functional recovery, while the intravenous injection did not fully rescue the compromised sphincter. Direct injection of BMSCs also increased, in the injured area, the expression of the RNA level of lysyl oxidase and TFG-Beta1, two genes involved in collagen, elastin, and matrix synthesis.

Some other significant studies were published in the last years. Salcedo and colleagues [141, 142], in two consecutive articles in 2013 and 2014 on animal model, with induced lesion of the anal sphincter, tested the efficacy of BMSCs via intramuscular or intravenous injected. In both studies, he reported a significant improvement in the anal pressure in BMSCs transplanted groups. However, in the first study, in which BMSCs were also injected into a group of rats with nerve injuries by pudendal crush, he did not report any functional improvement. Nevertheless, he also describes a marked decrease in fibrosis and scar tissue as effects of MSC transplantation.

The articles published in 2015 by a study group of Texas University examine the relationship between the muscular disruption and contractile force of sphincters after transection and repair of external anal sphincter. In intramuscular injection of the myogenic stem group, there was a substantial improvement in the generation of the contractile force, but there was no difference in the anal sphincter volume compared to the control. He suggests that stem cells might improve the contractile function through other cellular processes [143]. Montoya paper [144] reported an original study in which, after 2 weeks from a complete sphincter transection, rats were injected

Table 14.3 Summary of clinical trials of stem cells for urinary incontinence

	Author	Stem cell type	Patients number	Injection/cell number	Outcome	Conclusion
1	Carr et al. [101] (2008)	Autologous MDSCs	8 Women	Intrasphincteric (transurethral injection) (18–22 × 10^6 cells)	Improvement in SUI at follow-up of 12 mounts (mean/median 16.5/17) No adverse events	Therapy is safe and clinically feasible
2	Sebe et al. [126] (2011)	Autologous MDSCs	12 Women	Intrasphincteric (transurethral injection) (1–5 × 10^7 cells)	8 subjects improved symptoms of SUI at follow-up of 12 mounts No local complication were reported	Cell therapy seems clinically feasible and safe and shows promising results
3	Gotoh et al. [127] (2013)	Autologous ADSCs not expanded (Celution system)	11 men	Intrasphincteric (transurethral injection) 7.5 × 10^6–3.3 × 10^7 cells	SUI improved progressively in eight patients during the 1-year follow-up No significant adverse events were observed	Cell therapy might represent a safe and feasible treatment modality for male stress urinary incontinence
4	Carr et al. [132] (2013)	Autologous MDSCs	38 women	Intrasphincteric (transurethral injection) Low doses 1–16 × 10^6 High doses 32–128 × 10^6 for one or two times	Improvement of SUI symptoms and quality of life during the 1-year follow-up Improvement is related to cell dose for a greater percentage of patients in the high dose group. No major adverse events were reported	Cell therapy reduces SUI severity and improves quality of life A potential dose-dependent treatment effect was observed with a trend toward greater efficacy in patients who received doses of 32 × 10^6 or greater per treatment

(continued)

Table 14.3 (continued)

	Author	Stem cell type	Patients number	Injection/cell number	Outcome	Conclusion
5	Gras et al. [128] (2014)	Autologous minced skeletal Muscle (not expanded)	35 women	Periurethral injection	Significant decrease in the mean number of stress leaks and the impact of SUI symptoms during the 1-year follow-up	Treatment is simple and appears to be safe and moderately effective in women with uncomplicated SUI. The treatment compares well to a similar but more complicated regenerative therapy using in vitro expanded muscle-derived cells
6	Stangel-Wojcikiewicz et al. [134] (2014)	Autologous MDSCs	16 Women	Intrasphincteric (transurethral injection) $0.6–25 \times 10^6$ cells	Success rate 75 %, with 50 % of patients cured and 25 % with improvement during the 2-year follow-up No serious adverse side effects or complications were noted	Treatment is safe and effective. In contrast with other reports, a relatively small number of cells was needed for relieving SUI symptoms
7	Jankowski et al. [133] (2014)	Autologous MDSCs	126 Women* *(enrolled in 4 phase I/II clinical trials)	Intrasphincteric injection $1–200 \times 10^6$ cells	More patients are responsive to doses of 100 and 200 million AMDC at 12-month follow-up than to lower doses No adverse events attributed to MDSCs	Treatment is safe. Efficacy data suggest that more patients are responsive to doses of 100 and 200 million cells than to lower doses

ADSCs adipose-derived mesenchymal stem cells, *MDSCs* muscle-derived mesenchymal stem cells, *SUI* stress urinary incontinence

with a hydrogel matrix scaffold combined with myogenic stem cells. Neurophysiology tests and histologic examination, performed after 4 and 12 weeks, highlighted how, compared to the control groups, the addition of a biogel scaffold to the myogenic stem cells increases the contractile force and the histological evidence of sphincter restoration with steady improvement over time.

In Table 14.4 the studies on animal model of fecal incontinence reported in literature are summarized.

14.2.3.2 Clinical Study

Until today, only two pilot studies have been produced using MSCs to treat fecal incontinence in humans.

In 2013, Frudinger and colleagues published, for the first time, a study on ten women with damaged anal sphincter by obstetric trauma which were followed up for 1 year after treatment [145]. All patients, with a preventive endosonographic diagnosis of anterior defect of the external anal sphincter, were treated with autologous myoblast cells harvested from a pectoral muscle

Table 14.4 Stem cell studies in animal model of fecal incontinence

	Author	Stem cell type	Animal	Injury/injection	Outcome	Conclusion
1	Lorenzi et al. [135] (2008)	Rat BMSCs	24 male rat	Sphincterotomy and surgical repair of both internal and external anal sphincters 0.75×10^6 cells into each cut end of both sphincters at the same time	The area at the site of injury appeared rich in irregularly disposed muscle cells of different sizes Improved response of anal sphincters to electrical field stimulation compared to control group	BMSCs increases contractile function and improves muscle regeneration
2	Kang et al. [136] (2008)	Rat MDSCs	15 female rat	Anal cryoinjury. Intrasphincteric injection 5 min after injury 3×10^6 cells	Regenerating smooth and skeletal fibers in the area of MDSCs injection Contraction amplitude higher than in the control group but not significantly	Autologous MDSCs grafts may be used as a tool for improving anal sphincter contractility
3	Aghaee-Afshar et al. [138] (2009)	hUCM and rabbit BMSCs	35 male rabbits	External anal sphincterotomy Intrasphincteric injection 2 weeks after injury 10^4 cells	In BMSCs group decreased muscle fibrosis Improvement in the electrical activity at 2 weeks after transplantation compared to pretreatment values and controls	BMSCs may provide an effective tool for treating anal sphincter injuries in humans
4	Kajbafzadeh et al. [139] (2010)	Rabbit myoblast	21 male rabbits	Subtotal external sphincterotomy Intrasphincteric injection 3 weeks after injury 7×10^7 cells	Regenerated myotubes in the injection area. Significant decrease in interstitial fibrosis. Improvement in the mean resting pressure of anal canal at 4 weeks after cell injection	Autografting of muscle progenitor cells showed the potential for a myogenic procedure
5	White et al. [137] (2010)	Rat myoblast	120 female rat	External anal sphincter transection with or without surgical repair Intrasphincteric injection at the same time of the injury 3.2×10^6 cells	Myogenic stem cells enhanced contractile function at both 7 days and 90 day in sphincter repair group	Myogenic stem cells may serve as positive adjunctive therapy in the treatment of anal sphincter injury

(continued)

Table 14.4 (continued)

	Author	Stem cell type	Animal	Injury/injection	Outcome	Conclusion
6	Pathi et al. [140] (2012)	Rat heterologous BMSCs	204 female rat	External anal sphincter transection and surgical repair Intrasphincteric or Intravenous injection At the same time of the injury 4×10^6	Direct, not intravenous, resulted in full functional recovery of compromised sphincter at 21 days after cell injection Increased level of lysyl oxidase and TFG-Beta1	MSC may play an important role in increased collagen deposition in the injured site Directly injected MSCs, but not intravenously injected, not only may provide progenitor cells for new myoblasts but also may stimulate matrix production to orient and guide migration of the cells into the injured muscle
7	Salcedo et al. [141] (2013)	Rat BMSCs	70 female rat	Sphincterotomy or pudendal nerve crush Intrasphincteric or intravenous injection 24 h after injury	In sphincterotomy group, not in pudendal nerve crush group, significant increase in anal pressure and sphincter EMG frequency at 9 days after cell injection	MSC treatment either IM or IV resulted in improved anal sphincter pressures after a direct injury to the anal sphincter complex
8	Salcedo et al. [142] (2014)	Rat BMSCs	50 female rat	Excision of 25 % of the external and internal anal sphincter Intrasphincteric or intravenous injection 24 h after injury 5×10^5 cells	Significant improvement in anal pressure Marked decrease in fibrosis and scar tissue in both intramuscular and intravenous BMSCs transplanted groups, at 10 and 35 days after cell injection	The process of increased pressures after i.v. infusions can be explained by MSCs homing to the site of injury in response to the cytokine There is a possibility of a bulking effect of an i.m. injection that needs to be explored

	Author	Stem cell type	Animal	Injury/injection	Outcome	Conclusion
9	Fitzwater et al. [143] (2015)	Heterologous rat myoblast	40 female rat	External anal sphincter transection and surgical repair Intrasphincteric injection at the same time of the injury 3.2×10^6	Substantial improvement in contractile force; no difference in anal sphincter volume, compared to the control, at 7 and 90 days after cell injection	The study suggests that the myogenic stem cells can improve the contractile ability of the anal sphincter through more complex cellular mechanisms besides merely the volumetric or morphological findings
10	Montoya et al. [144] (2015)	Heterologous rat myoblast	80 female rats	External and internal anal sphincter transection Intrasphincteric injection of stem cells combined with *hydrogel matrix scaffold* 2 weeks after injury 3.2×10^6 cells	Increasing of contractile force and histological evidence of sphincter restoration at 4 and 12 weeks after injection	A biologically compatible matrix may facilitate stem cell survival, differentiation, or functions leading to recovery of tissue function

BMSCs bone marrow-derived mesenchymal stem cells, *MDSCs* muscle-derived mesenchymal stem cells

biopsy and cultured for 39 days. Muscle-derived stem cells were injected under ultrasonography guidance into external anal sphincter ends and also in the interposed scar tissue. Twelve to 14 individual injections of 0.5 ml for a total of 6–7 ml (the number of myoblasts is not specified) were administered, making sure not to treat directly the internal anal sphincter. No adverse events were observed, and the procedure was well tolerated. At 12 months, all patients stated that their symptoms had improved and the Rockwood Fecal Incontinence Quality of Life Scale [146] resulted significantly improved. The Wexner Incontinence Score [147] had a significant decrease from a mean value of 15.3–1.6. However, the initial significant increase in mean and maximal anal squeeze pressures seen at 1 and 6 months was transient and not sustained at 12 months. As matter of fact, between the 6 and 12 months assessment, also a significant decrease in mean and maximal anal resting pressure occurred. The author reported in an additional article published in 2015 the updates of the 5-year follow-up for the ten patients reporting significant improved symptoms of anal incontinence.

The second study on regenerative treatment in patients affected by fecal incontinence was produced by the group of Giori and coinvestigators. In this pilot study, performed according to the Declaration of Helsinki and approved by the ethics committee, they treated 15 patients (14 females and 1 male) with incontinence due to obstetric injury and anorectal-pelvic surgery. Preliminary results of this study were published in 2015 [148]. Actual experience of the authors in the use, for the first time, of Lipogems® technique to treat patients with fecal incontinence is described below.

14.2.4 Personal Experience with Technique Lipogems®

Lipogems® is a regenerative product by autologous lipoaspirated fat rich in mesenchymal stem cells, obtained in a completely closed system by a disposable device without using enzymes, additives, and other manipulations. Mild mechanical processes of microfracturing, washing, and filtration progressively reduce the size of the fragments of adipose tissue and remove oily substances and blood residues [149] (Fig. 14.5). Differently, from the mesenchymal cells expanded in laboratory, Lipogems micro-tissue is not a "pool" of individual stem cells, but it is composed of small adipose spherical clusters (400/900 μm) with micro-fragments of intact connective structure maintained viable by a stromal vascular fraction (SVF), particularly rich in pericytes and MSCs incorporated in their "natural niche tissue" [150, 151] and exposed on the surface of the vascular stroma. The micro-fragmented tissue enclosing stromal vascular fraction (SVF) can be ideally assimilated to a biologic matrix scaffold that facilitates the engraftment and the biological activity of MSCs, as evident in previous experience described by Montoya [144]. These properties contribute to make Lipogems® able to survive in a suffering tissue, facilitating the engraftment and the paracrine activity of the embedded cells when autologously inoculated in target tissues [152–154].

However, studies have shown that, when the Lipogems® product was cultured in vitro, it yielded a virtually pure population of hMSCs exhibiting the typical characteristics of surface markers isolated from other sources, including CD90, CD73, CD105, and CD44 [32, 155].

In clinical practice, Lipogems procedure is conducted in a single surgical session that includes three different steps: (1) harvesting of subcutaneous adipose tissue from abdomen or thigh of the patient, (2) processing of adipose tissue with Lipogems® device, and (3) reinjecting the product in the same patient under ultrasound guidance.

Unlike to Frudinger, who had injected MSC only in the area of the sphincter lesion [145], in our study, we injected Lipogems not only in the area of muscle defects but also in the intersphincteric space and around the external anal sphincter [148]. Moreover, because a lesion of the sphincter muscle that affects from outside, such as in childbirth, is always associated to a lesion of the peripheral nerve endings, we have found it useful to also stimulate a neural-regenerative effect injecting Lipogems® also along the course of

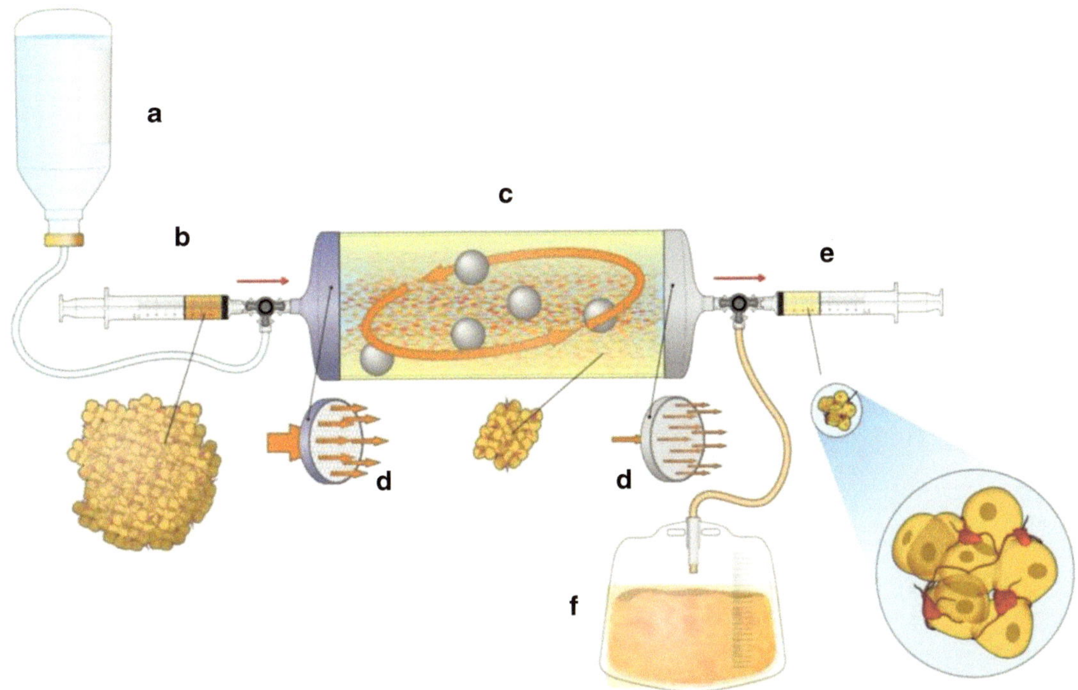

Fig. 14.5 Lipogems device is a disposable closed system filled with physiologic solution. It reduces the size of lipoaspirate clusters after washing of oil, blood, and cellular debris. (*A*) sac with saline solution; (*B*) syringe with lipoaspirate; (*C*) washing chamber containing marbles for the emulsion of fluid and elimination of oil and blood; (*D*) mechanical filters, (*E*) syringe with clusters of microfractured adipose tissue rich in MSCs; and (*F*) sac with waste oil and blood

peripheral pudendal nerve. An average of 340 cc of lipoaspirate was collected from subcutaneous fat of each patient. As a result of processing with the technique Lipogems®, an average of 87 cc of product was obtained, ready for injection in every patient. After treatment, the 15 patients of this series were followed up for 2 years. Wex ner Incontinence Score, Rockwood Fecal Incontinence Quality of Life Scale, digital exploration, proctoscopy, endoanal ultrasound, and anorectal manometry were used before treatment and after 3, 6, 12, 18, and 24 months from the injection of ADSCs, to assess fecal incontinence. The procedure has proven to be safe and well tolerated. In all patients, there were no adverse events related to ADSCs injection. Only in one patient occurred a hematoma at the site of harvesting in the subcutaneous adipose tissue, which resolved spontaneously. Improvement both short and long term was observed in all patients.

Patients' satisfaction for the treatment was very good, and the Fecal Incontinence Quality of Life Scale increased from a mean preoperative overall value of 53–102 after 3 months from treatment, essentially unchanged for the 2 years of follow up.

In the 15 patients, a significant improvement in the average values of the overall Wexner Incontinence Score was observed which decreased by a mean preoperative of 14.1 units to 3.4 units at 3 months and remained quite stable over the time of the study with a value of 4.1 at 24 months (Fig. 14.6). After treatment, the overall mean values of the anal pressure at rest and in squeeze improved in all the patients as reported in Fig. 14.7. In the graph, a remarkable increasing of the anal squeeze pressure during the entire second year of follow-up is evident. Ultrasound examinations showed a progressive reabsorption of the hyperechogenic Lipogems tissue from 3 to 12 months and increasing of muscle

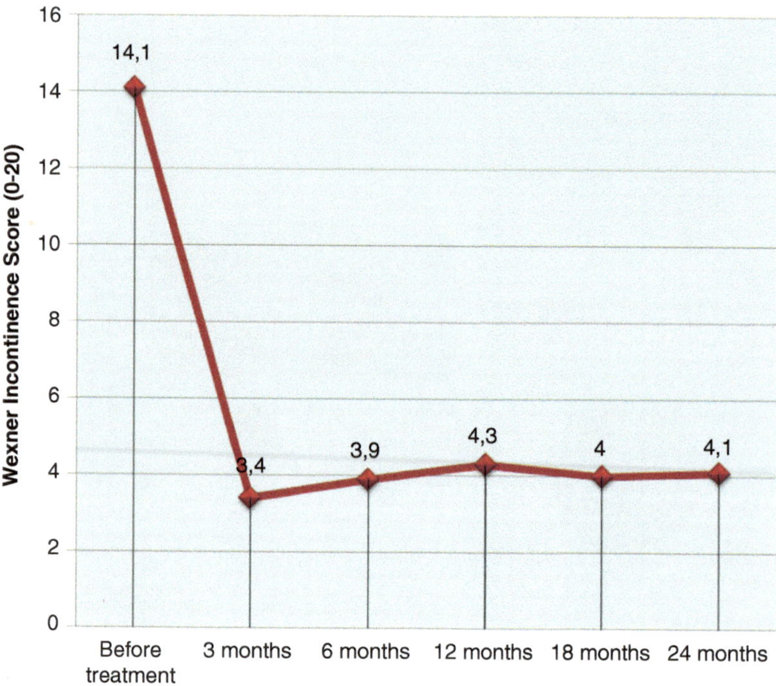

Fig. 14.6 Average values of the Wexner Incontinence Score (0–20) before and after treatment

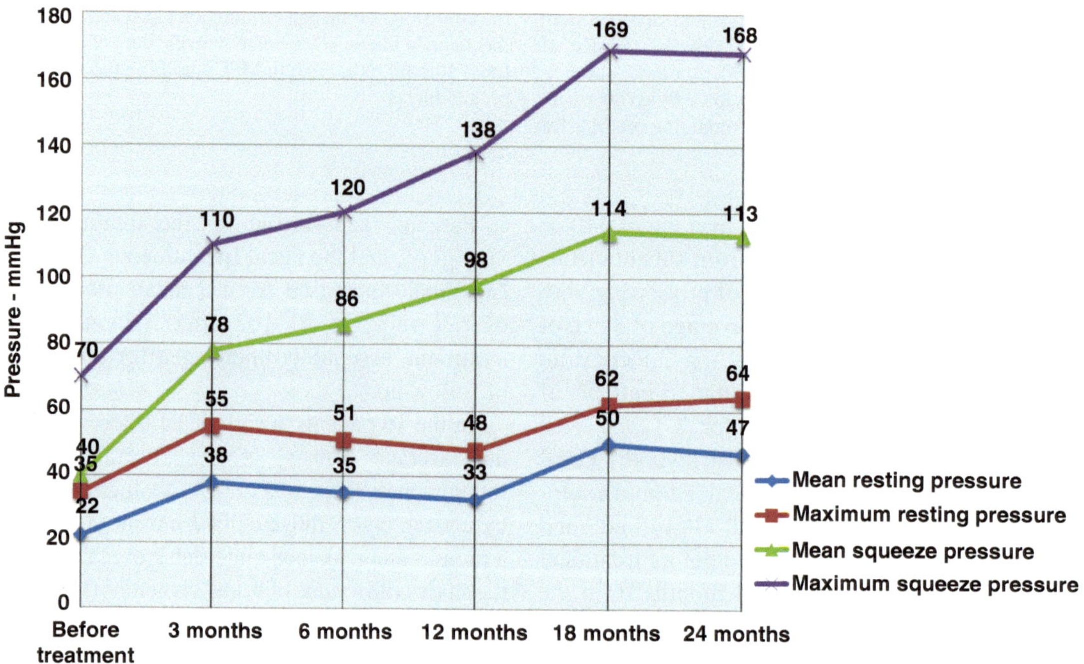

Fig. 14.7 Average values of anorectal manometry (mmHg) before and after treatment

fibers with images of sphincter restoration at 12 and 24 months in several patients (Fig. 14.8). After treatment, physical examination and proctoscopy did not show any new pathological findings of the anorectal complex. At palpation the enhancement in the contractile activity of the anal sphincters and

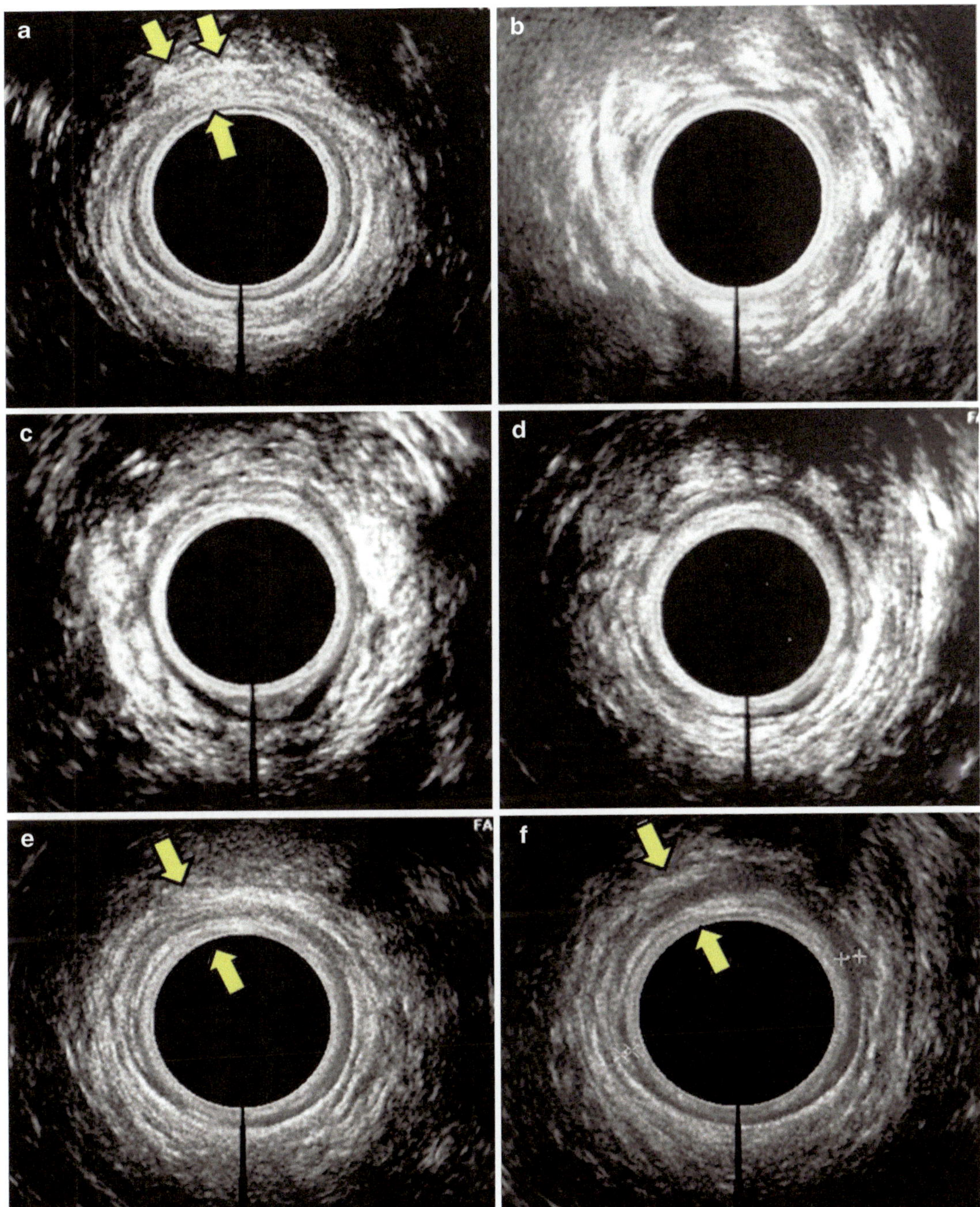

Fig. 14.8 Endoanal ultrasonography images of a representative patient at preoperative, intraoperative stage and at 3, 6, 12, 24 months after treatment. (**a**) Preoperative stage. Lesion of the external and internal anal sphincter localized in the anterior area, evidenced by arrows (**b**) Intraoperative stage. Diffuse hyperechoic spots at the sites of inoculation of Lipogems. (**c**) 3rd month. Partial resorption of hyperechoic spots of Lipogems. (**d**) 6th month. Aspect of the early development of new muscle tissue at the site of the lesion. Are still evident few hyperechoic spots of Lipogems. (**e**, **f**) 12th and 24th month respectively. The image shows muscle restoration in the area of previous lesion of the anal sphincters evidenced by arrows. No more evidence of hyperechoic depots of Lipogems

improvement of anocutaneous reflex, where it was lacking before treatment, was clearly observable.

From a detailed analysis of patients' data, between the 3rd and the 12th month, we have observed a slight decline of the resting pressure associated with mild worsening of the Wexner index. This feature is, in our opinion, attributed to a temporary bulking effect of the "not stem cells" component of Lipogems, which is reabsorbed in a period between 3 and 12 months from treatment, as it usually occurs with the traditional techniques of biological lipofilling [156]. Thus, the clear increase in the contractile ability of the anal sphincter recorded by anorectal manometry after 12 months (Fig. 14.8e, f), when deposits of material inoculated disappeared and ultrasound images showed muscle restoration, is attributable to the effect of mesenchymal cells.

This is also indirectly confirmed by the results of Frudinger, who obtained a temporary increase in anal squeeze pressures not sustained at 12 months as reported in her first article. However, the extension of the follow-up described in the second publication has proven a slow and gradual improvement of incontinence, which remained unchanged through all the 5 years of observation [145, 157].

14.2.5 Final Considerations

On the basis of preclinical studies and clinical trials conducted both in the field of urinary incontinence and fecal incontinence, the use of autologous MSCs revealed to be safe, minimally traumatic, well tolerated, and effective in improving the symptoms of incontinence. In particular, new techniques like Lipogems®, which uses autologous stem cells derived from adipose tissue easy to harvest and prepare the product using a device directly in the operating room in the course of a single surgical time, make the use of mesenchymal stem cells of simple execution and that are inexpensive and widely applicable in clinical practice. Further investigations are necessary to clarify the efficacy and the biological mechanism of this very simple regenerative procedure, but a future association together with surgical repair of damaged anal sphincters is also possible.

References

1. Ramalho-Santos M, Willenbring H. On the origin of the term "stem cell". Cell Stem Cell. 2007;1(1):35–8.
2. Wilson EB. The cell in development and inheritance. New York: The MacMillan Company; 1896.
3. Weissman IL, Anderson DJ, Gage F. Stem and progenitor cells: origins, phenotypes, lineage commitments, and transdifferentiations. Annu Rev Cell Dev Biol. 2001;17(1):387–403.
4. Smith AG. Embryo-derived stem cells: of mice and men. Annu Rev Cell Dev Biol. 2001;17(1):435–62.
5. Papaioannou V. Stem cells and differentiation. Differentiation. 2001;68(4–5):153–4.
6. Takahashi K, Yamanaka S. Induction of pluripotent stem cells from mouse embryonic and adult fibroblast cultures by defined factors. Cell. 2006;126(4):663–76.
7. Hussein SM, Nagy AA. Progress made in the reprogramming field: new factors, new strategies and a new outlook. Curr Opin Genet Dev. 2012;22(5):435–43.
8. Bayart E, Cohen-Haguenauer O. Technological overview of iPS induction from human adult somatic cells. Curr Gene Ther. 2013;13(2):73.
9. Rajasingh J. Reprogramming of somatic cells. Prog Mol Biol Transl Sci. 2012;111:51–82.
10. Robertson JA. Human embryonic stem cell research: ethical and legal issues. Nat Rev Genet. 2001;2(1):74–8.
11. Dhar D, Hsi-En Ho J. Stem cell research policies around the world. Yale J Biol Med. 2009;82(3):113–5.
12. Lee J-H, Lee JB, Shapovalova Z, Fiebig-Comyn A, Mitchell RR, Laronde S, Szabo E, Benoit YD, Bhatia M. Somatic transcriptome priming gates lineage-specific differentiation potential of human-induced pluripotent stem cell states. Nat Commun. 2014;5:5605.
13. Riggs JW, Barrilleaux BL, Varlakhanova N, Bush KM, Chan V, Knoepfler PS. Induced pluripotency and oncogenic transformation are related processes. Stem Cells Dev. 2012;22(1):37–50.
14. de la Morena MT, Gatti RA. A history of bone marrow transplantation. Hematol Oncol Clin North Am. 2011;25(1):1–15.
15. Martin PJ, Hansen JA, Storb R, Donnall Thomas E. Human marrow transplantation: an immunological perspective. Adv Immunol. 1987;40:379–438.
16. Chinen J, Buckley RH. Transplantation immunology: solid organ and bone marrow. J Allergy Clin Immunol. 2010;125(2):S324–35.
17. Bow EJ. Infection risk and cancer chemotherapy: the impact of the chemotherapeutic regimen in patients with lymphoma and solid tissue malignancies. J Antimicrob Chemother. 1998;41(4):1–5.
18. Vanichsetakul P. Clinical use of cord blood for stem cell transplantation. J Med Assoc Thailand. 2005;88:S93.
19. Goldstein G, Toren A, Nagler A. Transplantation and other uses of human umbilical cord blood and stem cells. Curr Pharm Des. 2007;13(13):1363–73.

20. Chen M, Przyborowski M, Berthiaume F. Stem cells for skin tissue engineering and wound healing. Crit Rev Biomed Eng. 2009;37(4–5):399–421.
21. Wei X, Yang X, Z-p H, F-f Q, Shao L, Y-f S. Mesenchymal stem cells: a new trend for cell therapy. Acta Pharmacol Sin. 2013;34(6):747–54.
22. Friedenstein A, Kuralesova AI. Osteogenic precursor cells of bone marrow in radiation chimeras. Transplantation. 1971;12(2):99–108.
23. Bianchi G, Borgonovo G, Pistoia V, Raffag hello L. Immunosuppressive cells and tumour microenvironment: focus on mesenchymal stem cells and myeloid derived suppressor cells. Histol Histopathol. 2011;26(7):941.
24. Prockop DJ. Marrow stromal cells as stem cells for nonhematopoietic tissues. Science. 1997;276(5309):71–4.
25. Granero-Molto F, Weis JA, Longobardi L, Spagnoli A. Role of mesenchymal stem cells in regenerative medicine: application to bone and cartilage repair. Expert Opin Biol Ther. 2008;8(3):255.
26. Salem HK, Thiemermann C. Mesenchymal stromal cells: current understanding and clinical status. Stem Cells. 2010;28(3):585–96.
27. Dezawa M, Ishikawa H, Itokazu Y, Yoshihara T, Hoshino M, S-i T, Ide C, Y-i N. Bone marrow stromal cells generate muscle cells and repair muscle degeneration. Science. 2005;309(5732):314–7.
28. Zuk PA, Zhu M, Mizuno H, Huang J, Futrell JW, Katz AJ, Benhaim P, Lorenz HP, Hedrick MH. Multilineage cells from human adipose tissue: implications for cell-based therapies. Tissue Eng. 2001;7(2):211–28.
29. Scherjon SA, Kleijburg-van der Keur C, de Groot-Swings GM, Claas FH, Fibbe WE, Kanhai HH. Isolation of mesenchymal stem cells of fetal or maternal origin from human placenta. Stem Cells. 2004;22(7):1338–45.
30. Anjos-Afonso F, Bonnet D. Nonhematopoietic/endothelial SSEA-1+ cells define the most primitive progenitors in the adult murine bone marrow mesenchymal compartment. Blood. 2007;109(3):1298–306.
31. Pittenger MF, Mackay AM, Beck SC, Jaiswal RK, Douglas R, Mosca JD, Moorman MA, Simonetti DW, Craig S, Marshak DR. Multilineage potential of adult human mesenchymal stem cells. Science. 1999;284(5411):143–7.
32. Bianco P, Robey PG, Simmons PJ. Mesenchymal stem cells: revisiting history, concepts, and assays. Cell Stem Cell. 2008;2(4):313–9.
33. Tsai MS, Hwang SM, Chen KD, Lee YS, Hsu LW, Chang YJ, Wang CN, Peng HH, Chang YL, Chao AS. Functional network analysis of the transcriptomes of mesenchymal stem cells derived from amniotic fluid, amniotic membrane, cord blood, and bone marrow. Stem Cells. 2007;25(10):2511–23.
34. Le Blanc K, Rasmusson I, Sundberg B, Götherström C, Hassan M, Uzunel M, Ringdén O. Treatment of severe acute graft-versus-host disease with third party haploidentical mesenchymal stem cells. Lancet. 2004;363(9419):1439–41.
35. Zappia E, Casazza S, Pedemonte E, Benvenuto F, Bonanni I, Gerdoni E, Giunti D, Ceravolo A, Cazzanti F, Frassoni F. Mesenchymal stem cells ameliorate experimental autoimmune encephalomyelitis inducing T-cell anergy. Blood. 2005;106(5):1755–61.
36. Kim J-M, Lee S-T, Chu K, Jung K-H, Song E-C, Kim S-J, Sinn D-I, Kim J-H, Park D-K, Kang K-M. Systemic transplantation of human adipose stem cells attenuated cerebral inflammation and degeneration in a hemorrhagic stroke model. Brain Res. 2007;1183:43–50.
37. Parekkadan B, Van Poll D, Suganuma K, Carter EA, Berthiaume F, Tilles AW, Yarmush ML. Mesenchymal stem cell-derived molecules reverse fulminant hepatic failure. PLoS One. 2007;2(9), e941.
38. Lee JW, Fang X, Gupta N, Serikov V, Matthay MA. Allogeneic human mesenchymal stem cells for treatment of E. coli endotoxin-induced acute lung injury in the ex vivo perfused human lung. Proc Natl Acad Sci. 2009;106(38):16357–62.
39. Amado LC, Saliaris AP, Schuleri KH, John MS, Xie J-S, Cattaneo S, Durand DJ, Fitton T, Kuang JQ, Stewart G. Cardiac repair with intramyocardial injection of allogeneic mesenchymal stem cells after myocardial infarction. Proc Natl Acad Sci U S A. 2005;102(32):11474–9.
40. Kharaziha P, Hellström PM, Noorinayer B, Farzaneh F, Aghajani K, Jafari F, Telkabadi M, Atashi A, Honardoost M, Zali MR. Improvement of liver function in liver cirrhosis patients after autologous mesenchymal stem cell injection: a phase I–II clinical trial. Eur J Gastroenterol Hepatol. 2009;21(10):1199–205.
41. Peng L, Xie D, Lin BL, Liu J, Zhu H, Xie C, Zheng Y, Gao Z. Autologous bone marrow mesenchymal stem cell transplantation in liver failure patients caused by hepatitis B: short-term and long-term outcomes. Hepatology. 2011;54(3):820–8.
42. Lu D, Chen B, Liang Z, Deng W, Jiang Y, Li S, Xu J, Wu Q, Zhang Z, Xie B. Comparison of bone marrow mesenchymal stem cells with bone marrow-derived mononuclear cells for treatment of diabetic critical limb ischemia and foot ulcer: a double-blind, randomized, controlled trial. Diabetes Res Clin Pract. 2011;92(1):26–36.
43. Rasulov M, Vasil'chenkov A, Onishchenko N, Krasheninnikov M, Kravchenko V, Gorshenin T, Pidtsan R, Potapov I. First experience in the use of bone marrow mesenchymal stem cells for the treatment of a patient with deep skin burns. Bull Exp Biol Med. 2005;139(1):141–4.
44. Yamada Y, Ueda M, Hibi H, Baba S. A novel approach to periodontal tissue regeneration with mesenchymal stem cells and platelet-rich plasma using tissue engineering technology: a clinical case report. Int J Periodontics Restorative Dent. 2006;26(4):363–9.

45. Lee RH, Pulin AA, Seo MJ, Kota DJ, Ylostalo J, Larson BL, Semprun-Prieto L, Delafontaine P, Prockop DJ. Intravenous hMSCs improve myocardial infarction in mice because cells embolized in lung are activated to secrete the anti-inflammatory protein TSG-6. Cell Stem Cell. 2009;5(1):54–63.
46. Zeng X, Y-s Z, Ma Y-h, Lu L-y, B-l D, Zhang W, Li Y, Chan WY. Bone marrow mesenchymal stem cells in a three-dimensional gelatin sponge scaffold attenuate inflammation, promote angiogenesis, and reduce cavity formation in experimental spinal cord injury. Cell Transplant. 2011;20(11–12):1881–99.
47. Goodwin M, Sueblinvong V, Eisenhauer P, Ziats NP, LeClair L, Poynter ME, Steele C, Rincon M, Weiss DJ. Bone marrow-derived mesenchymal stromal cells inhibit Th2-mediated allergic airways inflammation in mice. Stem Cells. 2011;29(7):1137–48.
48. Ortiz LA, DuTreil M, Fattman C, Pandey AC, Torres G, Go K, Phinney DG. Interleukin 1 receptor antagonist mediates the antiinflammatory and antifibrotic effect of mesenchymal stem cells during lung injury. Proc Natl Acad Sci. 2007;104(26):11002–7.
49. Roddy GW, Oh JY, Lee RH, Bartosh TJ, Ylostalo J, Coble K, Rosa RH, Prockop DJ. Action at a distance: systemically administered adult stem/progenitor cells (MSCs) reduce inflammatory damage to the cornea without engraftment and primarily by secretion of TNF-α stimulated gene/protein 6. Stem Cells. 2011;29(10):1572–9.
50. Alves H, Van Ginkel J, Groen N, Hulsman M, Mentink A, Reinders M, Van Blitterswijk C, De Boer J. A mesenchymal stromal cell gene signature for donor age. PLoS One. 2012;7(8), e42908.
51. Parolini O, Alviano F, Bagnara GP, Bilic G, Bühring HJ, Evangelista M, Hennerbichler S, Liu B, Magatti M, Mao N. Concise review: isolation and characterization of cells from human term placenta: outcome of the first international Workshop on Placenta Derived Stem Cells. Stem Cells. 2008;26(2):300–11.
52. Parolini O, Soncini M, Evangelista M, Schmidt D. Amniotic membrane and amniotic fluid-derived cells: potential tools for regenerative medicine? Regen Med. 2009;4(4):275.
53. Azuara-Blanco A, Pillai C, Dua HS. Amniotic membrane transplantation for ocular surface reconstruction. Br J Ophthalmol. 1999;83(4):399–402.
54. Solomon A, Espana EM, Tseng SC. Amniotic membrane transplantation for reconstruction of the conjunctival fornices. Ophthalmology. 2003;110(1):93–100.
55. Kubo M, Sonoda Y, Muramatsu R, Usui M. Immunogenicity of human amniotic membrane in experimental xenotransplantation. Invest Ophthalmol Vis Sci. 2001;42(7):1539–46.
56. Bailo M, Soncini M, Vertua E, Signoroni PB, Sanzone S, Lombardi G, Arienti D, Calamani F, Zatti D, Paul P. Engraftment potential of human amnion and chorion cells derived from term placenta. Transplantation. 2004;78(10):1439–48.
57. Magatti M, De Munari S, Vertua E, Gibelli L, Wengler GS, Parolini O. Human amnion mesenchyme harbors cells with allogeneic T-cell suppression and stimulation capabilities. Stem Cells. 2008;26(1):182–92.
58. Crisco JJ, Jokl P, Heinen GT, Connell MD, Panjabi MM. A muscle contusion injury model biomechanics, physiology, and histology. Am J Sports Med. 1994;22(5):702–10.
59. Carosio S, Berardinelli MG, Aucello M, Musarò A. Impact of ageing on muscle cell regeneration. Ageing Res Rev. 2011;10(1):35–42.
60. Tidball JG. Inflammatory processes in muscle injury and repair. Am J Phys Regul Integr Comp Phys. 2005;288(2):R345–53.
61. Karpati G, Molnar MJ. Muscle fibre regeneration in human skeletal muscle diseases. In: Schiaffino S and Partridge T editors. Skeletal muscle repair and regeneration. Dordrecht: Springer; 2008. p. 199–216.
62. Goetsch SC, Hawke TJ, Gallardo TD, Richardson JA, Garry DJ. Transcriptional profiling and regulation of the extracellular matrix during muscle regeneration. Physiol Genomics. 2003;14(3):261–71.
63. Kääriäinen M, Kääriäinen J, Järvinen TL, Sievänen H, Kalimo H, Järvinen M. Correlation between biomechanical and structural changes during the regeneration of skeletal muscle after laceration injury. J Orthop Res. 1998;16(2):197–206.
64. Nozaki M, Li Y, Zhu J, Ambrosio F, Uehara K, Fu FH, Huard J. Improved muscle healing after contusion injury by the inhibitory effect of suramin on myostatin, a negative regulator of muscle growth. Am J Sports Med. 2008;36(12):2354–62.
65. Huard J, Li Y, Fu FH. Muscle injuries and repair: current trends in research. J Bone Joint Surg. 2002;84(5):822–32.
66. Moore R, Silver R, Moore J. Physiological apoptotic agents have different effects upon human amnion epithelial and mesenchymal cells. Placenta. 2003;24(2):173–80.
67. Casey ML, MacDonald PC. Interstitial collagen synthesis and processing in human amnion: a property of the mesenchymal cells. Biol Reprod. 1996;55(6):1253–60.
68. Dominici M, Le Blanc K, Mueller I, Slaper-Cortenbach I, Marini F, Krause D, Deans R, Keating A, Prockop D, Horwitz E. Minimal criteria for defining multipotent mesenchymal stromal cells. The International Society for Cellular Therapy position statement. Cytotherapy. 2006;8(4):315–7.
69. Cawthorn WP, Scheller EL, MacDougald OA. Adipose tissue stem cells meet preadipocyte commitment: going back to the future. J Lipid Res. 2012;53(2):227–46.
70. Trayhurn P, Wood I. Signalling role of adipose tissue: adipokines and inflammation in obesity. Biochem Soc Trans. 2005;33(Pt 5):1078–81.
71. Zhang Y, Proenca R, Maffei M, Barone M, Leopold L, Friedman JM. Positional cloning of the mouse

obese gene and its human homologue. Nature. 1994;372(6505):425–32.
72. Rodbell M. The metabolism of isolated fat cells. J Biol Chem. 1964;239:375–80.
73. Gimble JM, Katz AJ, Bunnell BA. Adipose-derived stem cells for regenerative medicine. Circ Res. 2007;100(9):1249–60.
74. Mitchell JB, McIntosh K, Zvonic S, Garrett S, Floyd ZE, Kloster A, Di Halvorsen Y, Storms RW, Goh B, Kilroy G. Immunophenotype of human adipose-derived cells: temporal changes in stromal-associated and stem cell–associated markers. Stem Cells. 2006;24(2):376–85.
75. Yu G, Wu X, Dietrich MA, Polk P, Scott LK, Ptitsyn AA, Gimble JM. Yield and characterization of subcutaneous human adipose-derived stem cells by flow cytometric and adipogenic mRNA analyzes. Cytotherapy. 2010;12(4):538–46.
76. Bourin P, Bunnell BA, Casteilla L, Dominici M, Katz AJ, March KL, Redl H, Rubin JP, Yoshimura K, Gimble JM. Stromal cells from the adipose tissue-derived stromal vascular fraction and culture expanded adipose tissue-derived stromal/stem cells: a joint statement of the International Federation for Adipose Therapeutics and Science (IFATS) and the International Society for Cellular Therapy (ISCT). Cytotherapy. 2013;15(6):641–8.
77. Hicok KC, Hedrick MH. Automated isolation and processing of adipose-derived stem and regenerative cells. In: Gimble JM, Bunnell BA, editors. Adipose-derived stem cells. New York/Dordrecht/Heidelberg/London: Springer; 2011. p. 87–105.
78. Gimble JM, Bunnell BA, Casteilla L, Jung JS, Yoshimura K. Phases I–III clinical trials using adult stem cells. Stem Cells Int. 2011;2010:2.
79. Mesimäki K, Lindroos B, Törnwall J, Mauno J, Lindqvist C, Kontio R, Miettinen S, Suuronen R. Novel maxillary reconstruction with ectopic bone formation by GMP adipose stem cells. Int J Oral Maxillofac Surg. 2009;38(3):201–9.
80. Thesleff T, Lehtimäki K, Niskakangas T, Mannerström B, Miettinen S, Suuronen R, Öhman J. Cranioplasty with adipose-derived stem cells and biomaterial: a novel method for cranial reconstruction. Neurosurgery. 2011;68(6):1535–40.
81. Lendeckel S, Jödicke A, Christophis P, Heidinger K, Wolff J, Fraser JK, Hedrick MH, Berthold L, Howaldt H-P. Autologous stem cells (adipose) and fibrin glue used to treat widespread traumatic calvarial defects: case report. J Cranio-Maxillofac Surg. 2004;32(6):370–3.
82. Caplan AI. Adult mesenchymal stem cells: when, where, and how. Stem Cells Int. 2015:628767.
83. Santa María L, Rojas CV, Minguell JJ. Signals from damaged but not undamaged skeletal muscle induce myogenic differentiation of rat bone-marrow-derived mesenchymal stem cells. Exp Cell Res. 2004;300(2):418–26.
84. Bossolasco P, Corti S, Strazzer S, Borsotti C, Del Bo R, Fortunato F, Salani S, Quirici N, Bertolini F, Gobbi A. Skeletal muscle differentiation potential of human adult bone marrow cells. Exp Cell Res. 2004;295(1):66–78.
85. Feki A, Faltin D, Lei T, Dubuisson J-B, Jacob S, Irion O. Sphincter incontinence: is regenerative medicine the best alternative to restore urinary or anal sphincter function? Int J Biochem Cell Biol. 2007;39(4):678–84.
86. Tran C, Damaser MS. The potential role of stem cells in the treatment of urinary incontinence. Ther Adv Urol. 2014;7(1):22–40.
87. Lane FL, Jacobs S. Stem cells in gynecology. Am J Obstet Gynecol. 2012;207(3):149–56.
88. Wang H-J, Chuang Y-C, Chancellor MB. Development of cellular therapy for the treatment of stress urinary incontinence. Int Urogynecol J. 2011;22(9):1075–83.
89. Vaizey CJ, Norton C, Thornton MJ, Nicholls RJ, Kamm MA. Long-term results of repeat anterior anal sphincter repair. Dis Colon Rectum. 2004;47(6):858–63.
90. Baeten CG. Safety and efficacy of dynamic graciloplasty for fecal incontinence. Dis Colon Rectum. 2000;43(6):743–51.
91. Lehur P, Glemain P, des Varannes SB, Buzelin J, Leborgne J. Outcome of patients with an implanted artificial anal sphincter for severe faecal incontinence A single institution report. Int J Colorectal Dis. 1998;13(2):88–92.
92. Norderval S, Öian P, Revhaug A, Vonen B. Anal incontinence after obstetric sphincter tears: outcome of anatomic primary repairs. Dis Colon Rectum. 2005;48(5):1055–61.
93. Zorcolo L, Covotta L, Bartolo DC. Outcome of anterior sphincter repair for obstetric injury: comparison of early and late results. Dis Colon Rectum. 2005;48(3):524–31.
94. Dmochowski RR, Blaivas JM, Gormley EA, Juma S, Karram MM, Lightner DJ, Luber KM, Rovner ES, Staskin DR, Winters JC. Update of AUA guideline on the surgical management of female stress urinary incontinence. J Urol. 2010;183(5):1906–14.
95. Kuhn A, Eggeman C, Burkhard F, Mueller MD. Correction of erosion after suburethral sling insertion for stress incontinence: results and related sexual function. Eur Urol. 2009;56(2):371–7.
96. Kotb AF, Campeau L, Corcos J. Urethral bulking agents: techniques and outcomes. Curr Urol Rep. 2009;10(5):396–400.
97. Murphy MB, Moncivais K, Caplan AI. Mesenchymal stem cells: environmentally responsive therapeutics for regenerative medicine. Exp Mol Med. 2013;45(11), e54.
98. Patel DM, Shah J, Srivastava AS. Therapeutic potential of mesenchymal stem cells in regenerative medicine. Stem Cells Int. 2015: 496218.

99. Godara P, Nordon RE, McFarland CD. Mesenchymal stem cells in tissue engineering. J Chem Technol Biotechnol. 2008;83(4):397–407.
100. Chancellor MB, Yokoyama T, Tirney S, Mattes CE, Ozawa H, Yoshimura N, de Groat WC, Huard J. Preliminary results of myoblast injection into the urethra and bladder wall: a possible method for the treatment of stress urinary incontinence and impaired detrusor contractility. Neurourol Urodyn. 2000;19(3):279–87.
101. Carr L, Steele D, Steele S, Wagner D, Pruchnic R, Jankowski R, Erickson J, Huard J, Chancellor M. 1-year follow-up of autologous muscle-derived stem cell injection pilot study to treat stress urinary incontinence. Int Urogynecol J. 2008;19(6):881–3.
102. Lin AS, Carrier S, Morgan DM, Lue TF. Effect of simulated birth trauma on the urinary continence mechanism in the rat. Urology. 1998;52(1):143–51.
103. Kerns JM, Damaser MS, Kane JM, Sakamoto K, Benson JT, Shott S, Brubaker L. Effects of pudendal nerve injury in the female rat. Neurourol Urodyn. 2000;19(1):53–69.
104. Chermansky CJ, Cannon TW, Torimoto K, Fraser MO, Yoshimura N, de Groat WC, Chancellor MB. A model of intrinsic sphincteric deficiency in the rat: electrocauterization. Neurourol Urodyn. 2004;23(2):166–71.
105. Kefer JC, Liu G, Daneshgari F. Pubo-urethral ligament injury causes long-term stress urinary incontinence in female rats: an animal model of the integral theory. J Urol. 2009;181(1):397–400.
106. Liechty KW, MacKenzie TC, Shaaban AF, Radu A, Moseley AB, Deans R, Marshak DR, Flake AW. Human mesenchymal stem cells engraft and demonstrate site-specific differentiation after in utero transplantation in sheep. Nat Med. 2000;6(11):1282–6.
107. Sakaida I, Terai S, Yamamoto N, Aoyama K, Ishikawa T, Nishina H, Okita K. Transplantation of bone marrow cells reduces CCl4-induced liver fibrosis in mice. Hepatology. 2004;40(6):1304–11.
108. Chen J, Li Y, Wang L, Zhang Z, Lu D, Lu M, Chopp M. Therapeutic benefit of intravenous administration of bone marrow stromal cells after cerebral ischemia in rats. Stroke. 2001;32(4):1005–11.
109. Cruz M, Dissaranan C, Cotleur A, Kiedrowski M, Penn M, Damaser M. Pelvic organ distribution of mesenchymal stem cells injected intravenously after simulated childbirth injury in female rats. Obstet Gynecol Int. 2012;2012:612946.
110. Dissaranan C, Cruz MA, Kiedrowski MJ, Balog BM, Gill BC, Penn MS, Goldman HB, Damaser MS. Rat mesenchymal stem cell secretome promotes elastogenesis and facilitates recovery from simulated childbirth injury. Cell Transplant. 2014;23(11):1395–406.
111. Rombouts W, Ploemacher R. Primary murine MSC show highly efficient homing to the bone marrow but lose homing ability following culture. Leukemia. 2003;17(1):160–70.
112. Fischer UM, Harting MT, Jimenez F, Monzon-Posadas WO, Xue H, Savitz SI, Laine GA, Cox Jr CS. Pulmonary passage is a major obstacle for intravenous stem cell delivery: the pulmonary first-pass effect. Stem Cells Dev. 2009;18(5):683–92.
113. Chermansky CJ, Tarin T, Kwon D-D, Jankowski RJ, Cannon TW, de Groat WC, Huard J, Chancellor MB. Intraurethral muscle-derived cell injections increase leak point pressure in a rat model of intrinsic sphincter deficiency. Urology. 2004;63(4):780–5.
114. Fu Q, Song X-F, Liao G-L, Deng C-L, Cui L. Myoblasts differentiated from adipose-derived stem cells to treat stress urinary incontinence. Urology. 2010;75(3):718–23.
115. Kinebuchi Y, Aizawa N, Imamura T, Ishizuka O, Igawa Y, Nishizawa O. Autologous bone-marrow-derived mesenchymal stem cell transplantation into injured rat urethral sphincter. Int J Urol. 2010;17(4):359–68.
116. Lim J-J, Jang J-B, Kim J-Y, Moon S-H, Lee C-N, Lee K-J. Human umbilical cord blood mononuclear cell transplantation in rats with intrinsic sphincter deficiency. J Korean Med Sci. 2010;25(5):663–70.
117. Lin G, Wang G, Banie L, Ning H, Shindel AW, Fandel TM, Lue TF, Lin C-S. Treatment of stress urinary incontinence with adipose tissue-derived stem cells. Cytotherapy. 2010;12(1):88–95.
118. Xu Y, Song Y, Lin Z. Transplantation of muscle-derived stem cells plus biodegradable fibrin glue restores the urethral sphincter in a pudendal nerve-transected rat model. Braz J Med Biol Res. 2010;43(11):1076–83.
119. Zou XH, Zhi YL, Chen X, Jin HM, Wang LL, Jiang YZ, Yin Z, Ouyang HW. Mesenchymal stem cell seeded knitted silk sling for the treatment of stress urinary incontinence. Biomaterials. 2010;31(18):4872–9.
120. Kim S-O, Na HS, Kwon D, Joo SY, Kim HS, Ahn Y. Bone-marrow-derived mesenchymal stem cell transplantation enhances closing pressure and leak point pressure in a female urinary incontinence rat model. Urol Int. 2011;86(1):110–6.
121. Corcos J, Loutochin O, Campeau L, Eliopoulos N, Bouchentouf M, Blok B, Galipeau J. Bone marrow mesenchymal stromal cell therapy for external urethral sphincter restoration in a rat model of stress urinary incontinence. Neurourol Urodyn. 2011;30(3):447–55.
122. Imamura T, Ishizuka O, Kinebuchi Y, Kurizaki Y, Nakayama T, Ishikawa M, Nishizawa O. Implantation of autologous bone-marrow-derived cells reconstructs functional urethral sphincters in rabbits. Tissue Eng Part A. 2011;17(7–8):1069–81.
123. Wu G, Song Y, Zheng X, Jiang Z. Adipose-derived stromal cell transplantation for treatment of stress urinary incontinence. Tissue Cell. 2011;43(4):246–53.
124. Zhao W, Zhang C, Jin C, Zhang Z, Kong D, Xu W, Xiu Y. Periurethral injection of autologous adipose-

derived stem cells with controlled-release nerve growth factor for the treatment of stress urinary incontinence in a rat model. Eur Urol. 2011;59(1):155–63.
125. Chun SY, Kwon JB, Chae SY, Lee JK, Js B, Kim BS, Kim HT, Yoo ES, Lim JO, Yoo JJ. Combined injection of three different lineages of early-differentiating human amniotic fluid-derived cells restores urethral sphincter function in urinary incontinence. BJU Int. 2014;114(5):770–83.
126. Sèbe P, Doucet C, Cornu J-N, Ciofu C, Costa P, de Medina SGD, Pinset C, Haab F. Intrasphincteric injections of autologous muscular cells in women with refractory stress urinary incontinence: a prospective study. Int Urogynecol J. 2011;22(2):183–9.
127. Gotoh M, Yamamoto T, Kato M, Majima T, Toriyama K, Kamei Y, Matsukawa Y, Hirakawa A, Funahashi Y. Regenerative treatment of male stress urinary incontinence by periurethral injection of autologous adipose-derived regenerative cells: 1-year outcomes in 11 patients. Int J Urol. 2014;21(3):294–300.
128. Gräs S, Klarskov N, Lose G. Intraurethral injection of autologous minced skeletal muscle: a simple surgical treatment for stress urinary incontinence. J Urol. 2014;192(3):850–5.
129. Carr LK, Herschorn S, Birch C, Murphy M, Robert M, Jankowski RJ, Pruchnic R, Wagner D, Chancellor MB. Autologous muscle-derived cells as a therapy for stress urinary incontinence: a randomized, blinded, multi-dose study. J Urol. 2009;181(4):546.
130. Carr L, Herschorn S, Birch C, Murphy M, Robert M, Jankowski R, Pruchnic R, Wagner D, Chancellor M. Aautologous muscle-derived cells as therapy for stress urinary incontinence: a randomized, dose-ranging trial. J Urol. 2010;183(4):e587–8.
131. Peters K, Kaufman M, Dmochowski R, Carr L, Herschorn S, Fischer M, Sirls L, Nagaraju P, Biller D, Ward R. 1340 Autologous muscle derived cell therapy for the treatment of female stress urinary incontinence: a multi-center experience. J Urol. 2011;185(4):e535–6.
132. Carr LK, Robert M, Kultgen PL, Herschorn S, Birch C, Murphy M, Chancellor MB. Autologous muscle derived cell therapy for stress urinary incontinence: a prospective, dose ranging study. J Urol. 2013;189(2):595–601.
133. Jankowski R, Werner S, Snyder S, Chancellor M, Kultgen P, Pruchnic R. Cell therapy for treatment of stress urinary incontinence in women: potential dose effect of autologous muscle-derived cells for urinary sphincter repair (AMDC-USR). Cytotherapy. 2014;16(4):S91.
134. Stangel-Wojcikiewicz K, Jarocha D, Piwowar M, Jach R, Uhl T, Basta A, Majka M. Autologous muscle-derived cells for the treatment of female stress urinary incontinence: a 2-year follow-up of a polish investigation. Neurourol Urodyn. 2014;33(3):324–30.
135. Lorenzi B, Pessina F, Lorenzoni P, Urbani S, Vernillo R, Sgaragli G, Gerli R, Mazzanti B, Bosi A, Saccardi R. Treatment of experimental injury of anal sphincters with primary surgical repair and injection of bone marrow-derived mesenchymal stem cells. Dis Colon Rectum. 2008;51(4):411–20.
136. Kang S-B, Lee HN, Lee JY, Park J-S, Lee HS, Lee JY. Sphincter contractility after muscle-derived stem cells autograft into the cryoinjured anal sphincters of rats. Dis Colon Rectum. 2008;51(9):1367–73.
137. White AB, Keller PW, Acevedo JF, Word RA, Wai CY. Effect of myogenic stem cells on contractile properties of the repaired and unrepaired transected external anal sphincter in an animal model. Obstet Gynecol. 2010;115(4):815–23.
138. Aghaee-Afshar M, Rezazadehkermani M, Asadi A, Malekpour-Afshar R, Shahesmaeili A, Nematollahi-mahani SN. Potential of human umbilical cord matrix and rabbit bone marrow-derived mesenchymal stem cells in repair of surgically incised rabbit external anal sphincter. Dis Colon Rectum. 2009;52(10):1753–61.
139. Kajbafzadeh A-M, Elmi A, Talab SS, Esfahani SA, Tourchi A. Functional external anal sphincter reconstruction for treatment of anal incontinence using muscle progenitor cell auto grafting. Dis Colon Rectum. 2010;53(10):1415–21.
140. Pathi SD, Acevedo JF, Keller PW, Kishore AH, Miller RT, Wai CY, Word RA. Recovery of the injured external anal sphincter after injection of local or intravenous mesenchymal stem cells. Obstet Gynecol. 2012;119(1):134–44.
141. Salcedo L, Mayorga M, Damaser M, Balog B, Butler R, Penn M, Zutshi M. Mesenchymal stem cells can improve anal pressures after anal sphincter injury. Stem Cell Res. 2013;10(1):95–102.
142. Salcedo L, Penn M, Damaser M, Balog B, Zutshi M. Functional outcome after anal sphincter injury and treatment with mesenchymal stem cells. Stem Cells Transl Med. 2014;3(6):760–7.
143. Fitzwater JL, Grande KB, Sailors JL, Acevedo JF, Word RA, Wai CY. Effect of myogenic stem cells on the integrity and histomorphology of repaired transected external anal sphincter. Int Urogynecol J. 2015;26(2):251–6.
144. Montoya TI, Acevedo JF, Smith B, Keller PW, Sailors JL, Tang L, Word RA, Wai CY. Myogenic stem cell-laden hydrogel scaffold in wound healing of the disrupted external anal sphincter. Int Urogynecol J. 2015;26(6):893–904.
145. Frudinger A, Kölle D, Schwaiger W, Pfeifer J, Paede J, Halligan S. Muscle-derived cell injection to treat anal incontinence due to obstetric trauma: pilot study with 1 year follow-up. Gut. 2010;59(01):55–61.
146. Rockwood TH, Church JM, Fleshman JW, Kane RL, Mavrantonis C, Thorson AG, Wexner SD, Bliss D, Lowry AC. Fecal incontinence quality of life scale. Dis Colon Rectum. 2000;43(1):9–16.

147. Jorge JMN, Wexner SD. Etiology and management of fecal incontinence. Dis Colon Rectum. 1993;36(1):77–97.
148. Giori A, Tremolada C, Vailati R, Navone S, Marfia G, Caplan A. Recovery of function in anal incontinence after micro-fragmented fat graft (Lipogems®) injection: two years follow up of the first 5 cases. CellR4. 2016;3(2):e1544.
149. Bianchi F, Maioli M, Leonardi E, Olivi E, Pasquinelli G, Valente S, Mendez AJ, Ricordi C, Raffaini M, Tremolada C. A new nonenzymatic method and device to obtain a fat tissue derivative highly enriched in pericyte-like elements by mild mechanical forces from human lipoaspirates. Cell Transplant. 2013;22(11):2063–77.
150. Maioli M, Rinaldi S, Santaniello S, Castagna A, Pigliaru G, Gualini S, Cavallini C, Fontani V, Ventura C. Radio electric conveyed fields directly reprogram human dermal skin fibroblasts toward cardiac, neuronal, and skeletal muscle-like lineages. Cell Transplant. 2013;22(7):1227–35.
151. Carelli S, Messaggio F, Canazza A, Hebda DM, Caremoli F, Latorre E, Grimoldi MG, Colli M, Bulfamante G, Tremolada C. Characteristics and properties of mesenchymal stem cells derived from micro-fragmented adipose tissue. Cell Transplant. 2014;24(7):1233–52.
152. Tremolada C, Palmieri G, Ricordi C. Adipocyte transplantation and stem cells: plastic surgery meets regenerative medicine. Cell Transplant. 2010;19(10):1217–23.
153. Jiang X-X, Zhang Y, Liu B, Zhang S-X, Wu Y, Yu X-D, Mao N. Human mesenchymal stem cells inhibit differentiation and function of monocyte-derived dendritic cells. Blood. 2005;105(10):4120–6.
154. Le Blanc K, Tammik C, Rosendahl K, Zetterberg E, Ringdén O. HLA expression and immunologic properties of differentiated and undifferentiated mesenchymal stem cells. Exp Hematol. 2003;31(10):890–6.
155. Maurer MH. Proteomic definitions of mesenchymal stem cells. Stem Cells Int. 2011:704256.
156. Vaizey C, Kamm M. Injectable bulking agents for treating faecal incontinence. Br J Surg. 2005;92(5):521–7.
157. Frudinger A, Pfeifer J, Paede J, Kolovetsiou-Kreiner V, Marksteiner R, Halligan S. Autologous skeletal muscle-derived cell injection for anal incontinence due to obstetric trauma: a five-year follow-up of an initial study of ten patients. Colorectal Dis. 2015;9794–801.